NEONATAL INTENSIVE CARE HANDBOOK

third
EDITION

NEONATAL
INTENSIVE CARE
HANDBOOK

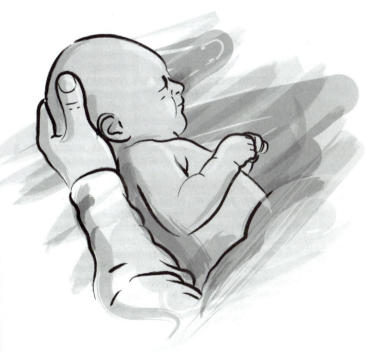

BOYD W. GOETZMAN / RICHARD P. WENNBERG

Mosby

Publisher	Laura De Young
Development Editor	Maria Stewart
Project Manager	Sarah Gray
Designer	Pete Wilder
Layout	Louise Bond
Illustration	Susan Tyler
Cover design	Deborah Gyan
Copyeditor	Colin MacNee
Proofreader	Heather Russell
Production	Susan Walby
Index	Nina Boyd

© Copyright 1999 Mosby International Ltd.
Published in 1999 by Mosby, an imprint of Mosby International Ltd.

ISBN: 0 3230 0814 3

Printed and bound by R.R Donnelly & Sons Company

Cataloging-in-Publication Data:
Catalogue records for this book are available from the US Library of Congress and the British Library

For full details of Mosby titles please write to:
Mosby International Ltd
Lynton House
7–12 Tavistock Square
London WC1H 9LB
UK

CONTENTS

The Neonatal Intensive Care Handbook had its inception in 1975 as a 'House Officer's Manual' for our Neonatal Intensive Care Unit at the University of California, Davis Medical Center in Sacramento. It had become apparent that many physicians in training, including residents in pediatrics, obstetrics, anesthesiology, and family practice, would have but a brief opportunity to learn the fundamentals of newborn stabilization and care, and a ready reference was needed to guide them. Since then, the knowledge about neonatal care has grown continuously, resulting in the need for a second edition and, now, this third edition. Future revisions can be anticipated as new information emerges.

This Neonatal Intensive Care Handbook is not a textbook; but is intended to be used as a quick reference for procedures and acceptable first approaches to problems encountered in the care of newborn infants. For the inexperienced, the handbook should facilitate orientation to newborn intensive care. For the more senior residents, it should serve as a refresher for common routines, drug dosages, and normal values as well as an immediate guide for managing problems not previously encountered. It should not be considered the totality of reading experience required to gain competence in newborn care.

While guidelines to the clinical management of neonatal disease have become relatively uniform between institutions in recent years, each nursery has its own unique resources and approach to specific problems. The handbook is, to a large extent, a distillation of our current practices. Unfortunately, many of the recommendations are of necessity based on 'clinical experience' rather than on the results of convincing clinical and basic research. We hope that the acquisition of new knowledge will eventually render both the problems and our recommended therapeutic approaches obsolete. In the meantime, we hope this handbook will prove to be a practical resource to facilitate patient care and teaching and would welcome suggestions which might improve future editions.

We are deeply indebted to the handbook's contributors who not only provided the written word but who also spent time in the Newborn Intensive Care Unit assisting in the care of our patients. Many others have contributed to the handbook by their review and comments. We would particularly like to acknowledge the current, and past Fellows in the Division of Neonatology for their help in developing our approaches to neonatal intensive care.

Boyd W. Goetzman, MD, PhD
Richard P. Wennberg, MD

CONTRIBUTORS

Charles E. Ahlfors, MD,
Department of Pediatrics
Pacific Presbyterian Medical Center
San Francisco, California.

Robert Cannon, MD,
Associate Professor, Department of
Pediatrics
University of California at Davis
Davis, California.

Michael Choy, MD,
Associate Professor, Department of
Pediatrics
University of California at Davis
Davis, California.

Matthew Connors, MD,
Associate Clinical Professor
Department of Pediatrics
University of California at Davis
Davis, California.

Christine Enstine, RN, MSN, NNP,
Neonatal Nurse Practitioner
University of Chicago Children's
Hospital
Chicago, Illinois.

William M. Gilbert, MD,
Associate Professor, Department of
Obstetrics/Gynecology
University of California at Davis
Davis, California.

Boyd W. Goetzman, MD, PhD,
Professor, Division of Neonatology
Department of Pediatrics, University
of California at Davis
Davis, California.

Sidney M. Gospe Jr, MD, PhD,
Associate Professor, Division of
Child Neurology
Departments of Neurology and
Pediatrics, University of California
at Davis
Davis, California.

Stephen Greenholtz, MD,
Clinical Professor, Department of
Surgery
University of California at Davis
Davis, California.

Linda Greve, RN, PHN,
Coordinator Newborn Screening
Department of Pediatrics
University of California at Davis
Davis, California.

Arthur W. Grix, MD,
Assistant Clinical Professor,
Department of Pediatrics
University of California at Davis
Davis, California.

Michael Haight, MD,
Assistant Professor
Department of Pediatrics
University of California at Davis
Davis, California.

Chrystie Halsted, MD,
Clinical Professor
Department of Pediatrics
University of California at Davis
Davis, California.

Hanne Jensen, MD,
Associate Professor in Residence
Department of Pathology
University of California at Davis
Davis, California.

Jack Lazerson, MD,
Professor of Pediatrics,
University of Nevada
Las Vegas, Nevada.

T. Allen Merrit, MD,
Director of NICU
Family Birthing Center
Bend, Oregon.

Jay M. Milstein, M.D.,
Clinical Professor
Division of Neonatology
Department of Pediatrics
University of California at Davis
Davis, California.

Fred Royce
Assistant Professor
Department of Pediatrics
University of California at Davis
Davis, California.

Dennis M. Styne, MD,
Professor, Department of Pediatrics
University of California at Davis
Davis, California.

Dena Towner, MD,
Assistant Professor,
Obstetrics/Gynecology
University of California at Davis
Davis, California.

Richard P. Wennberg, MD,
Professor Emeritus
Division of Neonatology
Department of Pediatrics
University of California at Davis
Davis, California.

Mark Wheeler, MD,
Pediatric Endocrinology,
Tucson, Arizona.

PRENATAL DIAGNOSIS

I. WHY DO PRENATAL DIAGNOSTIC SCREENING?

a. In the first month of life there is a 3–4% risk for each neonate to be identified with a birth defect or genetic condition.
b. By puberty 10–15% of children have a condition diagnosed with a genetic or developmental component.
c. 95% of these children will be born to families without risk factors.
d. Identification of affected fetuses gives families reproductive options.
e. Identification of affected fetuses may alter obstetrical management, site of delivery, and/or neonatal management.

II. QUESTION FOR KNOWN RISK FACTORS

A. FAMILY RISK FACTORS.

1. Parent or prior child with birth defect or genetic disease.
2. Mental retardation.
3. Seizure disorder.
4. Multiple spontaneous abortions (>3). One parent may carry a balanced translocation (5% chance).
5. Prior unexplained stillbirth or neonatal death.
6. Genetic disorders that run in the family.
a. Hemophilia.
b. Duchenne muscular dystrophy.
c. Myotonic dystrophy.

B. ETHNICITY.

1. Ashkenazi Jew.
a. Tay–Sachs disease.
b. Gaucher disease.
c. Cannivan disease.
2. African-American.
a. Sickle cell disease.
b. Hemoglobin C disease.
c. Thalassemias, α and β.
3. Asian.
a. Thalassemia, α.
b. Hemoglobin E.
4. Mediterranean.
a. Thalassemias, α and β.
b. Glucose-6-phosphatase deficiency.

5. Caucasian.
a. Cystic fibrosis.

C. MATERNAL AGE.

1. Trisomy.
a. Increasing risk for trisomic conceptions with increasing maternal age.
b. >95% of trisomy 21 and 18 are due to maternal meiotic nondisjunction.

D. MATERNAL MEDICAL CONDITIONS.

1. **Diabetes uncontrolled before pregnancy.**
a. 25% spontaneous abortions.
b. Three- to five-fold increased risk for major congenital anomalies.
c. CNS: holoprosencephaly, spina bifida.
d. Heart: transposition, coarctation of the aorta.
e. Renal: dysplasia, agenesis, horseshoe.

2. **Myotonic dystrophy.**
a. Congenital myotonic dystrophy.

3. **Seizure disorder.**
a. Two-fold increased risk for malformations.
b. Irrespective of medication use.
c. Cleft lip and heart defects primarily.

4. **Maternal autoimmune diseases.**
a. Anti-SSA or SSB antibodies.
b. Congenital heart block.
c. Myasthenia gravis.
d. Fetal akinesis and pulmonary hypoplasia secondary to the anti-acetylcholine receptor and neuromuscular blockade.

5. **Maternal PKU.**
a. Congenital heart defects.
    1) Coarctation of aorta
    2) Hypoplastic left heart
    3) VSD.
b. Mental retardation.

E. TERATOGEN EXPOSURE during embryogenesis.

1. **Prescription drugs.**
a. Retinoic acid.
    1) Hydrocephaly and microcephaly
    2) Cardiac defects
    3) Craniofacial anomalies, especially of the ear.
b. Methotrexate.
    1) Spina bifida
    2) Skeletal dysplasia.
c. Lithium.
    1) Heart defects, Ebstein's anomaly.

   d. Dilantin.
      1) Fetal hydantoin syndrome (10%)
      2) Intrauterine growth restriction, microcephaly
      3) Craniofacial dysmorphia
      4) Heart and cleft lip +/- palate anomalies.
   e. Tegretol: 1% risk for neural tube defect.
   f. Valproic acid.
      1) 1–2% risk for neural tube defects
      2) Cardiac defects
      3) Radial (thumb side) arm and hand anomalies.
   g. Chemotherapies.
      1) Growth restriction and possible childhood cancer risks (leukemia).

2. Infectious agents.
   a. CMV and toxoplasmosis.
      1) Microcephaly, mental retardation
      2) Lissencephaly and abnormal neuronal migration (CMV)
      3) Chorioretinitis; deafness
      4) Growth restriction.
   b. Varicella (up to 20 weeks gestation).
      1) 1% risk for limb scarring and hypoplasia.
   c. Rubella.
      1) Microcephaly, cataracts, deafness, heart defects.

3. Illicit drug use.
   a. Alcohol.
      1) Fetal alcohol syndrome
      2) Microcephaly
      3) Growth restriction
      4) Developmental delays.
   b. Cocaine.
      1) Vascular disruption events (e.g. porencephaly)
      2) GU anomalies.

4. Maternal hyperthermia. Fever or exposure (sauna) is associated with neural tube defects and possibly cleft lip and palate.

5. Radiation exposure.
   a. <10 rad is considered safe.
   b. High dose (>25 rad).
      1) Microcephaly and mental retardation
      2) Cataracts and micro-ophthalmia
      3) Growth restriction
      4) Leukemia.

III. SCREENING FOR LOW-RISK WOMEN

Women with no identifiable risk factor from history deliver 95% of babies with congenital birth defects. Analysis of three maternal serum biochemical markers is useful in identifying fetuses at risk for certain birth defects. 5–7% of these low-risk women will have an abnormal test warranting further testing.

A. BIOCHEMICAL MARKERS.

1. **AFP.**
2. **hCG.**
3. **Unconjugated estriol (uE3).**

B. DEFECTS IDENTIFIED (% detected).

1. **High maternal serum AFP.**
   a. Neural tube defects (70–95%).
      1) Anencephaly (95 + %).
      2) Spina bifida (80% of open and 70% of all).
      3) Encephalocele (70%).
   b. Gastroschisis (90%).
   c. Omphalocele (50%).
2. **Down syndrome** (up to 60%). Typical pattern is high hCG and low AFP and uE3.
3. **Trisomy 18** (up to 80%). Low levels of all three markers.

C. OTHER CONDITIONS IDENTIFIED.

1. **Wrong dates.**
2. **Twins (45%).**
3. **Renal anomalies.**
   a. Finnish nephrosis.
   b. Renal agenesis, dysplasia.
   c. Urinary obstruction.
4. **Fetal demise.**
5. **Fetomaternal hemorrhage.**

D. ELEVATIONS OF AFP AND HCG that are unexplained by a fetal defect place the pregnancy at risk for preterm delivery, growth restriction, stillbirth, and pre-eclampsia, presumably due to a placental abnormality.

IV. METHODS OF PRENATAL DIAGNOSIS

A. ULTRASOUND is useful for identifying major structural defects.

1. **Anencephaly, spina bifida, hydrocephalus.**
2. **Major heart defects.**
3. **Urinary tract anomalies.**
4. **Abdominal wall defects:** omphalocele and gastroschisis.
5. **Limb defects and skeletal dysplasias.**
6. **Nuchal thickening.**
7. **Echogenic bowel pattern.**

B. **AMNIOCENTESIS.** Aspiration of amniotic fluid for analysis after 12 weeks gestation.
1. **Karyotype.**
2. **Biochemical studies.**
a. Identification of some organic acidemias.
b. AFP and acetylcholine esterase for open neural tube defects.
c. Bilirubin (ΔOD_{450}) in hemolytic disease.
3. **Enzymatic tests,** e.g. Hurler syndrome.
4. **DNA tests.**
a. Myotonic dystrophy.
b. Duchenne muscular dystrophy.
C. **CHORIONIC VILLUS SAMPLING.**
a. Removal of a sample of chorionic villi at 10–13 weeks of pregnancy either through transvaginal or transabdominal aspiration of villi.
b. Same tests can be performed as with amniocentesis, except amniotic fluid levels of compounds can not be done (e.g. AFP).
D. **UMBILICAL CORD BLOOD SAMPLING** (cordocentesis or PUBS).
a. Removal of fetal blood from the umbilical cord guided by ultrasound.
b. Technically difficult prior to 18 weeks.
c. 1–3% loss of pregnancy.
d. Limited in amount removed (<5ml).
e. Direct testing of fetal samples.
    1) Blood gas
    2) Hemoglobin and hematocrit, platelets
    3) Chemistries: liver tests
    4) IgM for infections
    5) Rapid karyotype (2 days).

V. FETAL THERAPIES
A. **INTRAUTERINE TRANSFUSION.**
1. **Rh sensitized.**
2. **Other conditions producing severe anemia and hydrops.**
B. **OBSTRUCTIVE UROPATHIES:** double pigtail catheter drainage above obstruction into amniotic space.
C. **FETAL SURGERY** for some conditions, such as diaphragmatic hernia, sacral teratoma removal, and resection of chest masses such as cystic adenomatoid malformations, has been performed in some centers when poor outcome is predicted.

PRENATAL DIAGNOSIS   **1**

ASSESSMENT OF FETAL WELL-BEING

I. FETAL LUNG MATURITY ASSESSMENT

The following amniotic fluid tests are used to evaluate fetal lung maturity and the relative risk of neonatal RDS.

A. FOAM STABILITY INDEX.

a. Serial dilution of ethanol with constant quantity of amniotic fluid.
b. Adequate surfactant stabilizes a foam ring at the meniscus of a mixture of 47% by volume ethanol and amniotic fluid.
c. FSI value less than 44 indicates a >50% risk of RDS, while RDS is rare at FSI >47.
d. False-positive results are rare unless specimens are contaminated (blood, meconium, or vaginal secretions).
e. Many false-negative results are seen, for example in polyhydramnios.

B. LECITHIN/SPHINGOMYELIN RATIO.

a. Requires time and skilled technicians.
b. L/S ratio ≥ 2:1 is a reliable indicator of fetal lung maturity in the non-diabetic patient.
c. 2% false-positive results.
   1) With an L/S ratio <1.5, about 70% develop RDS.
   2) With an L/S ratio between 1.5 and 2.0, about 40% develop RDS.
d. Not reliable in specimens contaminated by blood, meconium, or vaginal secretions.

C. PHOSPHATIDYL GLYCEROL.

a. Aids in stabilizing surfactant membrane.
b. Virtually no false-positive findings.
c. Not affected by blood, meconium, or vaginal secretion contamination.
d. Lack of PG does not correlate well with presence of RDS. Presence of PG correlates well with absence of RDS.

D. FETAL LUNG PROFILE.

a. Combination of L/S ratio, percent lecithin, PG, and phosphatidylinositol (PI), improves both the false-positive and false-negative rates.
b. Costly and time consuming.

II. ELECTRONIC FETAL HEART RATE MONITORING

Monitoring the FHR by an external Doppler ultrasound or via an internal fetal ECG electrode applied to the fetal scalp has been widely applied in modern obstetrics despite lack of proven effectiveness in low-risk patients. Despite this, FHR monitoring does appear to be an indirect measurement of the activity of the fetal CNS, degree of fetal oxygenation, and acid–base status. The heart rate assumes greater importance in the fetus because of the relatively fixed stroke volume of the ventricles and the fetus's inability to regulate the respiratory function of the placenta. The CNS receives information about the PO_2, PCO_2, pH, tissue perfusion, intravascular volume and blood flow rates, which is integrated to regulate the FHR via the sympathetic and parasympathetic nervous systems.

A. BASELINE FETAL HEART RATE.

1. **Normal baseline** FHR is 120–160bpm.
2. **Tachycardia** is defined as a heart rate >160bpm and is often due to early hypoxia, fever (maternal or fetal), infection or fetal arrhythmia.
3. **Severe bradycardia** is a rate of <100bpm sustained longer than 10 minutes and may be due to persistent hypoxia, acidosis, or direct myocardial depression.

B. FETAL HEART RATE VARIABILITY. This is the variation or change in the baseline FHR with time; it appears as the 'chicken scratch' pattern and may be both constant and cyclical.

1. **Short-term** beat-to-beat variability is present in all normal records.
2. **Long-term:** 3–5 cycles per minute (amplitude of 5–20bpm is normal).
a. Reflected in 'waviness' of fetal heart rate tracing or the cyclic changes in the FHR over minutes to hours.
b. Decreased late in the course of hypoxemia/acidosis.

C. REACTIVITY.

1. **Acceleration** of the FHR above baseline is defined as a 15 beat acceleration for at least 15 seconds, occurring at least twice in 20 minutes.
a. This is a reassuring sign of fetal well-being because it is a highly integrated response to perceived stimulation (movement, sound, light).
b. It is also a product of CNS maturation, usually being absent in fetuses <30 weeks gestation due to CNS immaturity.
2. **Reactivity** may be decreased or absent as a result of:
a. normal fetal sleep cycles (lasting 20–90 minutes)
b. hypoxia/acidosis
c. CNS depressants (narcotics, barbiturates, phenothiazines)
d. congenital anomalies.
3. **Prolonged nonreactivity** due to hypoxia is associated with development of acidosis.

D. DECELERATION PATTERNS.

1. **Early decelerations.**
a. Caused by compression of the fetal head with reflex lowering of the heart rate.
b. Onset at the beginning of the contraction and return to baseline with completion of contraction. Deceleration shape mirrors the uterine contraction shape.

c.   Least common of periodic changes and uniformly benign but is important because of its similarity to late decelerations.

2.   **Variable decelerations.**

a.   Caused by umbilical cord compression with resultant reduction of flow through the umbilical vein. Hypoxia is not a contributory factor unless there is >50% reduction in umbilical vein blood flow over time.

b.   Abrupt onset and return to baseline during contraction, with highly variable shape to the deceleration.

c.   Mild to moderate variable decelerations are common and relatively benign.

d.   Severe variable decelerations are >45 seconds duration, smooth or blunted, deep (<80bpm), and may have a very slow return to the baseline. These are worrisome, since they may be associated with hypoxia and fetal compromise.

3.   **Late decelerations.** These decelerations are late relative to the contractions and are thought to be largely due to uteroplacental insufficiency. Any maternal condition which affects uterine blood flow, such as hypertension, end stage diabetes, or renal disease, may cause uteroplacental insufficiency.

a.   Caused by hypoxia with decrease in fetal PO_2 to 18–20 torr.

b.   They are an appropriate physiologic response generated by the CNS to intermittent hypoxia. As such, they are not intrinsically harmful but are important as markers for fetal hypoxia.

c.   The deceleration begins once the contraction is well established and uterine blood flow is compromised. It presents after the contraction ends and lasts until the fetus is reoxygenated (Figure 2.1).

III. FETAL MONITORING TECHNIQUES

A.   **EXTERNAL MONITORING** may be performed with either intact or ruptured membranes.

1.   **Advantages** are that it is noninvasive, it is technically easier to place the equipment, and the equipment is reusable.

2.   **Disadvantages** are that it is dependent upon Doppler technique to record the FHR and so it is an indirect FHR recording. The equipment may also be uncomfortable to the patient.

3.   **Contractions.** External uterine contraction monitoring records only the interval and duration of contractions, but not the strength.

B.   **INTERNAL MONITORING** requires rupture of the membranes.

1.   **Advantages.** Since they are obtained by direct and continuous fetal ECG via an electrode inserted in the fetal scalp, FHR reactivity, short- and long-term variability, and decelerations can all be assessed.

2.   **Contractions.** Placement of an intrauterine pressure catheter provides direct measurement of both the strength and duration of contractions as well as the uterine tone.

2

ASSESSMENT OF FETAL WELL-BEING

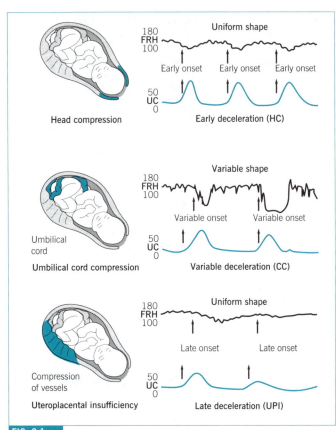

Head compression

180
FRH
100

Uniform shape

Early onset   Early onset   Early onset

50
UC
0

Early deceleration (HC)

Umbilical
cord

Umbilical cord compression

180
FRH
100

Variable shape

Variable onset   Variable onset

50
UC
0

Variable deceleration (CC)

Compression
of vessels

Uteroplacental insufficiency

180
FRH
100

Uniform shape

Late onset   Late onset

50
UC
0

Late deceleration (UPI)

FIG. 2.1
Basic patterns in electronic fetal heart rate monitoring. UC indicates uterine
contraction; HC, head compression; UPI, uteroplacental insufficiency; CC, cord
compression. (From Hon[1], with permission.)

IV. ANTEPARTUM

A. **NONSTRESS TESTING** is based on the observation that a healthy
nonstressed fetus will have an increase in heart rate in response to
fetal body movement. The NST is repeated at anywhere from 1- to
7-day intervals, based on the clinical situation.

1. **Reactive NST** – the presence of two accelerations of the fetal heart rate of at least 15 seconds duration and which reach at least 15 beats above the baseline in a 20 minute span.
2. **Nonreactive NST** – the absence of two accelerations in a 20 minute span. A nonreactive NST requires more prolonged monitoring to exclude a fetal sleep cycle (up to 90 minutes) and then further evaluations if still nonreactive with either a CST or biophysical profile.

B. CONTRACTION STRESS OR OXYTOCIN CHALLENGE TEST evaluates the effect of uterine contractions on FHR.

1. **Contractions can be spontaneous or induced** by oxytocin or breast (nipple) stimulation.
2. **CST should be preceded by an** NST to determine reactivity or non-reactivity.
3. **Interpretation:**
a. Negative CST – the absence of late decelerations.
b. Positive CST – late decelerations with >50% of contractions.
c. Suspicious CST – late decelerations present with <50% of contractions.
d. Hyperstimulation – decelerations present only with prolonged or hyperstimulated uterine contractions.
4. **Clinical significance:**
a. Reactive negative CST – very reassuring; repeat in 7 days.
b. Nonreactive negative CST – unusual; consider fetal cardiac or CNS abnormality, drug effect.
c. Reactive positive CST – generally associated with good outcome, but indicates fetal compromise and increased risk; specific management depends upon gestational age and the clinical situation.
d. Nonreactive positive CST – ominous, rare false positive, particularly if greater than 30 weeks gestation when reactivity should be present. Delivery regardless of maturity. If less than 30 weeks, may temporize with biophysical profile testing.

V. FETAL ULTRASOUND

A. GESTATIONAL AGE ASSESSMENT. The earlier in gestation the ultrasound examination is performed, the more accurate the dating of the pregnancy. Prior to 12 weeks, the accuracy will be ±5–7 days. From 12 to 20 weeks, the accuracy declines and becomes ±10 days. From 20 to 30 weeks, the accuracy is ±2 weeks. After 30 weeks the accuracy is ±3 weeks of gestation.

B. ESTIMATE FETAL WEIGHT.
1. **IUGR.** If there is no growth in the various fetal parameters over time, early delivery may be indicated.
2. **Macrosomia,** particularly with diabetics. If the diabetic fetus has an estimated fetal weight of >4250g, the risk of shoulder dystocia increases to >10%, and cesarean section should be considered.

2

ASSESSMENT OF FETAL WELL-BEING

C. AMNIOTIC FLUID VOLUME.

1. **Oligohydramnios.** Measurement of the amniotic fluid index (AFI) will suggest the diagnosis of oligohydramnios if the AFI <5cm. The AFI is the four-quadrant sum of the largest vertical pocket of amniotic fluid in each of four quadrants of the pregnant uterus. Oligohydramnios may be a good prediction of intrauterine growth retardation or renal agenesis.

2. **Polyhydramnios.** An AFI greater than the 95 percentile for gestational age implies polyhydramnios. It can be associated with diabetes, chromosome abnormalities, or tracheo-esophageal fistula.

D. ASSESSMENT OF STRUCTURAL ANOMALIES: e.g. hydrocephalus, cardiac, renal, or GI tract defects.

E. BIOPHYSICAL PROFILE.

1. **An ultrasound evaluation** of fetal physical parameters (breathing, movement, tone or posture, and amniotic fluid volume) included with the nonstress test.

2. **Indication.** It may be used as a primary surveillance tool or as a backup to heart rate testing. It is particularly useful in very premature fetuses (<30 weeks) with nonreactive heart rates.

3. **The timing of repeat tests** is controversial, ranging from hours to 7 days.

VI. DIRECT FETAL ACCESS

The fetus may be directly evaluated, either by sampling the amniotic fluid (amniocentesis) or fetal cord blood (PUBS). Each is an invasive procedure and therefore inherently limited in application.

A. PERCUTANEOUS UMBILICAL BLOOD SAMPLING.

1. **PUBS** is performed under direct ultrasound guidance to insert a needle into the fetal umbilical cord.

2. **Provides a fetal blood sample** for analysis.

a. Determination of fetal hemoglobin/hematocrit

b. Determination of fetal pH and blood gases

c. Rapid karyotyping

d. Testing for biochemical abnormalities

e. Evaluation of fetal WBC function

f. Fetal IgM determination for infection.

3. **Risks** are 1–2% for fetal demise, related to:

a. Cord bleeding or thrombosis

b. Infection.

B. AMNIOCENTESIS.

1. **Performed under ultrasound guidance** for insertion of a needle into a pocket of amniotic fluid.

2. **Provides amniotic fluid** for analysis of:

a. Fetal lung maturity

b. Bilirubin analysis (ΔOD_{450}) with erythroblastosis
c. Fetal karyotyping
d. Culture and Gram stain for infection.
3. Risk of complications is <0.5%.
a. Rupture of membranes
b. Labor
c. Bleeding
d. Fetal distress.

REFERENCE

1. Hon EH. *An atlas of fetal heart rate patterns.* New Haven, CT: Hartley Press; 1968.

FURTHER READING

ACOG Technical Bulletin # 188, *Antepartum fetal surveillance,* January 1994.
Cruikshank DP. Antepartum fetal surveillance. *Clin Obstet Gynecol* 1982; 25:633–804.
Freeman RJ, Garite TJ. *Fetal heart rate monitoring.* Baltimore: Williams & Wilkins; 1981.

ASSESSMENT OF FETAL WELL-BEING

2

PREMATURE DELIVERY

3

I. PREMATURE DELIVERY

Complications of preterm delivery are the major causes of perinatal morbidity and mortality in the United States today. The overall preterm rate is approximately 7–8% of all deliveries. Despite the development and widespread use of tocolytic agents to suppress uterine activity, the prematurity rate has not significantly decreased over the past 25 years. Many patients who present in premature labor are not candidates for tocolytic therapy, have advanced cervical dilatation (>4cm), or are unresponsive to tocolytic agents. Early identification and treatment of the pregnancy at risk for preterm delivery may ultimately improve the prematurity rate and perinatal outcome.

A. PRETERM LABOR.
1. **Diagnosis** is made by:
   a. Uterine contractions with documented cervical change or a cervix of at least 2cm dilatation and/or 80% effacement prior to term.
   b. Uterine contractions with rupture of membranes.

B. RISK FACTORS FOR PREMATURITY.
1. Lack of prenatal care.
2. Lower socioeconomic status.
3. Substance abuse.
4. Medical diseases.
5. Chronic hypertension.
6. Diabetes.
7. Renal disease.
8. Cardiac disease.
9. Autoimmune disease.
10. Urinary tract infection and asymptomatic bacteriuria.
11. **Repetitive abortion** (three or more consecutive spontaneous abortions).
12. Incompetent cervix.
13. Multiple gestation.
14. Abdominal trauma and surgery.
15. Iatrogenic prematurity.
16. Premature rupture of membranes.
    a. Diagnosis.
       1) History of leaking fluid.
       2) Vaginal pooling of amniotic fluid. Verify that it is amniotic fluid with positive nitrazine test result (amniotic fluid and blood are alkaline;

vaginal secretions are acid) and ferning pattern (arborization) on microscopic smear.

3) Ultrasound to evaluate intrauterine amniotic fluid volume.

b. Additional evaluation.

1) Amniocentesis for evaluation of fetal lung maturity and intrauterine infection.

2) Cervical culture for group B streptococcus, gonorrhea and chlamydia.

c. A management algorithm for patients with PROM is depicted in Figure 3.1. Antibiotics refers to a penicillin plus clindamycin or erythromycin.

17. Bacterial vaginosis.

a. This common vaginal condition may represent the most significant cause of idiopathic preterm delivery.

b. Diagnosis is by clinical signs of a discharge with increased vaginal pH >4.5, 'Clue cells' under microscopic examination in saline, and a positive 'whiff test' when KOH is placed on the microscope slide.

c. Vaginal cultures and stained smears are not diagnostic for bacterial vaginosis.

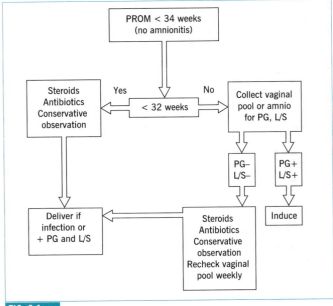

FIG. 3.1
Management algorithm for patients with premature rupture of membranes. FSI indicates foam stability index; L/S, lecithin/sphingomyelin ratio; PG, phosphatidyl glycerol.

C.   TOCOLYTIC AGENTS.
1.   Indications for tocolysis.
a.   Pregnancy between 20 and 35 weeks gestation.
b.   No chorioamnionitis or intrauterine infection.
c.   No maternal or fetal compromise.
d.   Cervical dilatation <4cm.
e.   Ruptured membranes are a relative contraindication.
2.   Bed rest.
a.   The first step in tocolytic therapy.
b.   Increase uterine perfusion with lateral uterine displacement. Left is preferable to right.
c.   Any hydration must be undertaken with care because of the potential for pulmonary edema with subsequent use of tocolytic drugs.
3.   Magnesium sulfate ($MgSO_4$) is often the agent of first choice.
a.   Interferes with calcium binding in myometrial smooth muscle.
b.   Maternal side effects.
    1)   Nausea, headache, palpitation
    2)   Respiratory depression
    3)   Hypothermia.
c.   Fetal side effects.
    1)   Hypotonia is common and often leads to lower Apgar scores
    2)   Respiratory depression is common with high magnesium levels.
4.   β-Adrenergic agents stimulate the β receptors of the sympathetic nervous system, producing uterine and bronchial smooth-muscle relaxation as well as peripheral vasodilatation and tachycardia. Ritodrine is the only agent currently approved by the FDA for use in inhibiting premature labor. However, it is rarely used, because of maternal side effects. The commonly used agent is terbutaline. (The following information holds for all β-mimetics.)
a.   Maternal side effects:
    1)   Restlessness
    2)   Tachycardia, palpitations, PVCs
    3)   Transient hypokalemia
    4)   Hyperglycemia
    5)   Hemodilution
    6)   Angina-like chest pain
    7)   Pulmonary edema.
b.   Fetal/neonatal side effects:
    1)   Tachycardia
    2)   Hypoglycemia
    3)   Hypocalcemia
    4)   Blood volume expansion.
5.   Indomethacin is the 'last line' of tocolytic therapy because of its fetal side effects associated with prolonged usage.

a. Inhibits synthesis of prostaglandins involved in initiation of labor.

b. Fetal urine output is decreased.

c. Potential for premature closure of ductus.

D. MATERNAL STEROID ADMINISTRATION. Multiple studies and the recent NIH Consensus study report state that steroids administered to the premature fetus via the mother to accelerate fetal lung maturation are effective at preventing or reducing neonatal RDS.

1. Betamethasone or dexamethasone are effective if delivery can be delayed for 48 hours after initiation of therapy and when given between 24 and 34 weeks of gestation. The data are less supportive for cases with PROM.

2. Regimens.

a. 48 hours of treatment are required to obtain the full maturational effect. Betamethasone and dexamethasone are used since they readily cross the placenta.

b. Betamethasone – 12mg i.m. q12h ×2 doses.

c. Dexamethasone – 6mg i.m. q12h ×4 doses.

3. Possible adverse effects have been reported mostly in animal studies and are described below.

a. Reduced lung growth.

b. Reduced brain weight secondary to brain growth inhibition.

c. Decreased immune responsiveness with risk for increased fetomaternal or maternal infection.

4. Sequelae. Long-term human follow-up studies have failed to expose any neurological, intellectual, or developmental sequelae attributable to steroid exposure in utero.

E. INTRAPARTUM MANAGEMENT.

1. Careful intrapartum management appears to have a significant influence on outcome for the premature fetus.

2. Continuous electronic monitoring should be used to detect fetal distress early in its development.

3. Cesarean section for premature infants.

a. Does not improve perinatal outcome in prematures unless specifically indicated.

b. Is indicated for breech presentation at <34–36 weeks gestation owing to the head being larger than the body and consequent risk of head entrapment.

c. Is indicated for any nonvertex-presenting twin at <34–36 weeks gestation.

d. At gestational ages <30 weeks, vertical uterine incisions may be required rather than low transverse uterine incisions because of the lack of development of the lower uterine segment. With these classical incisions, all future deliveries will need to be via repeat cesarean section.

RESUSCITATION OF THE NEWBORN

Cardiorespiratory depression (heart rate <100bpm, hypotension, hypoventilation, or apnea) may occur to some degree in 10–15% of newborn infants. Prompt therapy may be lifesaving and is necessary to minimize permanent CNS disability.

I. ETIOLOGY OF CARDIORESPIRATORY DEPRESSION

A. **DRUGS.** With few exceptions, anesthetic and analgesic drugs used in obstetrics cross the placenta and may affect the fetus.

B. **TRAUMA.** Rapid labor, mid-forceps, and breech delivery may be responsible for intracranial injury. Trauma has decreased in recent years, partly because of the more frequent use of cesarean section for breech presentations and cephalopelvic disproportion.

C. **HEMORRHAGIC SHOCK.** Fetal blood loss into the mother, placenta, or a twin, or from umbilical vessel rupture may be severe. Diagnosis of perinatal blood loss is frequently made retrospectively after noting a drop in the hematocrit.

D. **INTRINSIC CARDIAC, PULMONARY OR CNS DISEASE.** Anomalies, injury or fetal infection of these key organs can be responsible for depressed function at birth.

E. **ASPHYXIA.** One frequently considered cause of cardiorespiratory depression is asphyxia (decreased PO_2 and pH and increased PCO_2).

F. **UNKNOWN.** The cause of cardiorespiratory depression and low Apgar scores is frequently unknown.

II. ASPHYXIA

A. **CONDITIONS ASSOCIATED WITH ASPHYXIA.** A wide range of maternal, fetal, and placental conditions can lead to asphyxia in the newborn. A common factor seems to be marginal exchange of O_2 and CO_2 across the placenta, which becomes further compromised during labor. Antepartum tests as well as intrapartum fetal monitoring may detect some of those infants who cannot tolerate labor.

B. **PHYSIOLOGY.** Acute total asphyxia (8–15 minutes) of animals, followed by resuscitation, has not reproduced the acute clinical symptomatology or long-term CNS sequelae seen in human infants surviving perinatal asphyxia. Experiments in nonhuman primates indicate that more prolonged partial asphyxia (1–3 hours) is necessary to reproduce the clinical and pathologic condition most often seen in asphyxiated human infants. Acute cerebral ischemia can produce injury to the basal ganglia and brain stem in primates, but leaves the cerebral cortex relatively intact, a situation infrequently encountered in asphyxiated human newborns who survive. Injury to kidneys, gut, lung, and muscle typically precedes brain and myocardial injury when asphyxia is involved.

III. RESUSCITATION EQUIPMENT REQUIRED IN THE DELIVERY ROOM

A. CHECK PRESENCE AND FUNCTION PRIOR TO DELIVERY.

1. Overhead radiant warmer.
2. Suction source (wall and bulb).
3. Suction catheters.
4. Oxygen source.
5. Infant resuscitation bag.
6. Face masks (assorted sizes).
7. Laryngoscope (with Miller 0 and 1 straight blades).
8. Endotracheal tubes (2.5, 3.0, and 3.5mm diameters).
9. Umbilical catheterization tray.
10. Umbilical catheters (3.5 and 5.0 F).
11. Drugs.
12. Syringes, needles, and three-way stopcocks.
13. Gloves and goggles.

IV. RESUSCITATION TECHNIQUE

Prepare for receiving the infant by proper hand washing, donning scrub suits and gowns, and wearing protective rubber gloves and goggles.

A. **THERMAL PROTECTION.** Rapidly wipe the infant dry and place under a radiant heat source.

B. **POSITION FOR AIRWAY MANAGEMENT.** Place the infant in a left-lateral, head-down tilt position. The supine position can promote airway obstruction.

C. **PHARYNGEAL SUCTIONING.** Gently suction secretions from the pharynx with a bulb syringe or under direct vision (laryngoscope) with a whistle-tip catheter attached to wall suction. A DeLee Trap may be interposed. Avoid passing catheters through the nose and into the stomach for the first five minutes of life, as these maneuvers may induce bradycardia.

D. **AIRWAY SUCTIONING.** Thick secretions or meconium may require tracheal suction under direct vision (laryngoscope). On occasion, endotracheal tube replacement will be necessary to remove thick meconium from the trachea.

E. POSITIVE-PRESSURE VENTILATION. Infants with heart rates <100bpm need high-quality ventilation with oxygen-enriched gas immediately, as do infants who remain apneic for more than one minute after birth. With effective ventilation, the heart rate should increase to >100bpm within 15–30 seconds. The first few insufflations may require pressure of 30–50cm of water. Thereafter, lower pressures should suffice unless lung disease is present. The majority of infants with cardiorespiratory depression may be resuscitated by high-quality ventilation alone.

1. **Bag and mask ventilation.**
a. With the infant's head slightly extended, the mask is grasped with the thumb and first two fingers of the left hand and placed gently but firmly over the infant's mouth and nose. The other two fingers of the left hand are used to support the chin.
b. We usually use our continuous positive airway pressure (CPAP) device to deliver oxygen-enriched gas and to ventilate newborns. Self-inflating devices also work well.
c. A ventilatory rate of 30–50 per minute is usually adequate.
d. The effectiveness of ventilation is assessed by observation of chest motion and a prompt increase in heart rate. Auscultation of the chest should reveal air entry bilaterally.
e. Gastric distention should be watched for and may be relieved by passing a nasogastric or orogastric tube.
2. **Endotracheal intubation.** The need for intubation during resuscitation of newborn infants has often been an artifact of the supine position. In this position, the large occiput and tongue and small posterior pharynx combine to produce airway obstruction. Endotracheal intubation is indicated:
a. If bag and mask ventilation is ineffective.
b. If airway obstruction is suspected (e.g. goiter or micrognathia).
c. If meconium aspiration is suspected.
d. If external cardiac massage is necessary.
e. If prolonged ventilatory support is anticipated.
F. EXTERNAL CARDIAC MASSAGE. If the heart rate does not rise above 100bpm within 30 seconds of beginning ventilation, external cardiac massage should be started. Compression, with two fingers, should be over the middle one-third of the sternum (Figure 4.1). Lower positions are less effective and may lacerate the liver. A frequency of 120 compressions per minute is adequate. Depress the sternum 1.5–2.0cm with each compression. Coordinate chest compressions with ventilation in a 3:1 ratio. Assess effectiveness by palpating the femoral pulse and observing skin perfusion.

RESUSCITATION OF THE NEWBORN

4

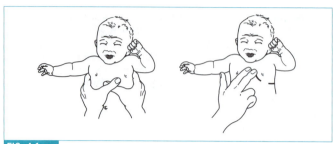

FIG. 4.1

External cardiac massage being performed on a newborn infant. (From Goetzman[1], with permission.)

G. PHARMACOLOGIC THERAPY.

1. **Epinephrine.** If the heart rate does not respond promptly to resuscitation efforts, administer epinephrine 1:10,000 (0.1mL/kg). May be repeated after several minutes. May be given via endotracheal tube or umbilical vein catheter.
2. **Catheterization** of the umbilical vein with a 5 F catheter advanced 3–4cm often provides the quickest vascular route for administering drugs and volume expanders.
3. **The endotracheal tube** is often the most accessible route for administering epinephrine and is clearly a preferred alternative to intracardiac injection. Dilute the epinephrine in 1–2mL of saline to facilitate delivery by this route.
4. **Hypovolemia.** If hypovolemia is suspected, administer 10–20mL/kg of 0.9% saline, type O Rh-negative blood cross-matched against the mother, heparinized placental blood, plasmanate or albumin (1g/kg) diluted to a 5% solution (1g/20mL) with saline.
5. **Metabolic acidosis.** If the infant remains pale and/or bradycardiac for four to five minutes after beginning ventilation, he or she probably has metabolic acidosis and will benefit from the administration of sodium bicarbonate as long as ventilation is adequate. Use a 0.5mEq/mL concentration and infuse 2–3mEq/kg at a rate of 1–2mEq/kg/min or less. Subsequent doses of sodium bicarbonate should be based on blood gas analysis. In general, metabolic acidosis with a base deficit of ≥ 10mEq/L should be corrected if the infant's condition remains unstable after resuscitation.

6. **Other drugs** such as atropine (0.01mg/kg) or 10% calcium gluconate (0.5mL/kg) are seldom used in the delivery room.
7. **Narcotic depression.**
a. Naloxone, 0.1mg/kg, should be administered for suspected drug depression only after appropriate initial resuscitation has taken place and the infant continues to hypoventilate. Too often, a narcotic antagonist is administered in lieu of assisting ventilation, and a wait-and-see attitude prevails to the detriment of the patient.
b. Knowledge of maternal heroin use is essential to avoid precipitation of acute narcotic withdrawal.
c. Maternal general anesthesia may result in an anesthetized newborn who requires 10–15 minutes (occasionally longer) of manual ventilation to recover from the anesthetic.

V. APGAR SCORE

The Apgar score provides a standard method for describing the condition of infants at birth. At 1 and 5 minutes after birth, five objective signs are evaluated and each is given a score of 0, 1, or 2 (Table 4.1). The sum of the five scores is the Apgar score. A score of 3 to 6 indicates moderate depression, and a score of 0 to 2 indicates severe depression. The 1 minute Apgar score and the 5 minute correlate best with survival, while those at 10 and 20 minutes seem to be better prognosticators of neurological damage at 1 year of age.

TABLE 4.1

APGAR SCORING SYSTEM

Sign	0	1	2
Heart rate (bpm)	Absent	<100	>100
Respiratory effort	Absent	Slow; irregular	Good crying
Muscle tone	Flaccid	Flexion of extremities	Active motion; well-flexed extremities
Reflex irritability	No response	Grimace	Vigorous cry
Color	Blue; pale	Body pink; extremities blue	Completely pink

VI. POSTNATAL MANAGEMENT OF ASPHYXIATED INFANTS

Apgar scores do not accurately predict asphyxia or metabolic acidosis. A cord blood gas analysis from the umbilical artery should be obtained from all depressed newborns to confirm asphyxiation. Problems to be anticipated include the following:

A. METABOLIC SEQUELAE.

1. **Lactic acidosis** (blood pH <7.2 and lactate >4.0mEq/L) may persist, indicating low cardiac output and poor peripheral perfusion. Alkali therapy or cardiotonic agents such as dopamine may be indicated.

2. **Hypoglycemia** (blood glucose level <40mg/dL in full-term infants or <30mg/dL in premature infants) is not uncommon and usually responds well to glucose infusion at rates of 8mg/kg/min.

3. **Hypocalcemia** (serum calcium level <8.0mg/dL in term infants or <7.0mg/dL in premature infants) frequently occurs during the second 24 hours of life in asphyxiated infants. The indications for therapy of hypocalcemia are not well defined and calcium administration is suspect for increasing tissue injury after hypoxemia/ischemia. Convulsions or heart failure caused by hypocalcemia should respond to infusion of 200mg/kg of calcium gluconate over 10 minutes followed by 400mg/kg/day.

B. CNS SEQUELAE.

1. **Cerebral edema** may lead to coma or convulsions. The syndrome of inappropriate antidiuretic hormone secretion may also occur. Assessments of fontanelle tension, cerebral suture width, and head circumference are helpful diagnostically. Fluid infusion in asphyxiated infants should be conservative initially, of the order of 50–60mL/kg/day. Serum sodium should be maintained in high normal ranges to inhibit cellular edema.

2. **Cerebral hemorrhage or infarction** may occur with catastrophic results. CT or ultrasound studies of the brain are usually indicated to evaluate presence of cerebral edema, hemorrhage, or infarction.

3. **Other interventions.** The use of hyperventilation alkalosis, glucocorticoids, depressive levels of phenobarbital, and/or osmotic agents is controversial. Mild hypothermia, certain calcium channel blockers and antioxidants show promise for decreasing CNS injury in experimental models.

C. RENAL SEQUELAE.
Acute renal failure is commonly caused by ATN, less frequently by medullary necrosis, renal cortical necrosis, or renal vein thrombosis. Careful fluid and electrolyte management is required. In ATN, renal function usually improves in 3–5 days. Occasionally, peritoneal dialysis is necessary.

D. URINARY BLADDER.
Bladder paralysis is common. It may be necessary to express urine manually from the bladder or to place a urinary catheter for 24–48 hours. Do not confuse this with posterior urethral valves in the male infant.

E. CARDIAC SEQUELAE.
Asphyxial cardiac damage may be lethal. Myocardial damage may produce hypotension, low cardiac output, and persistent metabolic acidosis. Radiographically, the heart is enlarged, and echocardiography reveals left or biventricular dysfunction. Careful

fluid management is required, and administration of oxygen, alkali, and, occasionally, cardiotonic agents may be necessary.

F. PULMONARY SEQUELAE. A variety of pulmonary problems may be precipitated by asphyxia, including pulmonary hypertension, RDS, and impaired lung fluid clearance. When seen together, the term 'shock lung' is often applied. Either sepsis or meconium aspiration may contribute to and complicate perinatal asphyxia. Pneumothorax may further complicate any of these pulmonary disorders.

G. OUTCOME. The mortality of severely depressed infants (5 minute Apgar 0 to 2) and significant metabolic acidosis (base deficit >12mEq/L) is significant. Survivors have an increased risk of CNS damage, but it must be remembered that more than 90% will develop normally. Thus, in the absence of serious congenital anomalies, it is prudent to begin resuscitation efforts in severely depressed infants. If an infant does not respond with a sustained increase in heart rate in 15–20 minutes, a decision to stop resuscitative efforts may be considered.

REFERENCE

1. Goetzman BW. Resuscitation of the newborn. In: Niswander KR, ed. *Manual of obstetrics.* Boston, MA: Little, Brown & Co; 1987:389–397.

FURTHER READING

Chameides L, the AHA/AAP National Resuscitation Steering Committee, eds. *Textbook of neonatal resuscitation.* Elk Grove Village, IL: American Academy of Pediatrics; 1994.

RESUSCITATION OF THE NEWBORN

4

ASSESSMENT OF GESTATIONAL AGE

5

I. CLASSIFICATION OF NEWBORNS

All newborn patients should be classified according to maturity and intrauterine growth.

A. **MATURITY.** Estimate gestational age using a physical/neurological assessment and lens examination.

1. **Premature.** Gestational age <37 weeks.
2. **Term.** Gestational age 37–42 weeks.
3. **Post-term.** Gestational age >42 weeks.

B. **INTRAUTERINE GROWTH.** Plot the weight, length, and head circumference vs the estimated gestational age on the intrauterine growth curve.

1. **Large for gestational age** – weight above the 90th percentile.
2. **Appropriate for gestational age** – weight between the 10th and 90th percentiles.
3. **Small for gestational age** – weight below the 10th percentile.

II. ASSESSMENT – PHYSICAL/NEUROLOGICAL

Using a combination of neuromuscular and external physical criteria, gestational age can be estimated independently of obstetric history (Figure 5.1). Accuracy is within 2 weeks for infants over 30 weeks gestation. Assessment of gestational age in babies under 30 weeks gestation is less precise. Very immature babies are frequently assigned too high a gestational age. Thus, heel to toe measurements have been added under 'plantar surfaces' in the Figure.

III. NOTES ON NEUROMUSCULAR EXAMINATION

1. **Posture.** Assess when the newborn is quiet and supine. Breech babies may have abnormal posturing of lower extremities.
2. **Square window.** Flex the hand between the thumb and index finger. Do not rotate the wrist.
3. **Arm recoil.** Hold the forearms flexed for 5 seconds, extend the forearms slowly and release.
4. **Popliteal angle.** Place the thigh in the knee–chest position with the pelvis flat on the mattress. Extend the lower leg from the knee until resistance is met and measure the angle.
5. **Scarf sign.** Grasp one hand and try to place it behind the contralateral shoulder, lifting the elbows across the body.
6. **Heel to ear.** Grasp the foot between thumb and index finger and attempt to touch the ipsilateral ear. Note the foot–ear distance and knee extension when resistance is met.

Neuromuscular maturity

	-1	0	1	2	3	4	5	Score	Weeks
Posture								-10	20
								-5	22
Square window (wrist)	>90°	90°	60°	45°	30°	0°		0	24
								5	26
Arm recoil		180°	140–180°	110–140°	90–110°	<90°		10	28
								15	30
								20	32
Popliteal angle	180°	180°	160°	130°	100°	90°	<90°	25	34
								30	36
Scarf sign								35	38
								40	40
Heel to ear								45	42
								50	44

Physical maturity

Skin	Sticky, friable, transparent	Gelatinous red, translucent	Smooth pink, visible veins	Superficial peeling, and/or rash, few veins	Cracking, pale areas, rare veins	Parchment deep cracking, no vessels	Leathery cracked wrinkled
Lanugo	None	Sparse	Abundant	Thinning	Bald areas	Mostly bald	
Plantar surfaces	Heel to toe 40–50mm: −1 <40mm: −2	>50mm No crease	Faint red marks	Anterior transverse crease only	Creases ant. 2/3	Creases over entire sole	
Breast	Imperceptible	Barely perceptible	Flat areola, no bud	Stippled areola 1–2mm bud	Raised areola 3–4mm bud	Full areola 5–10mm bud	
Ear/eye	Lids fused loosely: −1 tightly: −2	Lids open, pinna flat, stays folded	Sl. curved pinna, soft slow recoil	Well-curved pinna, soft but ready recoil	Formed and firm, instant recoil	Thick cartilage, ear stiff	
Genitals male	Scrotum flat, smooth	Scrotum empty, faint rugae	Testes in upper canal, rare rugae	Testes descending, few rugae	Testes down, good rugae	Testes pendulous, deep rugae	
Genitals female	Clitoris prominent, labia flat	Prominent clitoris, small labia minora	Prominent clitoris, enlarging minora	Majora and minora equally prominent	Majora large, minora small	Majora cover clitoris and minora	

FIG. 5.1

Scoring system for clinical assessment of maturation in newborn infants. (From Ballard et al[1], with permission.)

IV. ASSESSMENT BY LENS VASCULARITY

Examination of the anterior vascular capsule of the lens may help in estimating gestational age in the VLBW infant (<1500g) (Figure 5.2).

V. LGA INFANTS

Most LGA infants are simply genetically or nutritionally well endowed, but must be distinguished from IDMs or other conditions with hormonally induced excessive intrauterine growth (e.g. Beckwith syndrome). Infants of diabetic mothers have the following problems.

A. **HYPOGLYCEMIA** occurs with nadir at 1–2 hours.

a. In IDMs with marked obesity or a mother with poor control, start intravenous administration with 10% dextrose in water on admission to avoid panic when the reagent strip (e.g. Chemstrip™) indicates hypoglycemia.

b. IDMs have greater problems with glucose mobilization than with hyperinsulinism at birth, but do have β-cell hyperplasia and will overreact to a glucose bolus. Therefore, infuse glucose slowly, and wean from intravenous feedings when oral feedings are tolerated.

c. In general, the more the baby looks like an IDM, the more likely he or she is to have hypoglycemia and the more frequently the glucose should be monitored.

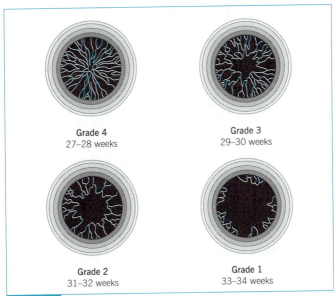

Grade 4
27–28 weeks

Grade 3
29–30 weeks

Grade 2
31–32 weeks

Grade 1
33–34 weeks

FIG. 5.2

Grading system for assessment of gestational age by examination of the anterior vascular capsule of the lens. (From Hittner et al[2], with permission.)

5 ASSESSMENT OF GESTATIONAL AGE

B. HYPERBILIRUBINEMIA IS COMMON. Both jaundice and hypoglycemia may be ameliorated or prevented by the early introduction of oral nutrition.

C. HYPOCALCEMIA is common in IDMs, may cause jitteriness and, rarely, seizures.

D. OTHER PROBLEMS. IDMs have an increased incidence of:

1. **Congenital anomalies.**
2. **Birth trauma:** e.g. Erb palsy, fractured clavicles.
3. **Respiratory disease,** particularly transient tachypnea and hyaline membrane disease.
4. **Cardiomyopathy** from increased cardiac glycogen.

VI. SGA INFANTS

A. CAUSES OF IUGR.

1. **Placental insufficiency and decreased oxygen/nutrient supply.** Effects of the following may be additive:
   a. Maternal hypertension.
   b. Abnormal uterine anatomy.
   c. Multiple birth with unequal placental size.
   d. Maternal smoking.
   e. Serious undernutrition.
   f. Premature aging of placenta.
2. **IUGR primarily due to fetal factors.**
   a. Fetal alcohol syndrome, cocaine abuse.
   b. Multiple congenital defects or syndrome.
   c. Chromosomal abnormality.
   d. Some inherited metabolic disorders.
   e. Intrauterine infection (e.g. TORCH group).

B. PROBLEMS ASSOCIATED WITH IUGR.

   a. Problems associated with primary condition if IUGR is due to fetal factors.
   b. Higher risk for congenital abnormalities and abnormal brain development.
   c. High risk for neonatal polycythemia and hypoglycemia.
   d. Frequently require high caloric intake for optimal growth.
   e. Infants with placental insufficiency may have decreased extracellular saline at birth, resulting in low urine output in the first day of life, and may benefit from saline supplementation.

REFERENCES

1. Ballard JL, Khoury JC, Wedig K, et al. New Ballard score, expanded to include extremely premature infants. *J Pediatr* 1991; 119:417–423.
2. Hittner HM, Hirsch NJ, Rudolph AJ. Assessment of gestational age by examination of the anterior vascular capsule of the lens. *J Pediatr* 1977; 91:455.

FURTHER READING

Dubowitz LMS, Dubowitz V, Goldberg C. Clinical assessment of gestational age in the newborn infant. *J Pediatr* 1970; 77:1–10.

TEMPERATURE REGULATION

I. SOURCES OF THERMAL STRESS

A. **EVAPORATION** may cause wet infants to undergo rapid heat loss.

B. **CONDUCTION** may cause heat loss in infants placed on a cold surface.

C. **RADIATION** causes infants to lose heat when exposed to (but not in contact with) surfaces such as incubator walls or windows with a lower temperature.

D. **CONVECTION** causes infants exposed to low ambient temperatures and drafts (e.g. open warmers) to lose heat.

E. **HYPERTHERMIA** may occur if infants are overwarmed, potentially resulting in dire metabolic consequences.

II. NEUTRAL THERMAL ENVIRONMENT

A. **DEFINITION.** Environment (temperature, humidity) at which infant's oxygen consumption is minimal (Figure 6.I).

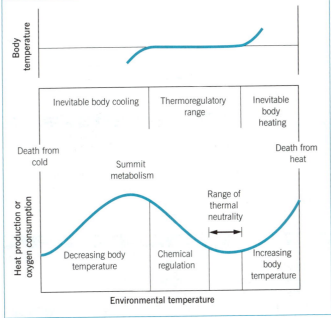

FIG. 6.1

Body temperature and oxygen consumption. (From Klaus & Fanaroff[1], with permission.)

B. **NEUTRAL THERMAL ENVIRONMENTAL TEMPERATURE** decreases with increasing gestational age and with postnatal age (Table 6.1).

C. **VERY VLBW INFANTS** may not increase metabolism in response to cold stress and behave as poikilotherms. Required environmental temperature to maintain normal skin temperature may exceed 37°C in babies less than 28 weeks gestation.

TABLE 6.1

APPROXIMATE NEUTRAL THERMAL ENVIRONMENT
TEMPERATURES

| | Weight (g) | | | |
| | (Temperature range °C) | | | |
Age	<1200 ±0.5° C	1201–1500 ±0.5° C	1501–2500 ±1.0° C	>2500 (>36 wks) ±1.5° C
0–12 h	35.0	34.0	33.3	32.8
2–24 h	34.5	33.8	32.8	32.4
24–96 h	34.5	33.5	32.3	32.0
4–14 days		33.5	32.1	32.0
2–3 wks		33.1	31.7	30.0
3–4 wks		32.6	31.4	
4–5 wks		32.0	30.9	
5–6 wks		31.4	30.4	

From Scopes and Ahmed[2], with permission.

III. MONITORING TEMPERATURE

A. **AXILLARY OR ABDOMINAL SKIN TEMPERATURES** correlate well with oxygen consumption (as opposed to rectal temperatures). A skin temperature of 36–36.5°C is generally satisfactory.

B. **THE RECTAL–SKIN TEMPERATURE** gradient may be useful in distinguishing cold stress from shock-like states. Foot–abdomen temperature gradient is usually >2°C if environment is too cold or if elevated temperature is due to fever.

IV. TEMPERATURE MODULATION

A. **TEMPERATURE REGULATION** may involve the following:
1. Vasodilatation and constriction.
2. Increased metabolism (including brown fat).
3. Increased activity.
4. Shivering and sweating. These are limited or absent in newborns, particularly in premature infants.

B. **ENVIRONMENT.** Infant should be placed in a crib, isolette, or under a radiant warmer as appropriate for the infant's size, gestational age, illness, and medical care requirements.

1. **Humidity** should be 40–60% or higher in cold infants or during the first days of life in micropremies with immature skin and high insensible water and heat loss.
2. **Swaddling.** Infants in cribs should be swaddled.
3. **Inner shields or double-walled incubators** to reduce radiant heat loss should be considered for infants weighing less than 1000g.
4. **Removal from incubators.** Infants should not be removed from incubators for extended periods of time (e.g. procedures, feedings) without providing for heat conservation.
5. **Servocontrolling incubator temperature** by a skin probe can mask temperature instability (e.g. sepsis) and is best reserved for older, stable newborns.

V. WITHDRAWAL OF TEMPERATURE SUPPORT

A. **WEIGHT.** Infants are usually larger than 1500g before they can maintain their temperatures in an open crib.
B. **TEMPERATURE.** Attempts to wean an infant who requires an incubator temperature >30°C usually are unsuccessful.

REFERENCES

1. Klaus MH, Fanaroff AA (eds). *Care of the high risk neonate,* 3rd edition. Philadelphia: WB Saunders; 1986.
2. Scopes JW, Ahmed I. Range of critical temperatures in sick and premature newborn babies. *Arch Dis Child* 1966; 41:417.

6

TEMPERATURE REGULATION

FLUID AND ELECTROLYTE BALANCE

I. GENERAL CONSIDERATIONS

A. **EXTRACELLULAR WATER.** Fluid requirements of term vs premature infants are different because of the variations of the amount and distribution of the total body water with gestational age (Table 7.1). Approximately 45% of birth weight in a term infant represents extracellular water (saline) compared with 60% or more in a 24–26 week edematous infant.

TABLE 7.1

DISTRIBUTIONS OF TOTAL BODY WATER
AS PERCENT OF BODY WEIGHT

Weeks gestation	Total body water (%)	ECW (%)	ICW (%)
24	86	60	26
28	84	57	26
30	83	55	28
32	82	53	29
34	81	51	30
36	80	49	31
Term	78	45	33

ECW, extracellular water; ICW, intracellular water. (Adapted from Friis-Hansen B[1].)

B. **NEONATAL DIURESIS.** Most newborn infants have abundant extracellular extravascular water. They are expected to excrete the excess and thus lose weight over the first 5–7 days of life. The normal saline diuresis may be delayed in patients with RDS. The approximate weight loss, as a percent of body weight, is related to gestational age (Table 7.2).

C. **INSENSIBLE WATER LOSS.** Normally 40–50 mL/kg/24h. Some infants (particularly those below 1000g birth weight) may have excessive water losses for the following reasons:

1. **High insensible water losses** may occur through immature or denuded skin, especially when placed under radiant warmers with low environmental relative humidity.

TABLE 7.2

GESTATION WEIGHT LOSS AS A PERCENT OF BODY WEIGHT (BW)

Gestation (weeks)	Weight loss (% of BW)
26	15–20
30	10–15
34	8–10
Term	5–10

2. **Phototherapy for hyperbilirubinemia** may increase insensible water losses from 40–50mL/kg/24h to as high as 100mL/kg/24 h.

II. GUIDELINES FOR INITIAL FLUID ADMINISTRATION

A. **FLUID RECOMMENDATIONS** for the first three days of life – the rates shown in Table 7.3 are based on experience with radiant warmers.
B. **HIGH INSENSIBLE WATER LOSSES** in very small infants under radiant warmers may necessitate parenteral fluid rates greater than 200mL/kg/24h. It may be desirable to limit insensible water losses using heat shields and vapor barriers.

TABLE 7.3

GUIDELINES FOR INITIAL FLUID ADMINISTRATION (mL/kg/24 h)

Birth weight Age	<1000g	1000–1500g	1500–2500g
1st 24h	100–150	80–100	60–80
2nd 24h	120–150	110–130	90–110
> 48h	140–180	140–180	120–140

C. **EXCESSIVE RATES OF FLUID** administration have been associated with hyperglycemia (due to glucose load), diuresis, and electrolyte loss, and, rarely, congestive heart failure.
D. **DECREASED EXTRACELLULAR WATER.** Occasionally an infant will be born with decreased extracellular water (e.g. some SGA and postmature infants). These babies will not lose weight in the first days and may become hyponatremic if not supplemented with NaCl on day 1–2.

III. ELECTROLYTE REQUIREMENTS

Sodium and potassium supplementation are not usually indicated during the initial (normal) obligatory saline diuresis. Begin at 48h depending on electrolyte measurements (Table 7.4). Routine calcium supplementation is not indicated during the first few days of life unless there is marked or symptomatic hypocalcemia.

TABLE 7.4

ELECTROLYTE REQUIREMENTS (mEq/kg/24 h)

Electrolyte	Parenteral	Oral
Sodium	3–5	8
Potassium	2–5	7
Calcium	2	2–3

IV. MONITORING INTRAVENOUS FLUID THERAPY

The following assessments of hydration should be obtained as frequently as needed (often every 8–12h in tiny infants with high insensible water loss):

A. BODY WEIGHT.

B. BLOOD CHEMISTRIES.

1. **Electrolytes.** Sodium tends to be lower in premature infants; 132mEq is acceptable. In very small infants, diuresis may exceed the ability of renal tubules to concentrate sodium, resulting in hypernatremia. Free water should be increased to maintain serum sodium <145mEq/L.

2. **Plasma osmolality.** 260–280mOsm/kgH$_2$O. In the first week of life it must be measured directly. After a week of age, it can be estimated by the following:

   Osm/kg water = 5 + 1.86 Na + 2.8 BUN + G/18
   (Na in mEq/L, BUN and glucose (G) in mg/dL).

3. **Serum creatinine and BUN** levels reflect both renal function and metabolism and may be elevated over the first 24h because of a normally low GFR and increased production.

C. URINE.

1. **Urine volume** is typically 2–5mL/kg/h (50–100mL/kg/24h).

2. **Urine electrolytes** do not assess hydration, but are useful in assessing requirements, e.g. by comparing sodium intake, output, and changes in serum sodium concentration.

3. **Osmolality** is typically 75–300mOsm/kg/24h if the renal solute load is between 7.5 and 15mOsm/kg/24h. (Assumes normal renal, adrenal, and posterior pituitary function.)

4. **Specific gravity** is proportional to osmolality if no protein or glucose is present in urine. Osmolality can be estimated by multiplying the decimal number of the specific gravity (sp gr) by 20:

   If sp gr = 1.003, mOsm = 20 x 3 = 60
   If sp gr = 1.015, mOsm = 20 x 15 = 300
   Normal range: 1.003–1.015.

V. INTERPRETATION OF DATA

A. AN APPROPRIATE MONITORING PERIOD should be decided upon depending on the patient's gestational age and condition (e.g. 6h, 12h, 24h, etc.).

7

FLUID AND ELECTROLYTE BALANCE

B. LABORATORY DATA should be obtained close to the time when fluids are to be assessed.

C. PREDICTED CHANGE IN WEIGHT. Predict (guess!) the expected change in weight over the monitoring period.

a. For a 1000 g infant at birth, expected to lose about 15% of its birth weight, one might predict a 2–4% weight loss over the first 12h.

b. Given a 1200g infant receiving 150mL/kg/24h, but only given 40kcal/kg/24h, one might expect a calorie deficit of about 20kcal/kg/24h. Since the infant has little fat, 4–5g of protein would need to be burned to make up the calorie deficit and thus 4–5g in weight would be lost over 24h even though fluid intake was adequate.

D. CONDITIONS THAT MAY ALTER FLUID REQUIREMENTS:

1. **ATN** following asphyxia may produce oliguria.
2. **Reduced GFR with HMD or RDS** decreases urine output.
3. **Shock, pituitary and renal dysfunction** can all affect urine output.
4. **Third spacing** after bowel surgery.
5. **Inappropriate antidiuretic hormone secretion.**
6. **Decreased extracellular saline** at birth.
7. **Adrenal insufficiency.**
8. **Phototherapy.**
9. **Extend losses:** e.g. nasogastric suction, diarrhea, external ventriculostomy.

VI. CORRECTION OF ABNORMALITIES

A. HYPONATREMIA may be due to excess sodium loss (usually renal or gut) or excess water gain (usually renal failure, or third spacing, or intracellular shifts).

a. Estimate extracellular volume (ECV) from Table 7.1, postnatal or recent weight change.

b. Calculate sodium deficit = $(140-[Na^+])$ x ECV (in liters), and estimate ongoing loss (or water gain if third spacing).

c. Replace deficit + anticipated loss over next 12–24h period.

d. If serum sodium is <120mEq/L, replace sodium with 3% NaCl solution (0.513mEq/mL) to achieve an estimated serum sodium of 125mEq/L.

e. Rarely, hyponatremia is due to excess free water administration, in which case fluid restriction is indicated.

B. HYPERNATREMIA may be due to excess insensible water loss, inability of kidney to concentrate sodium during postnatal diuresis (common in microprematures), or, infrequently, inadvertent excess sodium administration.

a. Estimate ECV (in liters).

b. Water deficit = (ECV x $[Na^+]$/140) − ECV.

c. If serum sodium >165mEq/L, correct slowly over 24h.

C. **HYPOKALEMIA** may be due to renal or intestinal loss or, rarely, intracellular shifts.

a. If K <2mEq/L, administer 0.5mEq/kg i.v. over 2h.

b. If patient is symptomatic, K may be given at a maximum infusion rate of 1mEq/kg/h.

D. **HYPERKALEMIA** may be due to renal failure, adrenal disease, injury, excess administration, or exchange transfusion.

a. Infants frequently tolerate potassium levels of 7.5–8.5mEq/L potassium without cardiac effects (peaked T waves, widened QRS complex).

b. Exchange resin (sodium polystyrene sulfonate-kayexalate) may be given as an enema, 1g/kg. One gram will exchange 2–3mEq sodium for 1mEq potassium, lowering the serum level by about 1mEq/L. Hypernatremia is a complication of excessive use. Exchange resins work slowly and are best used for potassium levels <7.0 in the absence of ECG changes.

c. Sodium bicarbonate, 2mEq/kg i.v., should be given if T waves are peaked.

d. Glucose, 3–5mL/kg of 10% dextrose, together with 0.2U insulin, will shift potassium intracellularly. Maintain GIR 3–5mg/kg/min higher than normally tolerated and add insulin, 0.2U/kg/h, monitoring glucose levels to prevent excessive hyper- or hypoglycemia.

e. Major electrocardiographic changes should be treated initially with 10% calcium gluconate (0.5mL/kg) given slowly, followed by sodium bicarbonate.

f. Dialysis is indicated if hyperkalemia with cardiotoxicity is not rapidly corrected by these means.

REFERENCES

1. Friis-Hansen BJ. In: Winters RW, ed.: *The body fluids in pediatrics.* Boston: Little, Brown & Co.; 1973:100.

7

FLUID AND ELECTROLYTE BALANCE

NUTRITION

The goal of neonatal nutrition is to provide sufficient substrate to promote optimal growth and development.

I. REQUIREMENTS

A. ENERGY.

1. **Special considerations.** Preterm infants have lower energy reserves, organs that are metabolically more active, and a greater growth velocity than term infants. Any infant who is ill is at risk of becoming catabolic.
2. **A comprehensive nutritional approach** for the preterm infant must be directed toward mimicking third-trimester accretion as well as facilitating the maturational changes in body composition.
3. **Total energy intake** should equal:
   a. Energy stored via fat and protein accretion.
   b. Energy expended in resting metabolism, thermoregulation, activity, and new tissue synthesis.
   c. Energy excreted owing to GI malabsorption with fat and protein loss in the stool, or urinary excretion.
4. **Caloric needs to maintain body weight.** In a neutral thermal environment with minimal physical activity, caloric needs to maintain body weight are 50–60kcal/kg/24h of parenteral intake or 60–80kcal/kg/24h if the intake is enteral.
5. **Caloric needs to support growth.** To support growth of the premature infant, a range of 120–130kcal/kg/24h is recommended. See Table 8.1.

B. PROTEIN

1. **Lean body mass.** The shorter the gestation, the lower the ratio of lean body mass to total body weight. Protein synthesis and the deposition of new tissue require energy. In addition, increase in lean body mass (protein gain) is linearly related to protein intake.
2. **Protein requirements** for the growing preterm are in the range 3–4g/kg/24h. Clinical trials comparing growth rates of infants on varying amounts of protein and energy intakes reveal 3–3.5g of protein per 120kcal to be most effective (Figure 8.1). Fortunately, preterm commercial formulas and fortified breast milk contain this protein–energy ratio.
3. **Optimal intake** must be assessed on an individual basis. Excessive intake of protein may result in metabolic acidosis and elevated BUN and ammonia levels.

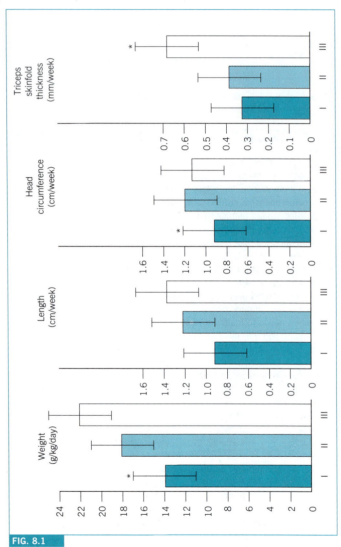

FIG. 8.1

Effect of protein–energy intake on growth. I: protein 2.24g/kg/day, energy 115kcal/kg/day; II: protein 3.6g/kg/day, energy 115kcal/kg/day; III, protein 3.6g/kgs/day, energy 149kcal/kg/day. * significant difference (p<0.05).

8

NUTRITION

4. **Inadequate intake** may result in a negative nitrogen balance, flattened growth curves (particularly length), and less than optimal mental and motor developmental outcome.
5. **Enzymes required** for amino acid metabolism are variably decreased in preterm infants, increasing the amount of essential amino acid intake needed.

C. CARBOHYDRATE.

1. **Nutritional significance.**
a. Direct source of energy for neural and other nervous tissue.
b. Calories to preserve protein for tissue synthesis.
c. Important effector for growth with stimulation of insulin secretion.
2. **Carbohydrate requirements.** Carbohydrates should constitute 40–60% of total calories (11–16g/kg/day at 3.4kcal/g).
3. **Assessment of adequate intake and tolerance.**
a. Calculate GIR of i.v. dextrose:
   GIR = (% dextrose x i.v. rate)/(6 x weight in kg).
b. A GIR of 4–6 mg/kg/min is an accepted beginning range.
c. Monitor blood glucose, urine for glucose, presence of osmotic diarrhea, and reducing substances in stool with enteral feeds.
d. Lactose intolerance is uncommon in the absence of gut injury, even in premature infants less than 28 weeks gestation.

D. FAT.

1. **Nutritional significance:**
a. Energy stores (as triglycerides in adipose tissue).
b. Good source of calories (9kcal/g), which contribute to a positive energy balance.
c. Structural component of membrane phospholipids, neurons and retina.
d. Precursor for prostaglandins and surfactant.
e. Vehicle for fat-soluble vitamins.
2. **Essential fatty acid deficiency.** Premature infants are at risk for essential fatty acid deficiency due to low stores, inefficient fat absorption, and rapid substrate utilization.

TABLE 8.1
DAILY CALORIC EXPENDITURE IN A GROWING PREMATURE INFANT

Item	kcal/kg/24h
Resting expenditure	40–50
Physical activity	15–30
Cold stress	10–70
Specific dynamic action	8
Fecal loss of calories	12
Growth allowance	25
Total	120

Modified from Sinclair et al[1], with permission.

3. **Fat requirements.** 35–50% of total calories should be from fat: i.e. 4–6g/kg/day (9kcal/g). Ketosis may occur if fat provides more than 60% of calories.
4. **Absorption of fatty acids.** Long-chain fatty acids are inefficiently absorbed in small preterm infants owing to decreased intraluminal bile salts. Medium-chain triglycerides (MCT) and fatty acids do not require micelle formation with bile salts for absorption. However, MCT do not provide essential fatty acids.

E. **VITAMINS.**
1. **Adequate intake.** Healthy term infants receive adequate vitamin intake if they consume 800–1000mL/24h of standard formula or breast milk.
2. **Factors placing preterm infants at risk for vitamin deficiency:**
a. Lack of third-trimester accretion.
b. Increased metabolic rate and rate of growth.
c. Inability to consume large quantities of formula or breast milk.
d. Decreased adipose tissue to store fat-soluble vitamins.
e. Compromised GI absorption interferes with the infant receiving the full complement of extra vitamins contained in preterm formulas or fortified breast milk.
3. **Suggested supplementation for preterms:**
a. Most multivitamin preparations (1mL/24h) will supply needed amounts of vitamins A, B, C, and D, when coupled with preterm formula.
b. Vitamin E deficiency may result in hemolytic anemia, thrombocytosis, and edema. Hemolysis may be potentiated by increased intake of iron and polyunsaturated fatty acids (PUFA) in the infant with low stores of vitamin E. We recommend that infants weighing <1500g at birth receive 12.5IU of vitamin E q12h). See Table 8.2.
c. 1mg of vitamin K should be given at birth (0.5mg to infants <1000g). If an infant is receiving only parenteral nutrition or antibiotic therapy for >1 week, we give vitamin K (1mg/week).

TABLE 8.2

NUTRITIONAL SUPPLEMENTATION OF PREMATURE INFANTS (1500G) RECEIVING ORAL FEEDS

Supplement	Recommendations
Polyvisol®, 1ml	Start when oral intake reaches 80kcal/kg/day
Vitamin E, 25IU/day	Start day 2–3 of life if tolerated; continue until infant weighs 1500g
Folate, 50mcg/day	Start day 2–7 of life when oral intake tolerated; continue until infant weighs 1800–2000g
Iron, 4–6mg/kg/day	Start at 2–4 weeks; continue supplementation for 3–4 months

d. If the chosen multivitamin preparation does not contain folic acid, 50mcg is the recommended supplementation.
e. Vitamin A supplementation, 5000 units i.m., 3 times a week for 4 weeks has been shown to maintain normal retinol levels and to decrease the incidence of chronic lung disease in infants <1000g with RDS.

F. MINERALS.

1. Iron

a. During the last trimester, the fetus accumulates 12.5–20.0mg/kg/day. Therefore, prematurely born infants have minimal iron stores.
b. Breast milk and 'Premature' formulas do not supply adequate iron for the growing preterm. We recommend supplementing growing premature infants with iron (4–6mg/kg/24h) after they are tolerating full enteral feeds at 10 days to 2 weeks of age.
c. Infants receiving erythropoietin therapy are placed on the higher end of the dosage range. Additionally, if infants are concurrently on vitamin E, each supplement should be administered on alternate days.

2. Calcium/phosphorus

a. Fluctuations in serum calcium level in the first days of life reflect metabolic or hormonal adaptations. During this time, administration is indicated only to prevent or treat symptoms of hypocalcemia rather than to promote skeletal growth and mineralization.
b. The accumulation of calcium by the fetus during the last trimester averages 130–150mg/kg/day. The calcium content of neither breast milk (35mg/dL) nor standard infant formulas (55mg/dL) is adequate to meet this accretion rate. 'Premature' formulas contain 165–180mg of calcium per deciliter.
c. Calcium and phosphorus absorption by the gut is inefficient (50–60% of intake), and loss of these minerals in the urine is increased by diuretics, especially furosemide.
d. Very small premature infants are at risk for development of osteoporosis and poor linear growth secondary to poor stores of calcium and phosphorus. Monitoring body length and serum alkaline phosphatase levels is helpful in assessing if intake of these minerals is adequate.

II. COMPOSITION OF MILK AND FORMULAS

A. COMMERCIALLY PREPARED formulas generally attempt to mimic human milk in terms of caloric density (67kcal/dL or 20kcal/oz) and distribution of calories between carbohydrate, fat, and protein.

B. STANDARD INFANT FORMULAS. SMA®, Similac PM 60:40®, Similac with whey, and Enfamil® contain a whey–casein ratio similar to that of human milk (60:40). Some standard formulas still contain protein with a ratio of whey to casein similar to that of cows' milk .

8

NUTRITION

C. **'PREMATURE' FORMULAS** contain a higher caloric density (8kcal/dL or 24kcal/oz), provide carbohydrates as a mixture of lactose and glucose polymers and provide higher levels of essential fatty acids, essential amino acids, electrolytes, calcium, and phosphorus. The protein content is higher than term formulas as well, and the protein–energy ratio is appropriate for the preterm infant.

D. **SUPPLEMENTATION OF BREAST MILK.** Despite the many nutritive and non-nutritive qualities of breast milk, supplementing it with commercially prepared human milk fortifier brings the content closer to the premature infant's nutritional requirements (compare listing of nutrients of breast milk and fortified breast milk in Table 8.3).

E. **SPECIAL FORMULAS** provide proteins as soy or casein hydrolysates, usually with a nonlactose source for carbohydrate. These formulas unfortunately fall short of meeting recommended nutritional guidelines for premature infants.

F. **CONCENTRATING FORMULA** beyond 24kcal/30mL is an option when an infant is fluid restricted or has poor pattern of growth. Adding MCT oil or polycose for extra calories is not recommended because the infant will not receive the optimum protein–energy ratio.

III. POSTNATAL INTRODUCTION OF NUTRIENTS

A. **INTRAVENOUS FEEDING.** SGA or premature infants should receive i.v. glucose by 2–6 hours of age if they cannot be fed orally. Infants with respiratory disease or feeding intolerance should receive supplemental protein, glucose, and lipids by peripheral vein or central venous line starting day 1–3 (see Chapter 9: Parenteral Nutrition).

B. **HYPOCALORIC (TROPHIC) FEEDINGS.**

a. Though protocols vary, trophic feeding is initiated on days 1–3 of life, at a volume of 15-20 mL/kg/24 h. Often, no advance in feeding volume is made for 3–5 days.

b. Positive findings in clinical trials of these hypocaloric feedings include:
   1) Infants reach full feedings sooner, with less feeding intolerance
   2) Gastric motility patterns are more mature, with a more rapid rise in serum gastrin levels
   3) Mean alkaline phosphatase levels are lower
   4) Fewer days of phototherapy are required
   5) Weight gain is improved, and hospital stay is shorter.

C. **MODE AND METHODS OF FEEDINGS.**

a. Most infants under 32 weeks gestation have immature suck/swallow patterns and require gavage feeding. For these infants, non-nutritive sucking should be encouraged. Additionally, infants who are not mature enough to breast-feed should be able to experience 'skin-to-skin' contact with their mothers. Such contact can have a positive effect on maternal breast-milk production.

TABLE 8.3

COMPOSITION OF INFANT FORMULAS

NUTRIENTS RECEIVED PER KG WHEN FED 150ML/KG

	Preterm Breast Milk	Breast milk + HMF (1pk/25mL)	Enfamil 20 (with Fe)	Similac 20 (with Fe)	SMA 20 (with Fe)	Enfamil Premature 20	Enfamil Premature 24	Similac Special Care 20	Similac Special Care 24
Energy (kcal)	100	120	100	101	101	100	122	101	122
Protein (g)	2.4	3.5	2.3	2.3	2.3	3.0	3.6	2.7	3.3
Carbohydrate	11	15	10.4	10.8	10.8	11.1	13.4	10.8	12.9
(source[a])	(a)	(a,b)	(a)	(a)	(a)	(a,b)	(a,b)	(a,e)	(a,e)
Fat (g)	5.3	5.4	5.7	2.3	5.4	5.1	6.2	6.2	6.6
(source[b])			(g,h)	(g,h)	(g,h)	(f,g,h)	(f,g,h)	(f,g,h)	(f,g,h)
Calcium (mg)	38	173	69	77	63	119	119	201	219
Phosphorus (mg)	22	90	47	59	42	60	60	101	110
Magnesium (mg)	5	6.5	7.8	6.2	6.8	10.2	10.2	8.3	15
Iron (mg)	0.14	0.14	0.17(1.9)	0.23 (1.8)	0.23 (1.8)	.26	0.26	.30	2.3
Zinc (mg)	0.56	1.63	0.78	0.77	0.75	1.7	1.0	.39	1.8
Sodium (mEq)	1.9	2.4	1.2	1.2	0.98	1.7	1.7	2.1	2.3
Potassium (mEq)	1.9	2.5	2.7	2.8	2.1	2.9	2.9	3.2	4.0
Chloride (mEq)	2.5	3.3	1.8	1.9	1.7	2.4	2.4	3.0	2.8
Vitamin A (IU)	72	1497	315	350	300	1215	1215	1455	828
Vitamin D (IU)	12	327	63	62	60	330	330	390	183
Vitamin K (mg)	3	9.6	8.7	8.1	8.3	13.2	13.2	15.9	15
Folate (mg)	5	43	16	15	7.5	35	35	44	45
Osmolality (mOsm/L)	290–300	390	278	290	300	240	240	300	300

8

NUTRITION

TABLE 8.3 (CONTD)

	Similac PM60/40	Similac 27	Isomil 20	Prosobee 20	Nutramigen 20	Pregestimil 20	Enfamil 24 (with iron)	Similac 24 (with iron)	Alimentum
Energy (kcal)	101	137	100	100	100	100	122	122	101
Protein (g)	2.4	3.7	3.0	3.0	2.9	2.9	2.7	3.3	2.8
Carbohydrate	10.4	14.4	10.2	10.4	13.7	10.3	12.5	12.8	6.9
(source[a])	(a)	(a)	(b)	(b)	(b,d)	(b,c,d)	(a)	(a)	sucrose tapioca starch
Fat (g)	5.6	7.2	5.5	5.4	3.9	5.6	6.8	6.4	5.6
(source[b])	(g,h)	(g,h)	(g,h)	(g,h)	(j)	(f,i,j)	(g,h)	(g,h)	(f,g,h)
Calcium (mg)	57	107	107	95	95	94	84	110	107
Phosphorus (mg)	29	77	77	75	63	63	57	86	77
Magnesium (mg)	6.2	7.7	7.7	11.1	11.1	10.5	9.5	8.6	7.7
Iron (mg)	0.23	1.8	1.8	1.9	1.9	1.9	0.20 (2.3)	0.27 (2.3)	1.8
Zinc (mg)	0.77	0.77	0.77	0.80	0.80	0.80	0.95	0.92	0.77
Sodium (mEq)	1.1	2.0	2.0	1.5	2.1	2.1	1.5	1.8	2.0
Potassium (mEq)	2.2	2.8	2.8	3.0	2.9	2.9	3.3	4.1	3.1
Chloride (mEq)	1.7	2.9	2.9	2.4	2.5	2.4	2.1	2.8	2.3
Vitamin A (IU)	350	305	305	315	315	315	375	336	305
Vitamin D (IU)	62	62	62	63	63	63	77	74	39
Vitamin K (mg)	8.1	15	15	15.9	15.9	15.9	10.5	9.8	15
Folate (mg)	15	15	15	16	16	16	19	18	15
Osmolality (mOsm/L)	280	250	250	200	320	320	360	380	370

[a]Sources of carbohydrates: a, lactose; b, corn syrup solids; c, glucose (dextrose); d, modified cornstarch; e, glucose polymers. [b]Sources of fat: f, MCT; g, soy oil; h, coconut oil; i, high oleic (safflower) oil; j, corn oil; k, palm oil. HMF, human milk fortifier.

b. Most VLBW premature infants tolerate either continuous (by pump) or bolus feedings. Residuals should be noted prior to each feeding, as well as measurement of girth. The pattern and consistency of stools should also be monitored, as well as the physical examination.

c. Bolus feedings should be delivered by gravity only. A 5 F polyethylene tube can be used, and should be changed every 12–24 hours. There are also softer Silastic NG and NJ (when NG feeds are not tolerated) tubes available, some of them designed to be indwelling. Placement of NJ tubes should be confirmed by radiograph.

d. In general, a feeding advance of 20mL/kg/24h is well tolerated. However, medical management styles in advancing enteral nutrition vary greatly, as does infant tolerance.

REFERENCE

1. Sinclair JC, Driscoll JM Jr, Heird WC et al: Supportive management of the sick neonate. *Pediatr Clin North Am* 1970; 17:863.

FURTHER READING

Kashyap S, Schulze K, Forsyth M, *et al.* Growth, nutrient retention, and metabolic response in low birth weight infants fed varying intakes of protein and energy. *J Pediatr* 1988; 113:713–721.

Pereira G, Georgieff M, eds. Neonatal/perinatal nutrition. *Clin Perinatol* 1995; 1–249.

Tsang R, Lucas A, Uauy R, eds. *Nutritional needs of the preterm infant.* Baltimore: Williams & Wilkins; 1993.

8

NUTRITION

PARENTERAL NUTRITION

Parenteral nutrition refers to the intravenous administration of amino acids, carbohydrates, and fats together with minerals, vitamins, and trace elements. It is an important form of therapy in infants with gastrointestinal problems and in premature infants. The latter have small energy reserves, as demonstrated by the calculated tolerance to malnourishment in newborns and adults (Table 9.1).

9

TABLE 9.1		
CALCULATED SURVIVAL TIME IN DAYS FOR STARVATION AND SEMISTARVATION		
	Water only[a]	10% dextrose[a]
Small premature infant	4	11
Large premature infant	12	30
Full-term infant	33	80
Adult	90	350

[a]75mL/kg/day for infant; 3L/day for adult. Adapted from Heird et al[1], with permission

I. INDICATIONS FOR PARENTERAL NUTRITION
a. Premature neonate (<1500g) in whom the combined oral and i.v. caloric intake is anticipated to be <90cal/kg by 1 week of age.
b. Any infant over 1 week of age who does not receive more than 80–90kcal/kg by combined oral and i.v. routes.
c. Infants with bowel atresia, short gut syndrome, intestinal dysmotility, and postoperative states where enteral nutrition is not expected to begin for 3–5 days.

II. ROUTE OF ADMINISTRATION
A. CENTRAL VEIN.
1. **Silastic Broviac catheters.** These are radiopaque catheters, 1.3mm o.d., placed by the pediatric surgeon.
a. Following a cutdown over the common facial vein, the catheter is threaded into the internal jugular vein and advanced into the superior vena cava. Placement is verified with radiography.
b. Complication rate is high in very small infants.
2. **Fine silicone elastomer catheters.** Introduced percutaneously or by cutdown into peripheral veins. Preferred in neonates weighing less than 1000g.
3. **Maximum concentration of dextrose** is 30% and of protein 4.5% for centrally positioned lines.
B. PERIPHERAL VEIN. Scalp vein needles and plastic cannulas are used for peripheral PN. Glucose concentrations should not exceed 12.5% and protein 2%. Care should be taken if large amounts of calcium are being administered (>100g/dL i.v. solutions).

C. UMBILICAL ARTERY CATHETER is not generally used for PN. This route is occasionally used for infants weighing <1000g.

III. CATHETER CARE

A. CENTRAL PARENTERAL-NUTRITION LINES should not be entered unless using aseptic technique.

B. BROVIAC CATHETER SITES are covered with gauze and a small amount of povidone-iodine ointment. Dressings are changed daily.

C. FINE SILASTIC DEEP LINES should be maintained with a dry dressing, if collodion is used as a stabilizer. Infusion of blood products should be avoided to prevent protein deposition and catheter obstruction.

D. PERIPHERAL LINES should be treated similarly to central lines.

E. LIPIDS (e.g. Intralipid®) may be infused simultaneously with amino acid solutions by using a 'Y' connector attached to the PN catheter. A 0.22m millipore filter unit is attached to the 'Y' connector arm leading to amino acid solutions. Lipids are administered through a 1.2m filter via the second arm. When PN is infused via the UAC, lipid should be administered peripherally.

IV. SOLUTION GUIDELINES

See Table 9.2. Standardized solutions may or may not be used. Special order sheets are commonly used.

A. GLUCOSE.

a. Infusion generally begins at 6–8mg/kg/min and is increased daily by 0.6–1.2mg/kg/min (approximately 1.0–2.0g/kg/day) as tolerated. Most infants do not tolerate more than 12–15mg/kg/min.

b. Dextrostix® readings may be obtained every 12 hours and more often if changes in glucose infusion are made, or if the infant's glucose level is elevated. If the serum glucose level is >180mg/dL, or urine glucose level is >2+, then glucose concentration should be decreased.

c. Insulin (0.25–0.5 units/kg) may be used if lowering the glucose concentration does not produce the desired effect.

B. AMINO ACIDS.

a. Begin at 0.5g/kg and increase by 0.25–0.5g/kg/day to a maximum of 3.0g/kg/day (3.5g/kg/day for BW <1000g).

b. Ratio of nonprotein to protein calories should be approximately 10:1.

c. Total protein, ammonia (NH_3), BUN, serum pH, ALT (alanine aminotransferase), AST (aspartate aminotransferase), and bilirubin values and urine output should be monitored.

d. The contents of amino acid solutions vary by manufacturer. Both FreAmine III® 10% and Travasol® 10% contain the percentages of essential amino acids required by neonates. Trophamine® 6% is specifically formulated for neonates and is preferred.

TABLE 9.2
GUIDELINES FOR GLUCOSE, AMINO ACID, AND LIPID INFUSION

	Starting amount (g/kg)	Maximum amount (g/kg)	Days to attain maximum	Laboratory monitoring	Maximum calories (cal/kg)
Glucose	11[a] (GIR 7.6mg/kg/min)	20	6–12[b]	Urine, serum, blood, glucose,	80
Amino acids	0.5	3.0	5–10	Total protein, ammonia, BUN, creatinine, pH, ALT[c], AST[c], bilirubin	10
Lipid	0.5	4	8–16	Serum turbidity; triglycerides orally with lung disease	44

[a]May need to start lower if glucose intolerant.
[b]May take longer if glucose intolerant.
[c]ALT, alanine aminotransferase; AST, aspartate aminotransferase.

1) Arginine is present in sufficient quantities to reduce the incidence of hyperammonemia.

2) Chloride contents are low, an important consideration with respect to metabolic acidosis. Travasol 10% contains 0.4mEq of chloride and 0.9mEq of acetate per gram of amino acid, and Freamine III 10% contains insignificant amounts of chloride and 0.7mEq of acetate per gram of amino acid. Supplementation with L-cysteine HCl, 2mmol/kg/day, is recommended.

3) Branched-chain amino acids are present and are anticatabolic. They provide the substrate to meet the necessary energy requirements that occur during stress.

4) Trophamine® plus L-cysteine has pH 5.5. Increases Ca and P solubility (Ca:P of 1.7:1).

5) Pharma Thera, Inc. of Memphis, Tenn., will formulate amino solutions to fulfill special needs of infants with inherited metabolic disorders. Nephramine® should be used for all urea cycle defects. Aminosyn® should be used for disorders of leucine metabolism (isovaleric acidemia, maple syrup urine disease, and hydroxy methyl glutamyl-CoA lyase deficiency. Trophamine® can be used for all other metabolic disorders as a protein source.

C. LIPID.

a. Intralipid® infusion is begun at 0.5g/kg/day and increased to 3g/kg/day for preterm and 4g/kg/day for term infants in increments of 0.5g/kg/day. The infusion rate should not exceed 0.8mL/kg/h (20% emulsion = 20g/100mL, 2kcal/mL) in preterm infants <33 weeks gestation and no more than 1.5mL/kg/h in other infants. The preferred 20% solution is cleared by premature infants better than the 10% solution.

b. Lipids should be given to avoid essential fatty acid deficiency. This may be accomplished by a dose of 2–4% of total calories by fat or 0.5g/kg/day 3–4 times per week, at a minimum.

c. Obtain a baseline serum triglyceride level before starting PN and weekly thereafter. Maintain <150mg/dL.

d. Heparin, 1 unit/mL, in TPN improves lipid clearance but may increase free fatty acid levels.

e. Calories from fat should not exceed 45% of the total daily caloric intake.

f. Risk for bacterial and fungal growth may increase when a lipid bottle is open longer than 12 hours. When it is not possible to infuse a daily requirement in 12 hours or less, then two 30mL bottles should be ordered and changed after 12 hours. When possible, infuse total dose over 20–24 hours.

g. Addition of lipids to PN solution in pharmacy is not practical. TPN solution compounding is not a standard practice because of concerns with solubility and the small catheter size used in neonates.

D. VITAMINS.

a. MVI-Pediatric concentrate solution provides the following per 5mL: vitamin A (0.7mg), vitamin B1 (1.2mg), vitamin B2 (1.4mg), vitamin B6 (1mg), niacin (17mg), vitamin C (80mg), vitamin D (10mcg), vitamin E (7mg), biotin (20mcg), folic acid (140mcg), vitamin B12 (1mcg), vitamin K1 (200 mcg) and pantothenic acid (5mg).

b. MVI-Pediatric daily dosage is based on infant size: 1.5mL for <1kg; 3.25mL for 1–3kg; 5mL for >3kg.

   1) Begin on Day 1 of PN.
   2) If other vitamin preparations are used, different volumes will need to be administered. Be aware of preservatives, i.e. propylene glycol, used in adult i.v. vitamin preparations. Neonates cannot tolerate high doses of these preservatives.
   3) Remember MVI-Pediatric contains vitamin K. If the patient is on coumadin, dosing may be difficult, especially if PN is cycled.

E. TRACE MINERALS.

a. For premature infants, zinc and copper, 0.3mg/kg/day, are added as the sulfates when caloric goals are being met or at about 2 weeks of age.

b. For term infants, the Zn and Cu requirements are less: 0.1mg/kg/day.

c. Selenium should be added at a dose of 2–3mcg/kg/day. It should be withheld if renal output is impaired or if renal failure is present.

d. Copper and manganese should be withheld in the presence of cholestasis: i.e. conjugated (direct) hyperbilirubinemia. They accumulate in the liver with impaired bile secretion and are hepatotoxic.

e. The addition of iron to PN is discouraged.

V. SPECIAL CONSIDERATIONS

A. FLUID, ELECTROLYTE, OR METABOLIC IMBALANCE may necessitate temporary (e.g. 24h) discontinuation of PN.

B. RENAL FAILURE may necessitate limiting amino acid administration to 0.5–1.0g/kg/day and eliminating selenium. Use the BUN concentration as a guide.

C. HEPATIC INSUFFICIENCY. Amino acid administration to an infant with hepatic insufficiency may result in serum amino acid imbalances, azotemia, and hyperammonemia. Discontinue PN if liver enzymes are markedly elevated in serum. Eliminate Cu and Mn if TPN is used with cholestasis.

D. CENTRAL VENOUS LINES should not be placed for PN when sepsis is suspected until the appropriate antibiotics have been administered for 24–48 hours. Parenteral nutrition during this time can be administered by a peripheral vein with appropriate considerations of solution osmolality, calcium content, etc.

9

PARENTERAL NUTRITION

VI. COMPLICATIONS

A. INFILTRATION of PN solutions in peripheral veins may cause subcutaneous tissue injury and skin sloughs. Hyaluronidase and/or sodium bicarbonate solution injected into the affected area may reduce injury.

B. METABOLIC.

1. **Hypoglycemia.** Discontinuation of i.v. solutions in infants receiving PN may cause the glucose level to fall rapidly. Therefore, the infusion must be restarted as soon as possible. If the daily infusion falls behind the expected rate, any effort to catch up must be done gradually without exceeding the infant's ability to tolerate glucose.

2. **Hyperglycemia.** Glucose administration is increased gradually to avoid hyperglycemia.

3. **Hyperammonemia** may be due to excessive amino acid administration. Decreasing, or temporarily discontinuing, protein administration will correct this problem. This now occurs infrequently since arginine in PN solutions has been increased. Ammonia levels should be monitored weekly but can be done less often if Trophamine® is used.

4. **Hyperlipidemia.** SGA infants are particularly prone to hyperlipidemia. Lipid should be used with caution, including avoidance in first week of life, in infants with severe lung disease. If increasing supplemental oxygen is required with no apparent cause, consideration should be given to decreasing or temporarily discontinuing lipid administration.

5. **Fluid or electrolyte imbalance.** Fluid and electrolyte status should be evaluated before ordering new solutions.

6. **Metabolic acidosis** is usually induced by hyperchloremia. It may be necessary to give more anions as acetate. The dose of amino acids should be checked. Sepsis must be ruled out.

7. **Liver damage.** Progressive cholestasis, with early elevation of serum bile acids and subsequently conjugated (direct) hyperbilirubinemia, portal tract fibrosis, and infiltration can occur with prolonged amino acid administration. Liver function usually returns to normal 1–4 months after discontinuation of PN. Delete copper and manganese during cholestasis.

C. INFECTION.

1. **Sepsis** should be considered if clinical deterioration occurs during PN.

2. **Catheters for PN** should be removed if blood cannot be sterilized after 48 hours of appropriate antibiotic therapy.

D. MECHANICAL.

1. **Catheter leakage.**
2. **Catheter clotting.**
3. **Catheter breakage.**
4. **Venous thrombosis.**
5. **Hydrothorax.**

VII. MONITORING INFANTS

1. **Body weight.** Usually once a day (depends on age and size of patient and duration of therapy).
2. **Laboratory.** See Table 9.3.

TABLE 9.3

LABORATORY TESTS FOR MONITORING INFANTS RECEIVING PARENTERAL NUTRITION

Test	Suggested frequency
Urine specific gravity, glucose, protein, and pH	Each shift until stable, then once a day
Glucose oxidase strip	As needed to check blood glucose STAT
Hematocrit	Once every 1–2 weeks, then every month when stable
CBC, platelets with differential	Once every 1–2 weeks, then every month when stable
CBG or ABG	As indicated
Serum Na, K, Cl, Ca, BUN	Daily first week, then twice a week when stable.
Total/direct bilirubin	Once a week. More often if jaundiced. Serum and urine osmolality as indicated
Magnesium	Once a week
Twenty-factor automated chemical analysis, particularly for liver enzymes, albumin, phosphate, creatinine, total protein	Once a week until stable then every 2–4 weeks
Blood glucose	Daily first week and if glycosuria 2+ and/or Chemstrip >130mg/dL
Serum triglycerides	Daily first week or with increased dosage of lipids, then once or twice a week

9

PARENTERAL NUTRITION

REFERENCE

1. Heird WC, Driscoll JH, Schullinger JN et al. Intravenous alimentation in pediatric patients. *J Pediatr* 1970; 80:351.

FURTHER READING

Kerner JA Jr, ed. *Manual of pediatric parenteral nutrition.* New York: Wiley; 1983.

INFECTIOUS DISEASES

I. INFECTIONS OF MATERNAL ORIGIN

Agents transmissible from the mother to the fetus and neonate include more than the traditional TORCH agents of toxoplasmosis, other (syphilis), rubella, cytomegalovirus, and herpes (Table 10.1). Some prenatal infections result in hepatosplenomegaly, jaundice, rashes, CNS signs, and intrauterine growth retardation. However, many newborns experiencing prenatal infection are asymptomatic.

TABLE 10.1

INFECTIOUS AGENTS TRANSMISSIBLE FROM MOTHER TO INFANT

Agent	Usual diagnostic methods
Rubella	Culture, IgM-specific antibody
Cytomegalovirus	Culture, IgM-specific antibody
Herpes simplex	Culture, immunofluorescence
Hepatitis A	IgM-specific antibody
Hepatitis B	Other serologic test or procedure.
Measles	Culture, acute and convalescent specific IgG titer
Varicella	Culture
Parvovirus B19	IgM-specific antibody
Echovirus	Culture
Coxsackie B	Culture
Treponema pallidum	IgM-specific antibody
Tuberculosis	Culture
Chlamydia	Culture
Gonorrhea	Culture
Listeria	Culture
Enteric bacteria	Culture
Hemophilus influenzae	Culture
Group B β-hemolytic streptococcus	Culture, latex agglutination
Candida albicans	Culture
Malaria	Cytology; immunofluorescence
Toxoplasma gondii	Culture, IgM-specific antibody

A. DIAGNOSIS.

1. **Ascertainment of infectious agent.**
a. Detection: immunofluorescence, PCR.

b. Pathology: cytologic findings.
c. Serology: immunodiffusion, CIE, ELISA.
d. Isolation: culture (most reliable).
2. **Persistence of specific IgG antibody** beyond the age of normal decline of maternal antibody (3–24 months, depending on maternal antibody value).
3. **Elevation of IgM-specific antibody** to >20mg/dL in cord or neonatal blood is suggestive, but it is occasionally normal in infants with intrauterine infection. IgA, absent in newborns, should also be measured to assure that the cord blood sample is not contaminated with maternal blood.

II. BACTERIAL INFECTIONS

Bacterial illnesses commonly encountered in the newborn include sepsis, meningitis, pneumonia, cutaneous infection, conjunctivitis, urinary tract infection, and, less commonly, arthritis and osteomyelitis.

A. **SIGNS AND SYMPTOMS.** Sepsis simulates many noninfectious conditions. Signs may include hypothermia, hyperthermia, poor sucking, vomiting, diarrhea, abdominal distention, apnea, respiratory distress, cyanosis, hepatosplenomegaly, jaundice, skin mottling, lethargy, hypotonia, and seizures. Since bulging fontanel and nuchal rigidity are not reliable signs of meningitis in the newborn, lumbar puncture must be considered when systemic neonatal infection is suspected.

B. **'SEPSIS WORKUP'.**
1. **Culture blood,** CSF, urine, tracheal secretions (if intubated), and infected sites.
2. **Gram stain,** CSF, urine, tracheal secretions, and infected sites.
3. **CSF culture,** Gram stain, cell count, protein, glucose.
a. Normal CSF findings are shown in Table 10.2.
b. Cloudy CSF may result from bacterial proliferation in the absence of pleocytosis. Less than 1% of infants with meningitis will have a totally normal initial lumbar puncture.

TABLE 10.2

NORMAL CSF FINDINGS IN HIGH-RISK NEWBORNS

	Term infant	Preterm infant
WBC count (cells/mm³)	0–32	0–29
% PMN[a]	~60%	~60%
Protein (mg/dL)	20–170	65–150
Glucose (mg/dL)	34–119	24–63
CSF/blood glucose (%)	44–248	55–105

[a]PMN indicates polymorphonuclear neutrophil leukocytes.
Adapted from Sarff et al[1].

c. Low CSF glucose level and PMN response may occur with intraventricular hemorrhage.

d. Ventricular tap may be necessary to document ventriculitis in patients with hydrocephalus – e.g. resulting from meningomyelocele – or in infants with failed response to antibiotics.

4. **Tracheal aspirate.** In the first hours of life, leukocytes and bacteria on Gram stain suggest congenital infection.

5. **White blood cell, differential, and platelet count.** Normal WBC and differential counts do not rule out sepsis. Leukopenia and neutropenia or an increase in the total band count, with ratio of bands to total neutrophils ≥ 0.2, suggest sepsis but may be present in nonseptic, stressed, premature infants. Thrombocytopenia occurs in sepsis with or without DIC.

6. **Chest radiograph.** Pneumonia may also look like HMD or wet lung.

7. **Suprapubic aspiration or bladder catheterization.**

a. Urine culture. On suprapubic aspirate cultures, any number of a single bacterium is considered significant.

b. Urinalysis. False-positive and false-negative results for pyuria are encountered. Finding >5 bacteria per HPF on Gram stain of unspun urine indicates urinary tract infection.

8. **Latex agglutination test or CIE** identify bacterial antigens in urine or CSF. Detectable neonatal infections include Group B β-hemolytic streptococcus, *Hemophilus influenzae* B, certain serotypes of *Streptococcus pneumoniae* and meningococci (may cross-react with *Escherichia coli*).

9. **ESR.** Capillary blood in a 75mm heparinized microhematocrit tube, ESR 15mm/h or higher, in septic infants. Normal values are age dependent: range, 1mm/h at 12 hours to 17mm/h at 14 days.

C. **MANAGEMENT.**

1. **Initial antibiotic therapy.** Obtain cultures and begin treatment with a combination of ampicillin and an aminoglycoside. Continue for 3 days or until sensitivity studies are completed on a recovered bacterium. Add an antistaphylococcal antimicrobic if *Staphylococcus aureus* is suspected. In infants with prolonged stays in the NICU, who have central lines, or who have received multiple courses of antibiotics for sepsis, initial antibiotic therapy may include vancomycin, often in combination with third-generation cephalosporin.

2. **Duration of treatment.**

a. Sepsis without focal involvement – 10–14 days.

b. Meningitis – 14–21 days

c. Pneumonia – 7–14 days for Group B streptococcus and usual enterics; up to 4 weeks for *S. aureus.*

d. UTI – usually 10–14 days.

10

INFECTIOUS DISEASES

3. **Meningitis.**
a. Consider ability of the antimicrobic to achieve bactericidal levels in the CSF. Third-generation cephalosporins (e.g. cefotaxime) have excellent CSF penetration.
b. Intrathecal administration of aminoglycoside is not effective. Intraventricular instillation of aminoglycoside has been associated with greater mortality and morbidity, but may be indicated in patients with meningomyeloceles depending on susceptibility of the organism. CSF shunt infections may require intraventricular vancomycin or aminoglycoside instillation.

4. **UTI.**
a. Repeat urine culture 48–72 hours after treatment is initiated, 2 weeks after treatment is completed, and at regular intervals for at least 1 year after infection.
b. Evaluate renal function (creatinine, BUN).
c. Ultrasound may be used initially to identify abnormalities of urinary tract which may predispose to infection. A voiding cystourethrogram is usually indicated to evaluate anatomic abnormalities.

5. **Adjuncts in overwhelming sepsis.**
a. Exchange transfusion. Efficacy is not established. In group B streptococcus sepsis, exchange transfusions with blood containing specific antibodies may improve outcome.
b. Granulocyte transfusion. Septic infants with neutropenia and depleted bone marrow reserves may have improved survival following granulocyte transfusion.
c. Intravenous human gamma globulin (IVIgG) remains experimental. It appears to be effective only if it contains high agent-specific antibody titer.

D. **CUTANEOUS INFECTION.**
1. **Etiology.** Varies with nature of skin lesion (Table 10.3). The possibility of herpes simplex infection should be considered in vesiculopustular lesions.

TABLE 10.3

BACTERIAL CAUSES OF SKIN LESIONS IN NEONATES

Type of lesion	Likely cause
Pustular–vesicular	S. aureus; Groups A and B β strep; other bacteria and candida are less common; erythema toxicum
Cellulitis	Groups A and B β strep; S. aureus; Gram-negative enterics
Abscess	S. aureus; Group B β strep; Gram-negative enterics
Omphalitis	S. aureus; Group B β strep; Gram-negative enterics
Scalded skin syndrome (Ritter's disease)	S. aureus.

2. **Diagnosis.** Culture and Gram-stain lesions, aspirate margin of cellulitis, scrape base of vesicular lesions for herpes direct fluorescent antibody (or PCR).
3. **Management.** Limited superficial pustules usually require local topical treatment only. Extensive pustules or involvement of compromised skin sites require systemic treatment with appropriate antimicrobics.
E. **CONJUNCTIVITIS.** See Table 10.4. Frequently bacterial; rare but important nonbacterial cause is herpes simplex virus.

TABLE 10.4

CONJUNCTIVITIS IN THE NEONATE

Time of onset	Likely cause	Order of frequency of infection
12–24h (typically improving in 24h)	Chemical conjunctivitis ($AgNO_3$)	–
2–5 days	*Neisseria gonorrhoeae*	2
5–26 days	*Chlamydia trachomatis*	1 (most common)
1st week – 1 month	*S. aureus*, Gram-negative enterics; other bacteria	3
Few days – few weeks	Herpes simplex	4

1. **Diagnosis.**
   a. Gram stain and culture discharge.
   b. Giemsa stain of conjunctival scrapings detects intracytoplasmic inclusions of chlamydial infection. Chlamydia may also be identified by culture.
   c. Consider viral culture, immune fluorescence, PCR, or Tzanck smear to look for multinucleated giant cells typical of herpes infection.
2. **Management and treatment.**
   a. Chemical conjunctivitis. No treatment indicated.
   b. Bacterial conjunctivitis (other than gonorrheal). Topical antimicrobics such as polymyxin–bacitracin combinations, sulfa, erythromycin, or tetracycline are usually sufficient.
   c. Gonorrheal conjunctivitis. Cetotaxime 50mg/kg/day (divided q12h) for 7 days. Topical treatment with saline washes followed by ophthalmic antibiotics every 2–4 hours.
   d. Chlamydial conjunctivitis. Oral erythromycin prevents onset of chlamydial pneumonia and effectively treats chlamydial conjunctivitis.
   e. Pseudomonas conjunctivitis may cause particularly virulent infection and requires treatment with parenteral gentamicin or tobramycin plus ceftazidine or piperacillin in addition to topical aminoglycoside therapy.

10

INFECTIOUS DISEASES

F.   ARTHRITIS AND OSTEOMYELITIS. Most episodes arise from bacteremic spread. Occasionally, local extension of osteomyelitis or direct inoculation occurs.

1.   **Etiology** includes *S. aureus*, Group B streptococcus, various Gram-negative enterics, *N. gonorrhoeae*, and Candida.

2.   **Signs and symptoms.** Failure to move extremity or pain on movement. Swelling, erythema, and increased warmth are occasionally present.

3.   **Diagnostic tests.**

a.   Radiograph of joint, bone; repeat after 10 days; radiographic findings in osteomyelitis are absent early.

b.   Bone scan can be useful in the neonate, but many false-negative findings occur.

c.   Blood culture.

d.   Bone and joint aspiration for Gram stain and culture.

4.   **Management.**

a.   Nafcillin plus cefotaxime or an aminoglycoside until results of culture and sensitivity are known. Intra-articular or intraosseous antimicrobials are unnecessary.

b.   Duration of antimicrobial treatment depends on the nature of the infection and the response to treatment.

    1)   About 2–3 weeks for arthritis and about 4–6 weeks for osteomyelitis.

    2)   Oral antimicrobials should not be considered unless monitoring of serum bactericidal levels can be accomplished and compliance with treatment can be assured.

    3)   The ESR is a useful guide to duration of treatment. Radiographic resolution of osteomyelitis lags behind clinical improvement and is not a useful guide.

c.   Surgical treatment.

    1)   Open drainage of hip is indicated to prevent ischemic necrosis and permanent damage to femoral head and joint.

    2)   Other joints may be managed by repeated aspiration.

    3)   Bone infection should be surgically drained if pus is recovered from needle aspiration.

III. SPECIFIC BACTERIAL PATHOGENS

A.   GROUP B β-HEMOLYTIC STREPTOCOCCUS.

GBS causes a variety of neonatal infections including sepsis, pneumonia, meningitis, empyema, cellulitis, arthritis, osteomyelitis, and impetigo. Two clinically and epidemiologically distinct forms of GBS sepsis are described (Table 10.5). Interestingly, the virulence of this organism may be decreasing.

1.   **Diagnosis.**

a.   Culture and Gram stain of appropriate specimens.

TABLE 10.5

FEATURES OF GROUP B β-HEMOLYTIC STREPTOCOCCUS INFECTIONS

	Early onset	Late onset
Time of onset	Birth to 3 days; often occurs within hours of birth	7–10 days to 4 weeks
Clinical manifestations	Fulminating onset: apnea, tachypnea, respiratory distress, hypoxemia, shock; meningitis uncommon	More insidious onset of symptoms: mild to moderately severe illness; meningitis frequently present
Delivery and maternal complications	High incidence	Low incidence
Group B serotypes	All 5 serotypes	Type III accounts for 90%
Prognosis	Poor; mortality 50–75%	Fair prognosis; mortality 10% with meningitis
Transmission	Maternal source	Maternal source, nosocomial source, community source

10

INFECTIOUS DISEASES

   b. Obtain latex agglutination or CIE tests on CSF to detect GBS antigen.

  2. **Maternal prophylaxis.** Vaginal/rectal cultures at 35–37 weeks gestation. Intrapartum intravenous antimicrobial therapy if:

   a. GBS+ colonization (offer intrapartum penicillin).

   b. Premature labor <37 weeks; maternal fever; PROM >18 hours (if not cultured); GBS bacteriuria during pregnancy; previously affected infant.

  3. **Newborn management.**

   a. If mother received intrapartum penicillin, follow American Academy of Pediatrics recommendations in Figure 10.1.

   b. If newborn is infected, treat initially with combination of ampicillin or penicillin and an aminoglycoside, since some GBS exhibits tolerance to penicillin-type drugs.

B. COAGULASE-NEGATIVE STAPHYLOCOCCUS

A common saprophyte of skin and mucous membranes, this Gram-positive coccus has emerged as a significant pathogen in the VLBW neonate, producing pneumonia and sepsis usually after the first week of life.

  1. **Diagnosis** may be suggested by deteriorating clinical course in association with glucose intolerance.

   a. Blood culture is definitive procedure.

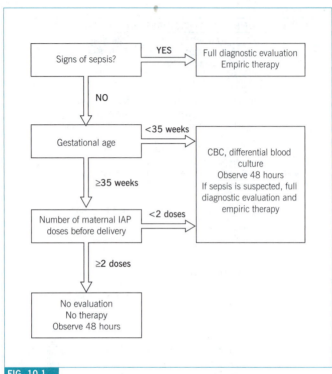

FIG. 10.1

Suggested management of newborns born to mother who received intrapartum antimicrobial prophylaxis (IAP) for GBS disease. (Adapted from AAP Red Book[2].)

    b. Endotracheal aspirate culture.

  2. **Management.**

    a. Removal of contaminated deep line is critical.

    b. Use vancomycin until antibiotic susceptibilities are available.

C. SYPHILIS. *Treponema pallidum* spirochetal infection. Spectrum varies from asymptomatic infection to serious multiorgan involvement. Clinical signs include rhinitis, rash, hepatosplenomegaly, jaundice, lymphadenopathy, nephrosis, pseudoparalysis, stillbirth, prematurity, failure to thrive, and unexplained hydrops fetalis.

1. **Diagnosis.**
a. Serological testing is the mainstay.
   1) Screening tests include so-called reagin (nonspecific) tests: e.g. VDRL or rapid plasma reagin (RPR).
   2) To establish the presence of infection, these positive screening tests must be confirmed with a positive result to a specific treponemal test such as the fluorescent treponemal antibody-absorption test (FTA-ABS) or microhemagglutination test for *T. pallidum* (MHATP).
   3) A positive FTA-ABS test in the neonate might represent transplacental passage of maternal IgG. The IgM FTA-ABS test, developed to confirm congenital neonatal syphilis infection, may not be reliable. Thus, infants with a negative IgM FTA-ABS finding should be followed with serial VDRL testing to confirm loss of serological reactivity.
b. Dark-field examination of appropriate lesions for spirochetes: e.g. nasal discharge.
c. Pathologic examination of placenta.
d. Radiograph of long bones to look for syphilitic changes: osteochondritis, periostitis, and osteomyelitis.
e. Lumbar puncture to exclude asymptomatic neurosyphilis.
f. A WBC count with differential; monocytosis occurs in infants with symptomatic congenital syphilis.
2. **Management.** The appropriate management of syphilis in the neonate involves consideration of history, prior antimicrobial therapy of mother, and the clinical and serological status of mother and infant (Table 10.6).
Current regimen for treatment of congenital syphilis is:
a. Penicillin G crystalline, 100,000–150,000U/kg i.v. twice a day for 10 days, or
b. Penicillin G procaine, 50,000U/kg i.m. daily for 10 days.
c. Benzathine penicillin should not be used to treat congenital syphilis.
D. LISTERIOSIS. The etiologic agent is *Listeria monocytogenes*.
1. **Presentation/clinical course.**
a. Infection in newborns has a bimodal distribution, with early-onset septicemic infection associated with low birth weight, obstetric complications, and maternal colonization. Intrauterine infection may produce a serious granulomatous interstitial pneumonia with high mortality rate. Late-onset disease tends to occur in infants with normal birth weight, with meningitis as a prominent finding, and is frequently associated with maternal colonization or obstetric complications.
2. **Management.**
a. Antimicrobial treatment with ampicillin plus gentamicin.
b. Duration of treatment depends on clinical syndrome: e.g. sepsis 7–10 days, meningitis 14 days.
c. Some authorities advocate treatment with penicillin or ampicillin alone.

TABLE 10.6
MANAGEMENT OF INFANT WITH POSSIBLE OR PROVEN SYPHILIS

Status of infant	Maternal status	Assessment	Management
Asymptomatic; positive VDRL; negative FTA-ABS[a]	Asymptomatic; positive VDRL; negative FTA- ABS; mother untreated	False-positive finding for syphilis in mother and infant	No treatment necessary
Asymptomatic; positive VDRL; positive FTA-ABS	Asymptomatic; positive VDRL; positive FTA-ABS	Syphilis in mother; syphilis possible in infant	Treat mother. For infant: (a) If FTA-ABS IgM positive, treat infant; if negative, follow VDRL; titer should disappear over time. (b) If FTA-ABS IgM unavailable, treat infant
Asymptomatic; positive VDRL; positive FTA-ABS	Asymptomatic; positive VDRL; positive FTA- ABS; mother treated appropriately with penicillin; maternal titer VDRL falling	Adequate treatment of maternal syphilis; adequate treatment of infant in utero	No treatment necessary for mother or infant; follow mother and infant serologically
Asymptomatic; positive VDRL; positive FTA-ABS	Asymptomatic; positive VDRL; positive FTA- ABS; mother treated with erythromycin; maternal titer VDRL falling	Adequate treatment of maternal syphilis but may be inadequate for infant in utero	No treatment of mother; may treat infant or follow serologically
Symptomatic; positive VDRL; positive FTA-ABS	Asymptomatic; positive VDRL; positive FTA-ABS; mother untreated	Syphilis in mother; syphilis in infant	Treat mother; treat infant; follow both serologically

[a]FTA-ABS, fluorescent treponemal antibody-absorption test.
Note: Rapid plasma reagin (RPR) or other reagin test may be substituted for VDRL. Microhemagglutination test for *T. pallidum* (MHATP) may be substituted for FTA-ABS.

d. Virtually all listeria exhibit tolerance to penicillin-type drugs, and the addition of an aminoglycoside is recommended for enhanced bactericidal effect initially.

E. ANAEROBIC INFECTION. *Bacteroides fragilis, Peptococcus* and *Peptostreptococcus, Veilonella* and *Clostridium perfringens* are most common. Infection is associated with PROM, maternal amnionitis, prematurity, fetal distress; perforated intestine in older neonate. Anaerobes may cause transient bacteremia. *Clostridium difficile* may cause diarrhea and PMC, particularly in the hospitalized neonate.

1. Presentation/clinical findings.
a. Indistinguishable from aerobic sepsis.
b. Foul odor of newborn may be clue.
c. Failure to respond to usual antimicrobic agents may also be a clue to anaerobic infection.

2. Diagnosis.
a. Culture – suitable specimens include blood, pus, and CSF.
b. Gram stain – the presence of organisms on Gram stain and no growth on routine culture supports the *possibility* of anaerobic infection.
c. Send stool for *C. difficile* toxin assay when PMC exists.

3. Management.
a. Ampicillin and gentamicin are of limited value.
b. Clindamycin may be used, but its failure to diffuse into the CSF makes it inappropriate for treatment of meningitis or brain abscess.
c. Metronidazole may be useful in some cases of *Bacteroides fragilis,* including CNS infection.
d. Penicillin is the drug of choice for clostridia and anaerobic streptococci.
e. Metronidazole orally is the drug of choice for *C. difficile* diarrhea.

F. TUBERCULOSIS.
1 **Neonatal tuberculosis is rare.**
2. Congenital tuberculosis is a devastating infection usually resulting in abortion or stillbirth.
3. Nonspecific findings. A surviving infant may show nonspecific findings: e.g. low birth weight, poor feeding, listlessness, and hepatomegaly.
4. Maternal infection. A more common problem is the management of an infant of a tuberculous mother, or mother with a positive purified protein derivative (PPD) result.
a. Diagnosis:
   1) Acid-fast stain and mycobacterial culture of tracheal aspirates, urine, gastric aspirates, and placenta.
   2) Pathologic examination of placenta.
   3) Intermediate (5 tuberculin units) PPD (often negative).
   4) Review maternal status and results of maternal tests.
b. Management. Consult Table 10.7.

10

INFECTIOUS DISEASES

TABLE 10.7

MANAGEMENT OF THE TUBERCULOUS OR POTENTIALLY
TUBERCULOUS INFANT

Status of infant	Maternal status	Management
Symptomatic	Active untreated disease or noncompliant	1. Treat infant with INH 2. Separate infant from mother 3. Assure maternal treatment
Asymptomatic	Active disease; untreated or noncompliant	1. Isolate infant from mother until latter is noninfectious then: 2a. INH prophylaxis 10mg/kg once daily for infant-apply intermed. tuberculin. If disease is absent, continue INH prophylaxis for 1 year; if disease is present, treat for disease with INH plus rifampin, or 2b. High-risk settings BCG infant; at birth; return to mother when 5TU PPD is positive (6–8 weeks)
Asymptomatic	On treatment for pulmonary tuberculosis	1. Separate infant from mother until latter is noncontagious 2. Follow infant; apply 5TU PPD at 3 months: if positive, evaluate for tuberculosis and treat accordingly, if negative, continue to follow and repeat PPD at 6–9 months
Asymptomatic	Adequately treated mother or mother with positive PPD only	1. Separation of infant from mother unnecessary 2. Follow infant with 5TU PPD at 3 months 3. INH prophylaxis in untreated, PPD-positive mother should be considered. 4. Treated mother should be followed to R/O relapse.

IV. ANTIMICROBIAL AGENTS

Special problems related to antimicrobial use in the neonate include differences in volume of distribution of drugs and immaturity of pathways involved in metabolism and excretion. Initial dosing is based on serum levels of antimicrobials in infants of similar age, weight, and maturity. Antimicrobials are generally given by the parenteral route (i.v. or i.m.) because of the need to ensure adequate serum levels. Intravenous treatment is preferred over i.m. injections because of the infant's limited muscle mass. Avoid occasional adverse reactions by infusing over 30 minutes rather than giving as a bolus.

A. RECOMMENDED INITIAL DOSES for antimicrobials commonly used in the neonate – consult Table 10.8. The following comments apply to dosage recommendations.

1. **When treating sepsis** of the newborn with penicillin or ampicillin, it is recommended that the 'meningitis' dose be used as the initial treatment pending results of CSF culture.

2. **Drug interactions.** Since chloramphenicol antagonizes the antibacterial effect of gentamicin, they probably should not be used together.

B. MONITORING OF ANTIMICROBIAL LEVELS.

1. **Measure serum and CSF antimicrobial levels** to ensure adequacy of dosage and avoid toxic reaction.

2. **When microbiologic assays** are used for serum antimicrobial determinations the laboratory must be aware of *all* antimicrobials the patient is receiving.

3. **Toxic levels** of commonly used drugs are noted in Table 10.9.

4. **Peak levels** generally are sampled 30 minutes after the conclusion of a 30 minute i.v. infusion or 1 hour after an i.m. injection.

5. **Trough levels** may be measured just before the next dose of antimicrobial.

6. **Special considerations.**

a. The doses of aminoglycosides and chloramphenicol should be based on serum levels at peak and trough times after the third dose.

b. Patients with shock or renal compromise should have serum levels monitored after the first dose to determine further dosing.

10

INFECTIOUS DISEASES

TABLE 10.8

DOSES AND SCHEDULES FOR ANTIMICROBIAL AGENTS

Antimicrobial agent	Route	Total daily dose (mg/kg/day) {number of doses per day}				Major route of elimination
		Infants <1 week of age		Infants 1–4 weeks of age		
		wt <2000g	wt >2000g	wt <2000g	wt >2000g	
Acyclovir	i.v.	30 {3}	30 {3}	30 {3}	30 {3}	R
Amikacin[a]	i.v./i.m.	15 {2}	15–20 {2}	15–20 {2}	20–30 {3}	R
Amphotericin	i.v.	0.25–1.0 {1}	0.25–1.0 {1}	0.25–1.0 {1}	0.25–1.0 {1}	H/R
Ampicillin						
Meningitis	i.v./i.m.	100 {2}	150 {3}	150 {3}	200 {4}	
Other infections	i.v./i.m.	50 {2}	75 {3}	75 {3}	100 {4}	R
Cefazolin	i.v./i.m.	40 {2}	40 {2}	40 {2}	60 {3}	R
Cefotaxime	i.v./i.m.	100 {2}	100 {2}	150 {3}	150 {3}	R/H
Ceftazidime	i.v.	60 {2}	100 {3}	100 {2}	150 {3}	R
Ceftriaxone	i.v./i.m.	50 {1}	50 {1}	50 {1}	75 {1}	R
Chloramphenicol[a]	i.v./i.m.	25 {2}	25 {2}	25–50 {3}	50 {4}	H
Clindamycin	i.v.	10 {2}	15 {3}	15 {3}	20 {4}	
Erythromycin	p.o.	20 {2}	20 {2}	30 {3}	30–40 {3}	H
Gentamicin[a]	i.v./i.m.	3 {1}	5 {2}	5 {2}	7.5 {3}	R
Imipenem	i.v./i.m.	40 {2}	50 {2}	50 {2}	60 {3}	R
Kanamycin	i.v./i.m.	15 {2}	20 {2}	20 {2}	30 {3}	R
Methicillin[b]	i.v./i.m.	50–100 {2}	100–150 {2–3}	100–150 {2–3}	100–200 {4}	R
Metronidazole[b]	i.v.	15 {2}	15 {2}	15 {2}	30 {2}	H
Mezlocillin[b]	i.v./i.m.	150 {2}	150 {2}	225 {3}	300 {4}	R
Nafcillin[b]	i.v.	50–100 {2}	75–150 {2–3}	75–150 {3}	100–200 {4}	H

TABLE 10.8 CONTD

Antimicrobial agent	Route	Total daily dose (mg/kg/day) {number of doses per day}					Major route of elimination
		Infants <1 week of age		Infants 1–4 weeks of age			
		wt <2000g	wt >2000g	wt <2000g	wt >2000g		
Penicillin G[b,c]	i.v./i.m.	50–100,000{2}	75–150,000 {3}	75–150,000{3}	100–200,000 {4}		R
Procaine penicillin[c]	i.m.	50,000 {1}	50,000 {1}	50,000 {1}	50,000 {1}		R
Piperacillin	i.v./i.m.	150 {2}	225 {3}	225 {3}	300 {4}		R/H
Rifampin	p.o.	10 {2}	10–20{2}	10–20 {2}	10–20 {2}		H
Ticarcillin	i.v./i.m.	150 {2}	225 {3}	225 {3}	300 {4}		R
Tobramycin[a]	i.v./i.m.	3 {2}	5 {2}	5 {2}	7.5 {3}		R
Trimethoprim (TMP) – i.v./p.o. sulfamethoxazole		not advised	not advised	TMP 2 {2}	TMP 2–6 {2}		H/R
Vancomycin[a]	i.v.	20 {1}	30 {2}	30 {2}	30–45 {2–3}		R

[a]Dosage depends on serum concentrations achieved.
[b]Use the higher dose for meningitis.
[c]Use units/kg/day for Penicillin G and Procaine penicillin.
R, renal; H, hepatic.

10

INFECTIOUS DISEASES

TABLE 10.9

TOXIC SERUM LEVELS FOR VARIOUS ANTIMICROBIAL AGENTS

Antimicrobial	Peak (mg/mL)	Trough (mg/mL)
Aminoglycosides		
Gentamicin	>10	>2
Tobramycin	>10	>2
Amikacin	>30	>10
Netilmicin	>10	>2
Vancomycin	>40	>5
Chloramphenicol	>25	>10

V. NONBACTERIAL NEONATAL INFECTION

A. CYTOMEGALOVIRUS.

1. **Incidence.** Common, occurring in 1–2% of all newborns. Higher rates in lower socioeconomic populations.

2. **Predisposing factors/pathogenesis.**

a. About 50% of fetuses will become infected during *primary* maternal CMV infection.

b. Infection occurs in about 10% of pregnancies with *recurrent* or reactivated maternal infection.

c. Significant neurological sequelae in offspring have been documented only following *primary* maternal infection.

d. CMV infection acquired during the birth process, via breast-feeding, or from blood or platelet transfusions has not been associated with neurological deficits.

e. The probability that a woman susceptible to CMV will develop a primary infection during a particular pregnancy is less than 1 in 100. If she does have a primary infection, the chances are 1 in 2 that her infant will have congenital infection and 1 in 14 that some residual damage will occur.

3. **Presentation/clinical course.**

a. Most infections are clinically inapparent. Late sequelae such as nerve deafness, learning difficulties, and neurological deficits may develop in 10–15% of clinically inapparent infections.

b. Syndrome of congenital CMV (cytomegalic inclusion disease) is uncommon and includes low birth weight, purpura, anemia, jaundice, hepatosplenomegaly, microcephaly, and chorioretinitis.

c. A more common symptomatic presentation is low birth weight, hepatosplenomegaly, and persistent jaundice.

d. Natal/postnatal disease – the incubation period of CMV is probably a minimum of 3 weeks, after which the infant may show signs of hepatosplenomegaly, lymphadenopathy, pneumonia, and atypical lymphocytes. Severe interstitial pneumonia, or transfusion-acquired

CMV, may be fatal in premature infants.

4. **Diagnosis.**
a. Infants with congenital infection excrete CMV in high titer in urine and saliva, making virus detection easy and rapid.
   1) Collect saliva in viral culture medium. Urine and other specimens should be sent to laboratory on ice.
   2) Do not freeze specimens, since that inactivates the virus.
b. Specific CMV IgM may be detected in cord or infant serum.
c. Look for typical large cells with inclusions by cytologic examination of urinary sediment or in liver tissue.
d. PCR can be used to detect viral antigen.
e. IgG CMV antibody in persistent high titer at 6–12 weeks of age supports diagnosis.
f. Additional diagnostic studies to determine extent of infection include skull film, head ultrasound or CT scan for detection of intracranial calcifications, liver function tests, long-bone films, and chest radiograph films.

5. **Management.**
a. No specific, effective, antiviral therapy exists. Guanciclovir efficacy in neonatal disease has not yet been demonstrated; studies are ongoing. Consideration of treatment of an infant with congenital CMV infection should be made in conjunction with a physician experienced in this area.
b. Newborn hearing screening is important: e.g. brain-stem auditory evoked response. Repeated evaluations are indicated, since postnatal development of deafness can occur.
c. Infants with congenital CMV infection may infect others. Universal precautions should be followed.
d. Prevention of neonatal CMV infection via transfusion in susceptible premature infants may be accomplished by use of CMV antibody-negative blood products.
e. Prevention of symptomatic congenital CMV infection is not possible. A live virus vaccine is under investigation.

B. **RUBELLA.** Congenital rubella syndrome (CRS) has become rare, reflecting the success of rubella vaccine. All personnel in contact with CRS should have antibody to rubella either as a result of prior infection or immunization.

1. **Signs and symptoms.** Developmental anomalies occur primarily as a result of infection in the first trimester and involve the heart (patent ductus arteriosus, peripheral pulmonic stenosis, ventricular septal defect, atrial septal defect), eye (glaucoma, cataracts, chorioretinitis), and ear (nerve deafness).
a. Vaccination should not be given during pregnancy, but inadvertent administration has not been demonstrated to cause fetal disease.

b. Sequelae of persistent viral infection are growth retardation, abnormal liver function, anemia, thrombocytopenia, CNS damage, immune deficiencies, and dental dysplasia.

c. Considerable overlap exists in clinical manifestations of CMV, herpes, toxoplasmosis, syphilis, and rubella.

2. Diagnosis.

a. Isolation of virus from urine and pharyngeal secretions. Infants with CRS may excrete virus for months to years.

b. Specific rubella IgM antibody or persistence of rubella IgG antibody in infant.

3. Management/prevention.

a. There is no specific antiviral chemotherapy.

b. Appropriate treatment of specific defects should be given.

c. Respiratory and enteric isolation of infants with CRS is required.

C. HERPES SIMPLEX VIRUS. Two serotypes are recognized: HSV 1 and HSV 2. Causes severe disease with high mortality and morbidity in the neonate.

1. Incidence. About 120 cases of neonatal HSV infection occur in the United States each year.

2. Predisposing factors/pathogenesis.

a. Primary infection of mother at time of vaginal delivery carries greatest risk.

b. Inoculation occurs at skin trauma sites: e.g. fetal scalp monitors. Nosocomial spread is possible.

c. Incidence in babies delivered by cesarian section within 4 hours of membrane rupture is very low.

d. Transplacental infection resulting in abortion or congenital malformations is rare.

3. Signs and symptoms vary with the type of disease. Asymptomatic infection is rare. Localized skin or eye involvement occurs. Disseminated disease may present with findings described for sepsis; localized CNS disease may present with fever, lethargy, poor feeding, hypoglycemia, DIC, and irritability followed by intractable focal or generalized seizures. Vesicular lesions, when present, are an important clue to diagnosis.

4. Diagnostic efforts.

a. Scrape the base of vesicles and lesions for direct immunofluorescent test for herpes simplex antigen.

b. Obtain a viral culture from vesicles, blood, throat, CSF, or eye lesions. Brain biopsy may be done in the appropriate setting. Vesicular fluid and CSF may be assayed by PCR for viral detection.

c. Examine the mother for vaginal, cervical, or other herpes lesions, but culture for virus even in the absence of lesions.

d. Tests for herpes simplex antibody in mother and infant have not proved helpful diagnostically.

e. Consider diagnosis in infant not responding to antibiotic treatment for sepsis.

5. **Management.**

a. Antiviral drug therapy is indicated for all forms of neonatal herpes infection, since even initially localized disease may disseminate with devastating effects. Currently available treatment consists of 30mg/kg/day of acyclovir divided in 3 doses given by infusion for 10–14 days. Encephalitis is treated for 14–21 days or longer.

b. Contact isolation precautions should be followed.

D. HEPATITIS. Neonatal hepatitis may have multiple infectious causes (Table 10.10). Hepatitis A, B, C, and E are discussed in this section.

1. **Hepatitis A** (HAV).

a. Incidence unknown. Transmission of HAV to the neonate is possible if the mother is in the incubation period, or is acutely symptomatic at the time of delivery, or by transfusion of infected blood. In the neonate, the virus is detectable in the stool for several weeks without obvious clinical illness. This poses a hazard to susceptible caretakers.

b. Diagnosis. HAV infection is established by finding anti-HAV-IgM antibody in serum specimens.

c. Management.

   1) Enteric precautions are recommended for duration of hospitalization.

   2) In the infant born to an acutely symptomatic mother, human immune serum globulin (0.02mL/kg) should be considered, although its effectiveness is unknown. The occurrence of HAV infection earlier in pregnancy is not an indication for withholding breast-feeding or administration of immune serum globulin.

2. **Hepatitis B** (HBV).

a. Incidence varies with ethnic origin of mother, the timing and type of maternal infection, whether or not mother is HBsAg and HBeAg positive.

TABLE 10.10	
CAUSES OF INFECTIOUS NEONATAL HEPATITIS	
Viral	**Other**
Hepatitis A, B, non-A, non-B	Bacterial sepsis
Rubella	Syphilis
Cytomegalovirus	Listeria
Herpes simplex	Tuberculosis
Enteroviruses	Toxoplasmosis
Coxsackie	
Echoviruses	
Adenovirus	
Varicella	

10

INFECTIOUS DISEASES

b. Predisposing factors/pathogenesis.
   1) Transplacental transmission is rare. Transmission to an infant by HBsAg-positive mothers occurs during or shortly after delivery. HBIG and hepatitis B vaccine are used to protect the infant from acute infection and subsequent chronic infection.
   2) A mother with acute (symptomatic) hepatitis late in pregnancy or shortly after delivery is much more likely to transmit infection to her infant than a mother with acute infection early in pregnancy or the mother who is a chronic carrier.
   3) The infected infant of a chronic carrier is more likely to develop severe chronic liver disease.
   4) Chronic liver disease is more common in Asians.
c. Presentation/clinical course.
   1) Most infants who develop HBV infection – i.e. become HBsAg positive as a result of maternal transmission – remain clinically well. Persistent antigenemia may develop (Table 10.11).
   2) Some infants (1–3%) may become icteric, have elevated liver enzyme levels, and otherwise do poorly; these are most likely to be the offspring of 'e' positive carrier mothers.
   3) Fulminant hepatitis in the newborn is rare.
   4) HBsAg carriers have increased risk for later development of hepatocellular carcinoma and cirrhosis.
d. Diagnosis – detection of specific antigens and antibodies.
   1) HBsAg positivity indicates either acute HBV infection or the presence of carrier state.
   2) HBeAg positivity, detectable only in the presence of HBsAg, indicates infectiousness and increased likelihood of transmission of HBV.
   3) Anti-HBs in serum indicates past infection and immunity to HBV.
   4) Anti-HBc in serum indicates recent, chronic, or remote HBV infection.

TABLE 10.11

RISK OF HEPATITIS B VIRUS TRANSMISSION FROM MOTHER TO INFANT AND OUTCOME FOR INFANT

Mother HB$_s$Ag positive	Infection rate for infant (%)	Chronic carrier risk in infant (%)
Acute hepatitis 3 months before to 1 month after delivery	80–90	
Acute hepatitis in early pregnancy	10–30	
Asymptomatic carrier mother	10	
HBeAg positive	90	85–90
HBeAg negative	30	Low
HBeAg negative, anti-HBe positive	Very low	Very low

e.   Management.
   1)   The hepatitis B status of all pregnant women should be evaluated.
   2)   Newborns of HBsAg-positive mothers (or high-risk mothers of unknown HBsAg status depending on local epidemiology) should receive 0.5mL i.m. of HBIG in the first hours of life.
   3)   HB vaccine (0.5mL i.m.) should be administered within 7 days, at 1 month, and at 6 months if mother is HBsAg positive.
   4)   Universal precautions are appropriate for infants with HBV infection.
   5)   After thorough bathing, isolation of a newborn born to a carrier is not necessary.
   6)   Strict isolation or separation of the carrier mother and/or her infant is not indicated. Breast-feeding is permitted.
   7)   Infants treated with HBIG and vaccine should be followed up at 12–15 months of age to determine the success of treatment.
   8)   The use of HBIG and vaccine can prevent approximately 90% of neonatal and subsequent HBV infections.

3. Hepatitis C (HCV)
a.   HCV causes most blood-borne cases of non-A, non-B hepatitis, resulting in chronic hepatitis. Transmission occurs via blood transfusion or perinatally (5% transmission for HIV negative, but higher transmission rate with HIV coinfection).
b.   Infection may be asymptomatic; however, infected individuals are at an increased risk for subsequent chronic hepatitis, cirrhosis, and hepatocellular carcinoma.
c.   Mothers with risk factors for HCV infection (i.v. drug users, blood product recipient before 1992) should be screened for HCV antibody. Infants of HCV-positive mothers should be tested for HCV antibodies after 12 months of age; a positive serology at this time represents infant infection (rather than passively acquired maternal antibody).
d.   HCV infection is not a contraindication to breast-feeding. However, since HCV may be transmitted in breast milk, the determination of feeding status should be individualized.

4. Hepatitis E (HEV)
a.   HEV causes epidemic hepatitis in subtropical and tropical countries. Transmission is commonly via contaminated water.
b.   Fulminant disease may occur, especially during pregnancy (with death rates of up to 25%).
c.   Premature labor and delivery may result from maternal HEV infection. In-utero or postnatal deaths may occur.
d.   Contact isolation is appropriate for those infected with HEV.

E.   ENTEROVIRUSES. Polio, Coxsackie viruses, and echoviruses.
1. Incidence undetermined. Seasonal occurrence in summer and fall, more common in males.

2. **Predisposing factors/pathogenesis.**

a. Infection may be acquired congenitally, natally, or postnatally. Onset of symptoms at birth suggests late-gestation congenital infection, onset of disease at 5–10 days suggests acquisition natally, and onset of disease beyond 10 days suggests postnatal acquisition.

b. Coxsackie infection during pregnancy may be associated with congenital malformation of cardiovascular, urogenital, and digestive systems in the neonate. Coxsackie B infections are more virulent than echoviruses or Coxsackie A.

3. **Presentation/clinical course.**

a. Fever and other nonspecific signs and symptoms are usual. Maculopapular or petechial rash may occur. Occasionally infants are asymptomatic.

b. More virulent infection causes hepatitis, meningitis, encephalitis, or myocarditis. Fulminant illness with jaundice, pulmonary infiltrates, diarrhea, DIC, and necrosis of adrenals and pancreas is less common.

4. **Diagnosis.**

a. Recovery of enterovirus from CSF, nasopharyngeal and rectal swabs, biopsy or autopsy tissue is suggestive of causal relationship to illness.

b. A documented rise in antibody titer to viral isolate supports the diagnosis.

5. **Management.**

a. No specific antiviral drug treatment.

b. Supportive care for myocardial, hepatic, and CNS involvement.

c. Vigorous infection control measures are indicated, including enteric isolation precautions, emphasis on hand-washing, and exclusion of personnel with symptoms of enteroviral disease from nursery.

F. **PARVOVIRUS (PV) B19** – the viral etiology of erythema infectiosum or fifth disease. Primary infection in a pregnant female may result in nonimmune hydrops fetalis and fetal death in approximately 5% of cases. Congenital anomalies do not result from this infection.

1. **Predisposing factors/pathogenesis.**

a. Approximately 50% of pregnant females are susceptible, i.e. nonimmune to PV B19.

b. Exposure of nonimmune pregnant females varies with setting: e.g. household exposure carries approximately 50% risk of infection and daycare or school exposure approximately 25% risk of infection.

c. For primarily infected pregnant females, fetal loss is estimated to be 1.5–4.5%.

2. **Presentation:** severe anemia, heart failure, hydrops, and death of fetus.

3. **Diagnosis.**

a. Paired sera in exposed pregnant female can confirm primary maternal infection.

b. Demonstration of PV B19 DNA in fetal tissue by in-situ hybridization

confirms infection.
4. **Management.** No treatment for affected fetus.
5. **Prevention.** Avoidance of exposure by susceptible pregnant females.

G. VARICELLA ZOSTER (VZ).

1. **Incidence.** 90% of women in the childbearing age are immune. Congenital varicella occurs in 2–3% of the offspring of mothers with varicella during the first 20 weeks of gestation. Neonatal varicella may occur if maternal varicella occurs in the perinatal period (5 days prior to delivery through 2 days postpartum).

2. **Presentation/clinical course.**
a. Maternal VZ infection in the first and second trimester has been associated with cutaneous scars, abnormalities of digits or a limb, defects of eye, brain, and low birth weight in newborns.
b. Newborns acquiring VZ infection during the perinatal period have a clinical illness varying from mild to fatal.

3. **Diagnosis.**
a. Congenital varicella-specific IgM VZ antibody or persistence of significant titers of VZ IgG.
b. Neonatal varicella.
   1) Characteristic diffusely disseminated skin lesions in varying states, from macules, papules, vesicles, pustules, to crusts.
   2) Recovery of VZ virus by culture.
   3) Immunofluorescent staining of scrapings.
   4) Tzanck smear of vesicle base scrapings will show multinucleated giant cells in both VZ and herpes simplex infections.
   5) Direct immunofluorescence of cells will differentiate VZ infection from HSV.

4. **Management.**
a. Infants with *congenital* varicella do not require isolation.
b. Infants with *neonatal* varicella should be placed in strict isolation for at least 7 days after onset of rash.
c. Infants born to mothers with onset of varicella 5 or more days before delivery require no specific treatment other than isolation if kept in hospital.
d. Infants whose mothers have onset of varicella from zero to 4 days before delivery, or within 2 days after delivery, should receive 1 vial (2.5mL) of VZ immunoglobulin (IG), preferably at birth or within 96 hours.
e. Infants who may be exposed to VZ infection as a result of contact with nursery personnel should have their immune status verified and, if susceptible, should receive VZIG, 2.5ml, within 96 hours of exposure. Premature infants are more susceptible.
f. Infants with active varicella in the first week of life should receive acyclovir 45mg/kg/day divided in 3 doses by infusion for a total of 10 days.

H.   HUMAN IMMUNODEFICIENCY VIRUS. HIV causes AIDS.
1.   Transmission.
a.   Vertical transmission from HIV+ mother to infant accounts for the majority of HIV-infected infants, occurring in 13–39% of untreated mothers. Risk is not affected by mode of delivery.
b.   May be transmitted by breast-feeding when mother is newly infected. Risk of breast-feeding in antenatal-acquired HIV is not clear.
c.   Transmission by transfusion of blood and blood products is now rare.
2.   Presentation/clinical course.
a.   Infected newborns are usually asymptomatic at time of birth.
b.   Recurrent infections, severe intractable diarrhea, candida infections, *Pneumocystis carinii* pneumonia, and failure to thrive are common clinical manifestations which may present shortly after birth or in the first 3 months of life.
3.   Diagnosis.
a.   Serology cannot be relied upon at birth, since maternal antibodies cross the placenta and may be detected for months. Verbal consent should be obtained to obtain HIV serology in infants at risk when mother's HIV status is unknown (e.g. i.v. drug abusers, prostitutes).
b.   Positive PCR detection of HIV genomic sequences, HIV culture, or HIV p24 antigen assay indicate presumptive infection in infant. Only 30–50% of infected infants will have a positive test at birth, but nearly all infected infants will be identified by 4–6 months of age. Results should be confirmed by a repeat PCR or culture (not p24 assay) before HIV infection is diagnosed. An exposed infant with negative tests at 1 month and >4 months of age and without clinical evidence of AIDS is presumed to be noninfected.
4.   Management of HIV-exposed infants[2].
a.   All HIV+ pregnant women should be treated with oral AZT (100mg q5h or 200mg q8h) throughout pregnancy, starting before 34 weeks gestation, and receive i.v. AZT (2mg/kg/h x1 hour followed by 1mg/kg/h) during labor. Exposed newborns should be treated with oral AZT (2mg/kg q5h) starting 8–12 hours after birth until 6 weeks of age. This protocol has resulted in about a 2/3 reduction in neonatal infection.
b.   HIV-infected mothers should be advised not to breast-feed their infants.
c.   Monitor PCR and/or viral cultures at 1, 3, 6 months in exposed infants.
d.   Monitor CD4+ T-lymphocyte counts. Count <1500 or 25% of total lymphocytes is evidence of immunosuppression.
e.   Live polio and varicella vaccines should not be given. Other immunizations are indicated.
5.   Management of infected infants. Strategies are evolving, and infectious disease consultation is advised.
a.   Good nutritional support.

b. *Pneumocystis carinii* prophylaxis beginning at 4–6 weeks of age.
c. Intravenous gamma globulin for antibody deficiency.
d. Antiretroviral treatment is indicated. Oral didanosine, AZT, or a combination are appropriate. Data on dosing, safety, and efficacy of protease inhibitors in infants are currently lacking.

I. *CANDIDA ALBICANS.*

1. Predisposing factors/pathogenesis.

a. Rarely, candidal infection may occur in utero by bloodstream invasion or, more likely, as the result of ascending infection.
b. Commonly, neonatal infection results from contamination during the birth process or nosocomial transmission.
c. Dissemination of candidal infection may occur postnatally in association with antibiotic usage, parenteral nutrition, or steroids. Incidence is high in VLBW infants with indwelling catheters.

2. Presentation/clinical course.

a. Superficial infection is common. Creamy white patches adherent to mucous membranes (thrush) or, in the diaper area, well-defined satellite erythematous vesiculopustules associated with confluent erythematous macules may be found.
b. Congenital disseminated candidiasis may involve kidney, lungs, liver, brain, eye, and other organs, or present as a localized infection, e.g. arthritis or meningitis. A generalized rash may be present. Course without treatment is ordinarily fatal.
c. Congenital cutaneous candidiasis is superficial and confined to skin and umbilical cord. It may occur with intact membranes. Manifestations include a diffuse maculopapular vesicular rash distributed over the face, trunk, neck, and limbs. Desquamation follows the acute phase. No constitutional symptoms are present and the infant thrives. Cutaneous candidiasis must be distinguished from erythema toxicum, congenital herpes, syphilis, or bullous impetigo.
d. Acquired candida sepsis is often associated with glucose intolerance, thrombocytopenia, or neutropenia. If blood culture is positive with hematological evidence of infection, urine should be cultured (bladder tap), kidneys surveyed with ultrasound for fungal balls, and a retinal examination performed.

3. Diagnosis.

a. Isolation on ordinary blood agar as well as fungal culture medium should be done. Recovery from blood culture may represent a transient candidemia or disseminated infection.
b. Gram stain may yield large, Gram-positive, watermelon seed-shaped yeast cells. Hyphae with budding yeast cells may be seen.
c. Tissue diagnosis from biopsy specimens should be done.
d. Ophthalmologic examination and renal ultrasound are indicated in suspected disseminated candidiasis.

10

INFECTIOUS DISEASES

4. **Management.**

a. Treatment of localized oral or GI tract candidiasis is with nystatin, 200,000 units orally 4 times daily for 1 week or longer.

b. Skin lesions may be treated with topical nystatin, topical clotrimazole solution or amphotericin B ointment applied 4 times daily for 1 week.

c. Invasive candidiasis should be treated with amphotericin B. Short-term therapy (7–10 days) may be adequate for catheter-associated infection if the catheter is removed. Treatment for systemic disease is usually 3–8 weeks following last positive blood culture, duration depending on rate of clearance, and nidus for recurrence (e.g. thrombus). Flucytosine (150mg/kg/day in 4 divided doses p.o.) should supplement amphotericin B in patients with persistent clinical or culture evidence of infection or CNS involvement. Flucytosine plateau plasma concentrations should be 40–60mg/mL. Patients with disseminated candidiasis failing amphotericin B therapy have responded to fluconazole. Experience in the premature is minimal.

J. TOXOPLASMOSIS is caused by a common obligate intracellular parasite, *Toxoplasma gondii*. Cats are the definitive host.

1. **Incidence.** Approximately 3000 cases of congenital infection occur yearly in the USA, or <1 per thousand births.

2. **Predisposing factors/pathogenesis.**

a. Only primary infection of the mother, which is usually asymptomatic, results in congenital infection. 90% of offspring of women who acquire infection during pregnancy appear normal, and 50% of these escape infection. Of the remaining 10%, most have minor problems, and only 3–5% have severe manifestations. Overall, 75% of congenitally infected infants are asymptomatic.

b. Transplacental transmission of maternal parasitemia increases from about 15% in the first trimester to about 65% at the end of the pregnancy.

3. **Presentation/clinical course.**

a. The classic triad of hydrocephalus, chorioretinitis, and intracranial calcification occurs in infants infected early in pregnancy.

   1) These infants may also appear septic and have jaundice, hepatosplenomegaly, purpura, and deafness.

   2) Differentiation from other congenital infections – e.g. herpes simplex, CMV, rubella, or syphilis – requires laboratory support.

b. Infants infected late in pregnancy usually appear clinically normal.

4. **Diagnosis.** A variety of serological procedures are available for diagnosis.

a. Sabin dye test. Sensitive and very specific, but the requirement for live parasites in the test has rendered it of historical interest only.

b. Indirect fluorescent antibody test (IFA). More readily available and most routinely used test.

c. IgM-IFA. Detects early antibody in acute infection, but not routinely available. Theoretically the test of choice for congenital toxoplasmosis. However, there are technical problems with the test, resulting in false-positive assays. Also, some congenitally infected infants lack IgM-IFA antibody.

d. A rising dye or IFA titer, the disappearance of IgM-IFA titer, or both of these occurring over an interval of several weeks generally establishes the diagnosis. A single high titer, while suspicious, does not establish the diagnosis.

e. Recovery of parasites from infected tissues, bone marrow, or blood is possible in tissue culture or after inoculation in mice (not routinely available).

5. Management.

a. Therapy for toxoplasmosis is evolving. Therefore, the following management should be undertaken in conjunction with a physician experienced with congenital toxoplasmosis.

b. Pyrimethamine/sulfadiazine combination.
1) Sulfadiazine, 100mg/kg/day in 2 doses for 1 year – not to exceed 4g daily.
2) A loading dose of pyrimethamine of 2mg/kg/day in 1 dose for 2 days is given.
3) This is followed by pyrimethamine, 1mg/kg/day for 2–6 months. Total daily dose should not exceed 25mg.
4) After 2–6 months, give pyrimethamine 1mg/kg three times per week until 1 year of age.
5) Folinic acid, 10mg three times per week, should also be administered to prevent hematologic toxic reaction.

c. Congenitally infected newborns should probably be treated to prevent progression of disease. In asymptomatic infants the prevention of debilitating sequelae is the aim of treatment. In face of a high stable titer of IgG antibody without clinical illness in early infancy, one may either treat or follow the patient carefully with monthly blood tests and examinations for evidence of disease (eye findings, failure to thrive).

10

INFECTIOUS DISEASES

REFERENCES

1. Sarff LD, Platt LH, McCracken GH Jr et al. Cerebrospinal fluid evaluation in neonates: comparison of high-risk infants with and without meningitis. *J Pediatr* 1976; 473–477.
2. Peter G, ed. *Red book: Report of the Committee on Infectious Diseases,* 24th edition. Elk Grove Village, IL: American Academy of Pediatrics; 1997.

FURTHER READING

Feigen RD, Cherry JD, eds. *Textbook of pediatric infectious diseases.* Philadelphia: Saunders; 1983.
Remington JS, Klein JO, eds. *Infectious diseases of the fetus and newborn,* 4th edition. Philadelphia: Saunders; 1995.

ACID–BASE PROBLEMS

Problems of respiratory acidosis, metabolic acidosis, and mixed respiratory/metabolic acidosis are common in the newborn. Alkalosis is uncommon and is usually iatrogenic. Significant respiratory acidosis is treated with assisted ventilation. Metabolic acidosis is treated with base replacement and correction, if possible, of the underlying cause. Although a lower-limit arterial blood pH value has not been established for well-being, we arbitrarily attempt to correct acute metabolic acidosis when the pH is below 7.15 and chronic acidosis below 7.20–7.25. Higher pH limits are desirable in the presence of hyperbilirubinemia since acidosis, particularly respiratory acidosis, may potentiate encephalopathy.

I. COMMON CAUSES OF METABOLIC ACIDOSIS
A. ACUTE ONSET.
1. Hypoxia.
2. Shock and hypoperfusion (e.g. sepsis, volume loss, heart failure, NEC).
3. Inborn errors of metabolism (lactic acidosis, organic acidemias).
B. SUBACUTE AND CHRONIC ACIDOSIS.
1. Renal tubular acidosis (usually due to immature renal function).
2. Hypoperfusion and inborn errors of metabolism may present with mild persistent acidosis.
3. Feeding acidosis in premature infants.

II. COMMON CAUSES OF RESPIRATORY ACIDOSIS
A. ACUTE ONSET.
1. Asphyxia.
2. Apnea.
3. Obstructed endotracheal tube.
4. Pneumothorax.
5. Bronchospasm (e.g. chronic lung disease, pneumonia).
B. SUBACUTE AND CHRONIC ACIDOSIS.
1. Pulmonary edema.
2. Central hypoventilation.
3. Chronic lung disease.

III. DIAGNOSTIC/THERAPEUTIC APPROACH

A. EVALUATE AND CORRECT CAUSE.

1. **Acute respiratory acidosis** can usually be treated by relief of airway obstruction and mechanical ventilation.

2. **If the cause of acute metabolic acidosis is corrected** (e.g. asphyxia), acids will usually be cleared by normal metabolism. Sufficient base should be given to raise pH, however, above 7.15 to protect cardiac function.

3. **If the cause of metabolic acidosis is not clear,** evaluate serum electrolytes, lactate, urine pH (renal tubular acidosis has lower threshold for acidification), evaluate possible source of hypoperfusion (e.g. sepsis, ischemic gut) or acid load (e.g. chloride, drugs), and obtain history of fetal drug exposure (e.g. salicylates). Obtain urine for organic acids if metabolic disease is suspected.

4. **Base therapy.** Except in severe cases, the value of base therapy in either acute or chronic metabolic acidosis is currently controversial.

B. SODIUM BICARBONATE (0.5mEq/mL pediatric injectable). Isotonic $NaHCO_3$ for simultaneous volume expansion and base correction may be prepared by diluting 3mL (1.5mEq) to 10mL with sterile water.

1. **Adequate ventilation** is a prerequisite for $NaHCO_3$ therapy since buffering requires pulmonary excretion of CO_2.

2. **Resuscitation.** In documented metabolic acidosis, give 2mEq/kg i.v. slowly over 2 minutes (1mEq/kg/min). If a blood gas cannot be obtained, prolonged hypoxia-ischemia is suspected, and the heart rate is <100bpm after epinephrine, $NaHCO_3$ may be given x2 at 5 minute intervals.

3. **Dose to correct measured base excess:**
    $NaHCO_3$ (mEq) = weight (kg) x 0.3 x base deficit (mEq/L).

4. **The $NaHCO_3$ volume of distribution** is roughly equal to the extravascular volume, which varies from 40% by wt in term infants to 65% by wt in edematous immature infants. Thus, response in base excess to an acid load and response to bicarbonate therapy may differ considerably depending on lean body mass (producing acid) and extracellular volume (distributing acid and bicarbonate).

5. **Rapid infusion of hypertonic $NaHCO_3$** will acutely increase plasma osmolality and has been incriminated as a possible cause of intraventricular hemorrhage. Although the relationship is unproven, $NaHCO_3$ should be infused slowly, preferably at a rate <0.5mEq/kg/min.

6. **$NaHCO_3$ may be given p.o.** 20–60% of orally administered dose can be recovered as expired CO_2. The dose must be adjusted for effect.

7. **Fluid expansion.** In acidotic patients requiring fluid expansion (usually given as normal saline), $NaHCO_3$ may be given rapidly as an isotonic solution: 3mL $NaHCO_3$ (1.5mEq) + 7mL sterile water. This minimizes sodium overload in patients requiring multiple treatments.

C.   TROMETHAMINE (THAM, tris-hydroxymethyl-aminomethane). THAM buffers hydrogen ions directly. The protonated THAM is rapidly excreted by the kidneys. Osmolality of 0.3M THAM is about 350mOsm/kg H_2O.

1.   **Indications.** THAM should be considered as an alternative base in patients with:

a. $PaCO_2$ >65 torr.

b.   Hypernatremia (Na >150mEq/L).

2.   **Dose and administration.**
     THAM (mL of 0.3M THAM) = weight (kg) x 1.1 x base deficit (mEq/L). As with $NaHCO_3$, THAM is hypertonic and should be administered by slow i.v. infusion (<1mL/kg/min). It is ineffective when given p.o.

3.   **Contraindications.** Renal failure, oliguria, hyperkalemia.

4.   **Complications and side effects.**

a.   Hypertonicity.

b.   Apnea.

c.   Left shift in oxygen–Hb dissociation curve (increased Hb–O_2 affinity).

d.   Hyperkalemia and hypoglycemia (particularly in patients with poor nutrition and relative dehydration). Must monitor potassium and glucose levels.

FURTHER READING
Roberts DJ. *Drug therapy in infants.* Philadelphia: Saunders; 1984:288–292.

11

ACID–BASE PROBLEMS

SHOCK AND HYPOPERFUSION

'Shock' in the newborn may present as hypotension or hypoperfusion with normal blood pressure. Shock is characterized by inadequate delivery and/or extraction of oxygen and other critical substrates such as glucose to meet the metabolic demands of the tissues. In general, the therapeutic approach is aimed at matching critical substrate delivery and demands until the underlying abnormality is corrected. Specific approaches vary depending on the underlying etiology.

I. CLASSIFICATION
A. HYPOVOLEMIC.
a. Blood loss may be external (including fetal–maternal and twin–twin transfusions) or internal (adrenal, intraventricular, or intraperitoneal hemorrhage).
b. Plasma loss may accompany major abdominal surgery or inflammation.
c. Extracellular fluid loss may result from vomiting, diarrhea, or high insensible water loss.
B. CARDIOGENIC.
a. Sequelae of severe asphyxia, hypoglycemia, acidemia, congenital heart disease, or myocardial dysfunction.
b. End stage of other forms of shock.
C. DISTRIBUTIVE. (Usually septic shock.)

II. BASIC PATHOPHYSIOLOGIC PRINCIPLES
A. **OXYGEN EXTRACTION** is enhanced to meet the tissue requirements when oxygen delivery to tissues becomes limited. When extraction cannot be increased enough to meet the oxygen requirements, the oxygen uptake is supply limited and oxygen consumption decreases, resulting in a metabolic acidosis.
B. OXYGEN CONSUMPTION ($\dot{V}O_2$) is equal to the product of systemic blood flow ($\dot{Q}$) and the arteriovenous oxygen content difference ($C_aO_2 - C_vO_2$), where $\dot{Q}$ is equal to the product of stroke volume (SV) and heart rate (HR) and where oxygen content (C_xO_2) is equal to the amount of oxygen bound to hemoglobin (Hb x O_2 sat% x 1.34mL/g) plus the amount of oxygen dissolved in the plasma, which is equal to the product of the partial pressure of oxygen (PO_2) and the solubility coefficient of oxygen (α). The dissolved oxygen is minute and can usually be ignored in assessing oxygen consumption

(α = 0.003mL/100mL plasma/mmHg).

$$VO_2 = Q (C_aO_2 - C_vO_2) \text{ and}$$
$$Q = SV \times HR$$
$$(C_aO_2) = (Hb \times O_2 \text{ sat}\% \times 1.34 \text{ mL/g}) + PaO_2 \times \alpha$$

C. **OXYGEN SUPPLY AND OXYGEN REQUIREMENTS** may be matched by decreasing the metabolic rate (oxygen requirements) or enhancing oxygen supply by increasing the blood flow, the arterial oxygen content, and/or the oxygen extraction (arteriovenous oxygen difference).

III. ASSESSMENT

A. **HISTORY.** Review for evidence of blood, plasma, or fluid loss, fetal distress, perinatal cardiorespiratory depression or other myocardial insults, as well as maternal infection.
B. **PHYSICAL EXAMINATION,** emphasizing cardiopulmonary status, including quality of pulses, perfusion and precordial activity, edema, peripheral circulation, blood pressure, and site of infection.
C. **BASIC MONITORING.**
1. **Blood pressure** using Doppler or, preferably, arterial line.
2. **Arterial blood gases** to assess acid/base status (respiratory and metabolic) and oxygenation.
3. **Urine output** should be monitored (bladder catheterization is often desirable), along with fluid intake and weights.
4. **Central venous pressure** is occasionally useful for management. This may be measured by an umbilical venous catheter above the diaphragm or by a central catheter placed via the external jugular or peripheral vein.
5. **Measurement of C_aO_2 and C_vO_2,** if a central venous line is present, may provide useful indicators of oxygen extraction and consumption, which serve as guides to management. Inspection of the arterial waveform may be helpful. The area under the systolic portion of the waveform is proportional to the stroke volume, while the rate of aortic diastolic pressure decay (runoff rate) may be useful in assessing systemic vascular resistance. Increased resistance produces a flattened diastolic pressure tracing, whereas decreased resistance, as in a PDA with left to right shunting, results in a very steep diastolic pressure tracing.
6. **Neutrophil count, platelet count, and clotting factors** should be monitored if infection or ischemia is suspected.
D. **INDICATORS OF BLOOD VOLUME.**
1. **Change in hematocrit readings.**
2. **Response to a fluid challenge** of 10mL/kg of saline (monitor BP, CVP, and urine output).
3. **Kleihauer–Betke acid elution test** on mother if fetal–maternal transfusion is suspended.

E. INDICATORS OF CARDIAC FUNCTION.

1. **Assessment of cardiopulmonary patterns** and other vital organ functions, BP, and perfusion.

2. **Echocardiogram.** Used to rule out anatomical defects, and to assess abnormal shunting, cardiac filling (left ventricular end diastolic diameter, LVEDD, may be measured to assess LV filling) and myocardial function (left ventricle shortening fraction, [LVEDD – LVESD]/LVEDD, may be utilized to assess contractility); further, systolic time intervals on the right and left may be utilized to assess pulmonary and systemic vascular resistance.

3. **ECG, CVP, and diastolic pressure analysis.**

F. INDICATORS OF SEPTIC SHOCK.

1. **Evidence of sepsis.**

2. **Hypoperfusion** usually prominent, often with normal central BP.

3. **Capillary leak** of protein and fluid with edema or sclerema.

4. **Oliguria, proteinuria,** with or without hypotension.

5. **Pulmonary hypertension** is common.

IV. TREATMENT

A. BLOOD VOLUME AND RED CELL MASS. Increase to maintain BP and to maximize blood oxygen content. Use BP, arterial waveform inspection, CVP, peripheral perfusion, and metabolic acidosis as guidelines for volume to be transfused. Adult hemoglobin releases oxygen more readily than fetal hemoglobin.

B. MAXIMIZE CARDIAC OUTPUT. Inotropes should be introduced early in septic shock, when there is evidence of oliguria, hypotension, or acidosis.

1. **Dopamine**, 5–20mcg/kg/min i.v.

2. **Dobutamine**, 5–20mcg/kg/min may be added concurrently.

3. **Digitalis** should be used selectively, since it may be hazardous in face of hypoxia or toxic myocardiopathy.

4. **Other inotropic agents.**

C. MAXIMIZE OXYGENATION. Various pulmonary vasodilators may be useful when pulmonary hypertension produces hypoxemia. Unfortunately, most of the agents utilized are not selective for the pulmonary vascular bed. In septic shock, tolazoline, for example, should be used cautiously and in conjunction with inotropic agents and volume expansion, since systemic hypotension is likely. Selective delivery to the pulmonary vascular bed is difficult even with delivery into the main pulmonary artery, because of right to left ductal shunting. Potential pulmonary vasodilatation without systemic vasodilatation may be possible with agents such as nitric oxide inhalation.

D. METABOLIC ACIDOSIS. Correct with $NaHCO_3$ or THAM.

E. DECREASE METABOLIC RATE. Sedation.

12

SHOCK AND HYPOPERFUSION

V. CONTROVERSIAL THERAPIES

A. CORTICOSTEROIDS may prevent adrenal insufficiency, stabilize lysosomal membranes, and inhibit complement-induced granulocyte aggregation. Massive doses, 2–6mg/kg, of dexamethasone every 4–6 hours have been advocated by some in the early stage of disease. Steroids may reverse potential α-adrenergic insensitivity which may be present, thus enhancing the response to inotropic agents which may have some α-adrenergic activity. Glucocorticoids may be helpful in hypotensive newly born micropremature who are unresponsive to fluid and vasopressor administration.

B. INDOMETHACIN inhibits cyclooxygenase activity and potentiates lipoxygenase activity; it may block pulmonary artery pressure changes in experimental septic shock. In infants with a PDA with left to right shunting, the peak systolic pressure may be increased due to increased LV stroke volume whereas the diastolic pressure may be decreased due to the runoff into the pulmonary vascular bed. Indomethacin may elevate the diastolic component by leading to PDA closure. Since indomethacin results in decreased levels of PGE_1, which has generalized vasodilatory properties, even in the absence of a PDA, the systemic blood pressure may increase.

C. NALOXONE competitively inhibits effects of endorphins and stimulates catecholamine release. May be effective in hemorrhagic and endotoxic shock and, rarely, in perinatal hypoxic–ischemic shock. Excessive endorphins may produce pinpoint pupils.

D. EXCHANGE TRANSFUSION may be effective in scleremic septic newborns and in group B β-hemolytic streptococcal sepsis when a donor with type-specific antibody is identified.

E. LEUKOCYTE TRANSFUSION may be effective in patients with severe neutropenia and bone marrow depression. Use of irradiated buffy coat concentrates is preferable.

F. HUMAN GRANULOCYTE-COLONY STIMULATING FACTOR (G-CSF). May also be effective in neutropenic patients as a hematopoietic hormone which promotes the proliferation and differentiation of neutrophils.

CARDIAC DISEASE

Some newborns with acyanotic heart disease will present with a heart murmur within the first week of life. Others may present with CHF, and a few may develop cyanosis and/or cardiovascular collapse. Critical pulmonary stenosis, critical aortic stenosis, and critical coarctation of the aorta are ductal dependent lesions and require prompt diagnosis and treatment. In the immediate newborn period pulmonary vascular resistance is high and, thus, pulmonary artery and right ventricular pressures are elevated. Left-to-right shunting through the PDA or VSD will usually be minimal during this time. As pulmonary vascular resistance falls over the next few days to weeks, left to right shunting usually increases.

A. CAUSES OF HEART MURMURS IN INFANTS

1. Presenting immediately after birth.

a. Semilunar valve stenosis.
   1) Aortic stenosis
   2) Pulmonary stenosis.
b. Peripheral pulmonary stenosis.
c. Atrioventricular valve regurgitation.
   1) Tricuspid regurgitation.
   2) Mitral regurgitation.
d. Hyperdynamic states.
   1) Anemia.
   2) Arteriovenous malformations.

2. Presenting 1–6 weeks of age.

a. VSD.
b. PDA.

B. APPROACH TO ACYANOTIC HEART DISEASE.

Table 13.1 describes a general approach to the diagnosis of acyanotic heart disease.

C. MANAGEMENT.

Acyanotic heart disease often does not require any medical or surgical intervention but requires follow-up with pediatric cardiology. If the patient is presenting with congestive heart failure, medications will be necessary and, for a ductal dependent lesion, prostaglandin E_1 will be indicated (see cyanotic heart disease management section below for dose and side effects).

TABLE 13.1

ACYANOTIC HEART DISEASE

Left to right shunts [a]	
1.	VSD
2.	ASD
3.	PDA

Obstructive lesions [b]	
1.	Aortic stenosis
2.	Coarctation of the aorta
3.	Pulmonary stenosis

Regurgitant lesions [c]	
1.	Tricuspid regurgitation
2.	Mitral regurgitation
3.	Pulmonary regurgitation
4.	Aortic regurgitation

[a]These lesions present with volume overload usually a few weeks after birth, which on physical exam will include an active and displaced impulse. The patient may have congestive heart failure and the chest radiograph will show increased heart size and increased pulmonary vascular markings.

[b]If mild to moderate obstruction, these patients may present with only a heart murmur. Critical aortic stenosis or coarctation may reveal pulmonary edema while critical pulmonary stenosis may reveal decreased pulmonary markings on chest radiograph.

[c]These lesions present with a heart murmur. Ebstein anomaly, which usually causes tricuspid regurgitation, also may present with cyanosis.

II. EVALUATION OF CYANOSIS IN THE NEWBORN

If a cyanotic heart defect is present, the fetus is usually not adversely affected, since oxygenation of the blood occurs in the placenta rather than the lungs. However, the newborn will have some degree of hypoxemia, and the diagnosis should be made expeditiously. The first consideration is to decide whether the cyanosis is central or peripheral. Peripheral cyanosis will appear as a slight bluish discoloration of the perioral region, hands, or feet. This type of cyanosis is generally benign and the arterial oxygenation is normal. In central cyanosis (Table 13.2) the mucus membranes, lips, and nail beds will be blue. Systemic oxygenation is abnormally low.

A. HEART DISEASE OR LUNG DISEASE.

Differentiating heart disease from lung disease is often the initial concern.

1. **History and physical exam.**
   a. Chest wall retractions often minimal in heart disease.
   b. Heart murmur often present in cardiac disease.
2. **Hyperoxia test.** In cyanotic heart disease, blood returning from the lungs is usually fully saturated with oxygen, in contrast to respiratory disease. If a neonate with cyanotic heart disease breathes 100% oxygen, the oxygen content in pulmonary venous blood changes little and, thus, the increase in systemic arterial oxygen saturation is minimal.

TABLE 13.2

DIFFERENTIAL DIAGNOSIS OF CENTRAL CYANOSIS

Respiratory disease	Seizures
Persistent pulmonary hypertension	Hypoglycemia
Heart disease	Polycythemia
Sepsis and/or meningitis	Methemoglobinemia
	Shock

13

CARDIAC DISEASE

a. Technique. Measure systemic oxygenation in room air or the lowest FiO_2 the baby can tolerate. After leaving the baby on 100% oxygen for 10–15 minutes, the systemic oxygenation measurement should be repeated from the same site.
b. Heart disease is unlikely if one of the following is noted:
   1) The Po_2 increases by more than 30mmHg or O_2 saturation increases by more than 20 percentage points
   2) The Po_2 is >100mmHg.
c. Often the differential diagnosis list is reduced to persistent pulmonary artery hypertension versus cyanotic heart disease. In pulmonary hypertension, oxygen saturation in the right hand will be greater than in the foot if the ductus arteriosis is patent. Also hyperventilation may raise the systemic Po_2 to >100mmHg. Echocardiogram is useful to quantitate pulmonary hypertension and to differentiate it from cyanotic congenital heart disease.

B. APPROACH TO CYANOTIC HEART DISEASE.

Table 13.3 describes a general approach to the diagnosis of cyanotic heart disease using the physical examination and chest radiograph. Pulmonary blood flow is a key factor in this approach. The three most common cyanotic heart defects presenting in the newborn period are as follows.

1. Transposition of the great arteries.
a. Cyanosis and possibly dyspnea.
b. Heart silhouette is an 'egg on a string'.
c. Pulmonary vascular markings may be increased.
2. Tetralogy of Fallot.
a. Systolic heart murmur and possibly cyanosis.
b. Heart silhouette is 'boot shaped'.
c. Pulmonary vascular markings are decreased.
3. Hypoplastic left heart syndrome.
a. Cyanosis, dyspnea, and vascular collapse.
b. Heart silhouette is enlarged.
c. Pulmonary edema.

C. MANAGEMENT.

1. **Monitor oxygen.** Some supplemental oxygen may be helpful to maintain oxygen saturation >75%. However, too much oxygen may cause PDA closure in a ductal dependent lesion.

TABLE 13.3		
CYANOTIC HEART DISEASE		
Increased pulmonary vascular markings[a]		
Increased venous markings		
1.		Hypoplastic left heart syndrome
2.		Total anomalous pulmonary venous return
Increased arterial markings		
1.		Transposition of great arteries
2.		Truncus arteriosus
3.		Single ventricle
Decreased pulmonary vascular markings[b]		
1.		Tetralogy of Fallot
2.		Pulmonary atresia
3.		Critical pulmonary stenosis
4.		Tricuspid atresia
5.		Ebstein anomaly
6.		Complex cyanotic heart disease stenosis

[a]Presents with dyspnea, retractions, hyperdynamic precordium, and possibly some component of CHF.
[b]Presents with tachypnea and a quiet precordium.

2. **Correct metabolic acidosis.**
3. **Keep hematocrit above 45%.**
4. **Prostaglandin E_1.**
a. Possible indications if noncardiac causes of cyanosis are ruled out and heart disease is suspected:
   1) Cyanotic term infant with a heart murmur or poor pulses
   2) Critically ill term infant with poor pulses or cyanosis.
b. Starting dose is 0.05mcg/kg/min i.v., and this can be increased to 0.1mcg/kg/min.
c. Side effects:
   1) Apnea – assisted ventilation is indicated
   2) Hyperthermia
   3) Hypotension
   4) Jitteriness leading to seizures.

III. CONGESTIVE HEART FAILURE IN THE NEWBORN

CHF is defined as the inability of the heart to meet the metabolic demands of the body. The general pathogenic mechanisms involve increased preload, increased afterload, impaired contractility, or chronotropic abnormalities. The newborn myocardium has an inadequate response to pressure and volume loads because of immaturity of contractile elements and sympathetic innervation. CHF in the newborn is often a high-output failure and usually presents as a mixed right-sided and left-sided failure.

A. CAUSES.
1. **Immediately after birth.**
a. Anemia.
b. Myocarditis.
c. Arteriovenous malformations.
d. Dysrhythmias:
   1) Supraventricular tachycardia
   2) Bradyarrhythmias.
e. Atrioventricular valve regurgitation.
f. Semilunar valve regurgitation.
2. **2–7 days of age.**
a. Coarctation of the aorta.
b. Interrupted aortic arch.
c. Aortic stenosis.
d. Shone's complex.
e. Hypoplastic left heart syndrome.
3. **2–6 weeks of age.** VSD.

B. RECOGNITION.
1. **History.**
a. Easy fatigue.
b. Tachypnea.
c. Diaphoresis.
d. Irritability.
e. Excessive weight gain (edema).
2. **Physical exam and chest radiograph.**
a. Increased heart rate (>160/min).
b. Increased respiratory rate (>60/min).
c. Increased liver size.
d. Increased heart size (cardiac/thoracic ratio >60%).
e. Others:
   1) Gallop rhythm
   2) Rales and/or wheezing
   3) Increased pulmonary vascular markings
   4) Pulmonary edema.

C. MEDICAL TREATMENT.
1. Mild to moderate congestive heart failure.
a. Positive nitrogen balance.
b. Correction of any significant anemia.
c. Diuretics
d. Consider digoxin or afterload reduction agents such as hydralazine.
2. **Suggested drug regimen.**
a. Lanoxin (digoxin), 5mcg/kg/dose p.o./NG q12h or 4mcg/kg/dose i.v. q12h (digitalizing dose is generally not recommended).
b. Aldactazide (thiazide and aldosterone antagonist), 1mg of each agent/kg/dose p.o. q12h. If enteral administration is not advised, use Lasix.

13

CARDIAC DISEASE

   c. May increase Aldactazide to 1.5mg/kg/dose q12h.
   d. May add Lasix (loop diuretic) 1mg/kg/dose i.v. or 1–3mg/kg/dose p.o.
      q48h, q6h, or q12h.
   e. May add hydralazine if afterload reduction beneficial,
      0.1–0.25mg/kg/dose p.o. q6h.
   f. Side effects.
      1) Diuretics.
      a) Thiazides and loop diuretics: hyponatremia, hypokalemia,
         hypochloremia, alkalosis, and hyperuricemia. Loop diuretics may
         be ototoxic.
      b) Aldosterone antagonists: hyperkalemia and gynecomastia.
      2) Digoxin: nausea, vomiting, second or third degree heart block,
         other dysrhythmias, and hyperkalemia.

3. Severe CHF.
   a. Loop diuretics.
   b. Intubation with assisted ventilation.
   c. Dopamine or dobutamine by intravenous infusion.
   d. Digoxin.

IV.   PATENT DUCTUS ARTERIOSUS IN THE PREMATURE
The incidence of clinically significant PDA increases with decreasing
gestational age and is often associated with resolving lung disease.
A. CLINICAL.
1. Respiratory deterioration (usually CO_2 retention), fluid retention,
   feeding intolerance, and apnea.
2. Active precordium.
3. Systolic murmur at the upper left sternal border that may extend into
   early diastole.
4. Bounding pulses with wide pulse pressure and rapid diastolic pressure
   decay.
5. Hepatomegaly occasionally occurs.
B. DIAGNOSTIC TESTS.
1. ECG may be normal.
2. Chest radiograph shows cardiomegaly and increased vascularity.
3. Doppler echocardiography with color flow is the most useful technique
   for demonstrating ductal left-to-right shunt.
C. TREATMENT
1. Medical management including fluid restriction and maintenance of a
   normal hemoglobin level may be attempted first if the premature infant
   is stable with improving respiratory status.
2. Indomethacin may be given if there are no clinical or laboratory
   findings suggesting renal failure, hepatic failure, GI tract or other
   bleeding, coagulation problems, thrombocytopenia, or NEC.
   a. Serum creatinine level should be <1.5mg/dL, platelet count
      >80,000/cm, and urine output normal.

b. Most effective in infants >800g and <2 weeks of age.
c. Medication (Table 13.4) is given i.v. q12–24h for 3 doses.
d. Prophylactic indocin in very small premature is used in some centers.
3. **Surgical closure** of PDA is a safe alternative, indicated in cases where indomethacin therapy fails or is contraindicated.

TABLE 13.4

INDOMETHACIN (MG/KG) FOR TREATMENT OF PATENT DUCTUS ARTERIOSUS

Age of infant	1st dose	2nd dose	3rd dose
<48 h	0.20	0.10	0.10
2–7 days	0.20	0.20	0.20
>7 days	0.20	0.25	0.25

IV. NEONATAL ECG INTERPRETATION

A. P WAVES.
a. P waves are normally upright in leads I, II, and AVF. Inverted P waves may indicate an ectopic atrial rhythm or dextrocardia.
b. Peaked P waves >2.5mm may indicate right atrial enlargement.
c. Broad notched P waves >0.08 seconds may indicate left atrial enlargement.

B. PR INTERVAL.
a. PR interval should not exceed 0.11 seconds.
b. Prolonged PR interval is seen in primary AV conduction defects, endocardial cushion defects, digitalis effect, and bradycardia.

C. QRS.
a. Duration: 0.10 seconds (<0.04 seconds in premature infants).
b. Frontal axis and amplitude. See Table 13.5.

D. QTC: CORRECTED QT INTERVAL.
a. QTC, which equals QT interval/R–R interval, should not exceed 0.44 seconds.
b. Prolonged QTC is seen in hypocalcemia, hypokalemia, quinidine effect, or metabolic derangements. It may represent a primary inherited disorder associated with dysrhythmias and sometimes deafness.

E. T WAVES.
a. Birth to 5 days – normally upright in V_1 and V_2
b. 5 days to adolescence – normally inverted in V_1 and V_2, and upright in V_5 and V_6.
c. Elevated and peaked in hyperkalemia.

F. VENTRICULAR HYPERTROPHY.
Neonatal ECG is normally characterized by right ventricular dominance.
1. **RVH** is suggested by the following.
a. R-Wave amplitude in right precordial leads in excess of normal (see Table 13.5).

b.   Upright T waves in V_1 beyond 5 days of age.
2.   LVH is suggested by the following.
a.   R-wave amplitude in left precordial leads in excess of normal.
b.   Sum of S-wave amplitude in V_2 and R-wave amplitude in V_5 is >55mm.
c.   Deep Q wave in precordial leads V_5 and V_6.

G.   CONDUCTION DISORDERS.

1.   Atrioventricular (AV) node block.
a.   First-degree AV block. PR interval >0.12 seconds.
b.   Second-degree AV block.
    1)   Type I (Wenckebach): progressive lengthening of the PR interval until there is blocked AV node conduction and a dropped ventricular beat. Rhythm usually occurs with periodicity.
    2)   Type II: constant PR interval with occasional dropped ventricular beats.
c.   Complete AV block: no conducted atrial impulses. Atrial rate is greater than ventricular rate and ventricular rhythm is either junctional or idioventricular. Consider maternal lupus.
2.   Bundle-branch block. Unusual in newborns.
a.   Complete left bundle-branch block:
    1)   QRS duration >0.10 seconds
    2)   Broad monophasic R wave in lead I, and a wide S in V_1 and V_2
    3)   Left axis deviation.
b.   Complete right bundle-branch block:
    1)   QRS duration >0.10 seconds
    2)   An RSR' complex in the right precordial leads
    3)   Broad S wave in leads I, V_5, and V_6
    4)   Right axis deviation.

H.   RHYTHM DISTURBANCES.

1.   Premature contractions.
a.   Premature atrial contractions are very common in healthy newborns. Premature P wave may be blocked, conducted with an aberrant QRS, or conducted normally.
b.   Premature junctional contractions are marked by early QRS with either inverted, absent, or retrograde P wave. Again, these may be found in healthy newborns.
c.   Premature ventricular contractions are marked by broad complex QRS occurring before the expected atrial beat. They may be unifocal or multifocal (variable QRS morphology). Beats are usually followed by compensatory pause (the distance between the QRS complexes before and after the PVC is twice the underlying R–R interval).
2.   Bradyarrhythmia. Slow heart rate.
a.   Sinus arrhythmia. Normal P waves but P–P interval varies with respiration: i.e. sinus rate increases during inspiration and decreases with expiration. This is a normal finding.

TABLE 13.5

NORMAL NEONATAL ELECTROCARDIOGRAPHIC VALUES

Age (days)	Heart rate (bpm)	Frontal QRS axis (degrees)		QRS amplitudes – chest leads (mm)			
		Mean	Range	Right: V_1, V_2		Left: V_5, V_6	
				R	S	R	S
0–1	100–200	135	60–180	4.3–21.0	1.1–19.1	3.2–16.6	2.4–18.5
1–7	100–180	125	80–160	3.3–18.7	0.0–15.0	3.8–24.2	2.8–16.3
8–30	120–180	110	60–160	3.3–18.8	0.0–15–0	3.8–24.6	2.8–16.3

Adapted from Moss et al[1].

   b.   Sinus bradycardia. Normal P waves, but rate is less than expected for
        age. May be caused by both cardiac and extracardiac disorders.
   c.   Sinus node block and arrest. Very rarely seen in newborns. Long pause
        with no atrial beats.
3. **Tachyarrhythmias.** The tachyarrhythmias that require therapy are as
        follows.
   a.   Supraventricular – narrow QRS.
        1)   Paroxysmal SVT. If asymptomatic, perform diving reflex maneuver
             or administer adenosine 0.1–0.375mg/kg rapidly i.v. (blocks AV
             node conduction for several seconds). Digoxin may be necessary
             for recurrent SVT. If symptomatic with heart failure or shock,
             cardiovert with 2W-s/kg, then follow with prophylactic digoxin.
        2)   Atrial flutter and fibrillation. Cardioversion if symptomatic, then add
             digoxin and possibly propranolol.
   b.   Ventricular.
        1)   Ventricular tachycardia must be differentiated from SVT with
             aberrancy. Ventricular tachycardia is supported by the presence of
             fusion beats, capture beats, and AV dissociation. If cardiac output
             is good, give a lidocaine bolus, 1mg/kg. If successful, follow by
             lidocaine drip, 10–30mcg/kg/min. If the patient is symptomatic,
             use cardioversion 2W-s/kg followed by lidocaine drip.
        2)   Ventricular fibrillation is life threatening and treated by defibrillation
             2–4W-s/kg.

V. ECHOCARDIOGRAPHY
A. **NORMAL CARDIAC CHAMBER SIZES** are listed in Table 13.6.
B. **CARDIAC FUNCTION.** Left ventricular contractility is determined by
        the shortening fraction percentage (SF):
        $SF = ([LVEDD - LVESD]/LVEDD) \times 100$.
        The normal range is 27–42%.

REFERENCE
1.   Moss AJ, Adams FH, Emmanoulides GC, eds. *Heart disease in infants,
     children and adolescents,* 2nd edition. Baltimore: Williams & Wilkins;
     1977:32–40.

TABLE 13.6

NORMAL ECHOCARDIOGRAPHIC VALUES FOR THE NEWBORN

Weight (g)	LAD (cm)	Aorta (cm)	LVEDD (cm)	RVEDD (cm)	IVS (cm)
750–1249	0.72±0.07	0.63±0.06	1.26±0.15		0.20±0.06
1250–1749	0.85±0.10	0.73±0.06	1.33±0.12		0.26±0.06
1750–2249	0.96±0.08	0.84±0.05	1.52±0.15		0.26±0.06
2250–2749	1.03±0.09	0.89±0.08	1.73±0.22		0.28±0.04
2750–3249	1.08±0.10	0.93±0.06	1.79±0.21		0.29±0.06
3250–3749	1.16±0.10	0.99±0.06	1.83±0.20	1.00±0.19	0.28±0.05
3750–4249	1.20±0.10	1.03±0.06	1.93±0.24	1.00±0.19	0.28±0.05
4250	1.25±0.07	1.06±0.08	2.12±0.23	1.00±0.19	0.30±0.06

LAD, left atrial diameter; LVEDD, left ventricular end diastolic diameter; RVEDD, right ventricular end diastolic diameter; IVS, intraventricular septal thickness.

13

CARDIAC DISEASE

PULMONARY DISEASES

I. RESPIRATORY DISTRESS SYNDROME

RDS, also known as HMD, is the most common cause of respiratory failure in newborns. It occurs in infants with immature lungs who produce or release inadequate amounts of pulmonary surfactant. Diffuse atelectasis and reduced lung compliance are the major pathophysiological features. The incidence of RDS increases with decreasing gestational age. Infants who are asphyxiated, hypovolemic, or IDM are at increased risk.

A. DIAGNOSIS.
1. Clinical findings.
   a. Signs of respiratory distress are tachypnea, chest wall retractions, nasal flaring, expiratory grunting, and cyanosis.
   b. Other findings include systemic hypotension, oliguria, hypotonia, temperature instability, ileus, and peripheral edema.
   c. Prematurity on physical examination.
2. **Chest radiograph.** Characteristic reticulogranular or ground-glass pattern and air bronchograms indicating diffuse atelectasis.
3. **Biochemical findings.**
   a. Amniotic fluid L/S ratio <2.0 and/or a negative FSI using amniotic fluid. Infants of diabetic mothers may develop RDS at L/S ratios >2.0.
   b. Absence of phosphatidyl glycerol from the amniotic fluid.

B. NATURAL HISTORY.
1. **Pulmonary insufficiency** worsens during the first 24–48 hours and then plateaus for 24 hours.
2. **Resolution** takes 5–7 days and is frequently preceded by increased urine output beginning between 60 and 90 hours of age.

C. MANAGEMENT.
The goal of therapy in RDS is to inflate the atelectasis-prone lung adequately and to provide general support until spontaneous resolution occurs. Oxygen consumption and CO_2 production may be minimized by maintaining the patient in a neutral thermal environment. Since renal function may be impaired, and insensible water loss may be transiently high, careful fluid and electrolyte management is critical.
1. **Airway management.**
   a. Position the infant to allow slight hyperextension of the head. Periodic rotation from supine to lateral to prone position promotes tracheobronchial drainage. Retractions and work of breathing may be less in the prone position because of chest wall splinting.

b. Tracheal suctioning is usually necessary in babies on assisted ventilation in order to remove thick secretions during the exudative phase, which begins at about 48 hours of age.

2. Oxygen administration.

a. Warmed, humidified, oxygen-enriched gas mixtures are delivered into lucite hoods placed over the infant's head or via masks, nasal prongs, nasal cannulae or endotracheal tubes.

b. Maintain the P_aO_2 between 50 and 80 torr and/or the oxygen saturation between 85% and 95%.

3. Vascular catheters.

a. Place UAC in infants requiring frequent ABG and blood pressure monitoring.

b. An UVC with its tip placed above the diaphragm may be useful for CVP monitoring and infusion of pharmacologic agents.

4. Hypovolemia and anemia.

a. Measure central hematocrit and BP serially, beginning as soon after birth as practical.

b. Maintain the hematocrit reading above 40% by transfusion during the acute phase of the illness. During resolution, a hematocrit >30% should suffice.

5. Acidosis.

a. Metabolic acidosis (a base deficit $\geq$ 6mEq/L or HCO_3^- $\leq$18mEq/L) requires evaluation for the possible causes.

b. Base deficits $\geq$ 8mEq/L are usually treated to maintain the pH above 7.25.

c. When the pH falls below 7.25 on a respiratory basis, assisted ventilation is usually indicated.

6. Feeding.

a. Attempt to start enteral feeding via orogastric tube between 24 and 72 hours of age if the cardiovascular system is stable and pulmonary disease is under appropriate management.

b. Avoid nipple feeding in infants with respiratory rates above 70 per minute to minimize the risk of aspiration.

c. Consider parenteral nutrition on day 2 of life if full enteral feeding will be delayed. Usually indicated in infants <250g.

d. Vitamin A, 2–5000IU parenterally every other day until feedings are established, may reduce the incidence of CLD.

7. Chest radiographic studies are important:

a. To diagnose and assess the course of the disease.

b. To document the position of endotracheal tubes, chest tubes, and umbilical catheters.

c. To evaluate lung expansion (especially on high-frequency ventilation).

d. To detect complications such as pneumothorax, pneumopericardium, and NEC.

8. **Irritability.**
a. Abnormal P_aO_2 and P_aCO_2 may cause, or may be caused by struggling and agitation. Minimal handling and clustered care will help to minimize agitation.
b. Sedation is usually indicated for infants on ventilators.
c. Paralysis may be indicated in infants on ventilators who cannot be soothed and whose ventilation is being adversely affected.

9. **Infection.**
a. All infants with respiratory distress deserve evaluation for sepsis and pneumonia, and initial coverage with antibiotics is indicated until culture results are known.
b. Early onset group B β-hemolytic streptococcus infection may mimic RDS both clinically and radiographically.

10. **Respiratory failure – management.**
a. Exogenous surfactant administration (see Chapter 32) is indicated in infants with RDS requiring mechanical ventilation.
   1) Artificial and animal preparations are available. The latter appear to be more effective.
   2) Administered prophylactically in delivery room to selected infants or later to rescue infants diagnosed as RDS.
   3) Administered as saline suspension via the airway according to the manufacturer's recommendations.
   4) RDS is less severe, pneumothorax is decreased, and survival improves by 30%. Mechanical ventilation is still required, and incidence of CLD (BPD) is unchanged, but severity may be lessened.
b. In RDS it is important to minimize lung trauma. Tidal volume breathing with underinflated surfactant-deficient lungs may begin the pulmonary injury sequence leading to BPD.
   1) Trials of nasal CPAP may avoid endotracheal intubation.
   2) The decision to intervene with pulmonary support techniques should be documented in the chart according to the criteria in the NICU.
   3) Optimal pulmonary function with minimal trauma is achieved by optimizing lung volume and preventing microatelectasis on expiration. This is achieved by manipulating PEEP and PIP to achieve normal lung expansion on chest radiograph.
   4) A short inspiratory time, 0.25–0.35 seconds, appears to be important in minimizing lung barotrauma.
c. Try to maintain oxygen saturation 88–95% and P_aCO_2 40–55 torr. However, permissive hypercapnia to a P_aCO_2 of 60 torr is well tolerated and may reduce barotrauma.
d. Monitor the effect of change in ventilator settings or fractional inspired oxygen (FiO_2) by blood gas analysis 20–30 minutes following the change or by using oximetry to monitor O_2 saturation. Intervals may be longer during high-frequency ventilation.

14

PULMONARY DISEASES

e. Ventilator weaning.

   1) In severe RDS, try to wean PIP to 24–26cmH$_2$O before weaning oxygen. Then try to wean FiO$_2$ <30% before lowering mean airway pressure. (See Chapter 31 on ventilatory assistance.)

   2) Unless the P$_a$O$_2$ is >100 torr, oxygen concentrations are lowered by small increments, or about 5% (e.g. from 65% to 60%).

   3) In general, if the FiO$_2$ >0.6 reduce the inspired oxygen. If FiO$_2$ is between 0.4 and 0.6, reduce the ventilator parameter that is considered most hazardous to the patient.

   4) When the FiO$_2$ reaches 0.3–0.4, the major emphasis should be to reduce ventilator rates and pressures.

   5) Adjust ventilator rate and inspiratory pressure to change P$_a$CO$_2$.

   6) When therapeutic attempts to correct an abnormality fail, consult the neonatal fellow or attending physician.

   7) Extubation is usually accomplished when the FiO$_2$ is <0.3 and PIP and rate are <16–18.

11. **Deterioration** in clinical condition may be due to:

a. Alveolar rupture and the development of PIE and/or pneumothorax or pneumopericardium.

b. Loss of continuity of the oxygen delivery or ventilatory system.

   1) Check the connections in the oxygen and pressure delivery systems.

   2) Consider obstruction of the endotracheal tube, accidental extubation, or advancement of the endotracheal tube into the right main-stem bronchus. The last is common in infants under 1000g.

3) When in doubt about obstruction of endotracheal tubes or occult extubation, remove the tube, and ventilate the infant with a bag and mask. The endotracheal tube can be replaced when the infant's condition is stabilized.

c. When RDS is very severe, a right-to-left shunt may occur through the foramen ovale and/or ductus arteriosus (see Section IV on pulmonary hypertension).

d. With improvement in respiratory function, pulmonary vascular resistance may fall dramatically, allowing a left-to-right ductal shunt, most common in sub-1000g infants.

e. Less common conditions that may cause sudden deterioration include hypovolemia, intracranial hemorrhage, septic shock, hypoglycemia, kernicterus, transient hyperammonemia, or inherited metabolic disorders.

D. SURVIVAL.

See Table 14.1 .

TABLE 14.1		
RDS SURVIVAL UCDMC[a] 1990–1996		
Birth weight (g)	Number	Survival (%)
501–750	72	68
751–1000	81	80
1001–1,250	101	89
1251–1500	74	98
1501–1,750	51	98
1751–2000	31	96
>2001	56	98

[a]UCDMC, University of California Davis Medical Center

II. RETAINED LUNG FLUID SYNDROME, RDS SYNDROME TYPE II, TRANSIENT TACHYPNEA

Failure to clear the pulmonary fluid present at birth or, more likely, failure of the lung to stop producing lung fluid at the intrauterine rate, impairs pulmonary adaptation. This occurs most frequently following intrapartum asphyxia, excessive maternal medication, cesarean section, and in IDM.

A. **NATURAL HISTORY.**

1. **Retained lung fluid.** Clinically may resemble RDS early in its course, but severe retractions are uncommon. The chest radiograph shows hilar streaking, fluid in the minor fissure, and increased vascular and interstitial markings. Most infants improve dramatically by 24–48 hours.

2. **RDS Type II.** Occasionally, the clinical course is severe and similar to RDS. This condition is sometimes referred to as RDS Type II.

3. **Transient tachypnea** of the newborn. Associated with an essentially normal chest radiograph and may be the mildest form of the above-mentioned disorder. Hypocarbia is often present.

B. **THERAPY** is aimed at correcting pulmonary insufficiency by the least invasive techniques possible and avoiding iatrogenic problems. Administration of a β-adrenergic agonist, such as salbutamol, has been suggested to stimulate fluid absorption in the lung. A tracheal aspirate to rule out pneumonia may be indicated, and antibiotics are usually administered until pneumonia is ruled out.

III. MECONIUM ASPIRATION

10–15% of newborn infants have passed meconium before birth. A small percentage of these aspirate meconium into their airways. While potentially fatal pulmonary failure may accompany meconium aspiration, controversy exists about the etiology of this pulmonary insufficiency, since longstanding hypertrophy of pulmonary vascular smooth muscle has been observed in fatal cases. However, if airway obstruction plays a role, this aspect may be preventable, and treatment for this condition should begin in the delivery room. Fetal asphyxia may also complicate this condition.

A. PREPARATION depends on communication between obstetrics and neonatology after recognition of meconium-stained amniotic fluid. Thick particulate meconium is of more concern than thin meconium staining. Amnioinfusion with saline may be used to irrigate the amniotic sac before delivery if thick meconium is seen when membranes rupture. This reduces meconium aspiration but not pulmonary hypertension.

B. PHARYNGEAL SUCTIONING. As soon as the head is delivered, meconium is suctioned from the nose and pharynx by the obstetrician.

C. TRACHEAL SUCTION. Visualize and suction the trachea under direct vision immediately after birth if particulate meconium is present and infant is depressed.

1. Technique.

a. Intubate immediately and suction the trachea before ventilating. Meconium aspirators are commercially available. Use oxygen-enriched gas for ventilating.

b. Withdrawal and replacement of the endotracheal tube may be necessary, in some instances, to remove thick meconium.

c. If the newborn is crying vigorously and struggling, intubation may do more harm than good and may promote deep aspiration of meconium.

d. Tracheal toilet.

    1) If no meconium is suctioned from the trachea, stabilize patient and transport to nursery.

    2) If meconium is suctioned from the trachea, ventilate for 1–2 minutes and then instill 1–2mL of sterile saline into the endotracheal tube. After a spontaneous breath or a brief puff on the ventilating bag, suction the tube and again ventilate for 1–3 minutes. May repeat this procedure several times. Extubate if spontaneous respirations and oxygenation are adequate. At this time there are no controlled clinical studies to demonstrate that tracheal lavage is therapeutically effective.

D. FOLLOW-UP CARE.

1. Observation and treatment.

a. Transport to intensive care nursery for immediate chest radiograph and observation.

b. If infiltrate is present on chest radiograph or signs of respiratory distress develop, consider chest physiotherapy every 3–4 hours.

c. Be prepared for emergency treatment of pneumothorax.

d. Use blood gases to guide oxygen and ventilator therapy.

e. Consider the possibility of pulmonary hypertension, which can be associated with meconium aspiration.

f.   Corticosteroids and antibiotics are of controversial value.
g.   Use of exogenous surfactant to aid in removal of meconium is experimental.

IV. PULMONARY HYPERTENSION IN THE NEWBORN

This entity is also referred to as persistent fetal circulation (PFC). PHN may lead to right-to-left shunting through the foramen ovale, ductus arteriosus, or both. Severe hypoxemia may result. When it is due to intense pulmonary vasospasm of normal or thickened arteriolar smooth muscle, therapy with hyperventilation, vasodilator drugs, or both may be useful. In severe cases, ECMO may be lifesaving. Fatal cases seem to have a marked increase in pulmonary vascular smooth muscle or marked decrease in the number of small pulmonary arteries – i.e. pulmonary hypoplasia.

A. CLINICAL FEATURES.
1. **Patients.**
a.   Pulmonary hypertension occurs in term or post-term infants without lung disease and at any gestational age as a complication of pulmonary disease. It may be associated with:
   1) Meconium aspiration
   2) Congenital pneumonia
   3) Severe RDS
   4) Diaphragmatic hernia
   5) Hypoplastic lung
   6) Chromosomal disorders.
b.   Pulmonary vasospasm may be responsible for the 'flip-flop' phenomenon sometimes seen during the acute phase of RDS, e.g. a marked decrease in P_aO_2 following a small decrement in oxygen concentration or ventilator pressure.
c.   Acidosis and hypoxia worsen the disease by promoting pulmonary vasoconstriction which can alter both lung compliance and pulmonary blood flow.
2. **Course** varies from mild (with spontaneous resolution) to death from intractable hypoxemia.
3. **Duration** of illness is usually 1–10 days.

B. DIAGNOSIS.
1. **Clinical.**
a.   Suspect when the clinical severity of pulmonary insufficiency is greater than the radiographic findings suggest.
b.   Suspect when pulmonary insufficiency is refractory to ventilatory therapy: e.g. increased inspiratory pressures and PEEP.
2. **Other.**
a.   Echocardiographic evidence of a large pressure gradient across pulmonic valve, triscuspid insufficiency, and right-to-left atrial shunt is usually present. Absence of structural heart disease is considered

essential for diagnosis. However, PHN may be associated with transposition of the great vessels. Left ventricular dysfunction is also noted in some 30% of cases.

b. Simultaneous right radial (or temporal artery) and aortic P_aO_2 with difference >10 torr, or upper and lower extremity O_2 saturation difference by oximetry. These are only present if there is a major right-to-left shunt through a PDA.

c. A triscuspid insuffiency murmur is often present.

d. P_aO_2 may increase with hyperventilation or pulmonary vasodilator therapy.

C. **MANAGEMENT** is aimed at supporting oxygen delivery and promoting pulmonary vasodilatation.

1. **Correction** of conditions which potentiate PHN: acidosis, hypoglycemia, hypocalcemia, hyperviscosity, and systemic hypotension.

2. **High-frequency ventilation.** Oscillatory or jet ventilation may dramatically improve P_aO_2.

a. Mechanism may involve release of prostacyclin.

b. Reduces barotrauma.

c. May rescue 25–40% of infants who would go on to meet ECMO criteria.

3. **Alkalosis.** Regulating the pH at >7.5 by hyperventilation or by infusion of $NaHCO_3$, or THAM, can be effective, but may result in hypernatremia or fluid retention and edema. Initial rate 0.5–1.0mEq/kg/h. Reduce rate after desired pH is achieved.

a. Decreased coronary and cerebral blood flow and hypocalcemic tetany have not been documented as problems secondary to hyperventilation alkalosis in newborn infants.

b. Long-term complications of prolonged alkalosis are currently unknown.

4. **Surfactant.** Administration of exogenous surfactant (Chapter 32) appears to overcome surfactant inhibitors present in the alveoli of infants with pulmonary hypertension. May rescue 30–40% of infants who would meet ECMO criteria.

5. **Pharmacologic pulmonary vasodilator.**

a. Inhaled nitric oxide at 5–20ppm is selective and may become the standard vasodilatior used in this condition when approved by the FDA. We sometimes use tolazoline, but other vasodilators such as sodium nitroprusside or nitroglycerin are used in other centers.

b. Infuse tolazoline, 1–2mg/kg, over 10 minutes via scalp vein or arm vein.

c. Monitor BP continuously and be prepared to treat systemic hypotension with volume expanders or by increasing dopamine infusion rate. We routinely begin dopamine, 5–10mcg/kg/min, prior to tolazoline infusion.

d. Monitor ABG and O_2 saturation to assess the response to tolazoline.
e. If cutaneous flushing does not occur, repeat bolus dose.
f. A positive response is an abrupt rise in P_aO_2 of $\geq$ 15 torr (usually 50–100 torr).
g. Begin tolazoline infusion in scalp vein at rate of 2mg/kg/h.
h. Increase tolazoline infusion rate (up to 4–6mg/kg/h) as indicated by BGA.
i. When FiO_2 can be reduced to 0.6, begin to decrease tolazoline infusion rate.
j. Complications:
    1) Systemic hypotension
    2) Systemic hypertension
    3) Gastric distention
    4) GI tract bleeding
    5) Transient renal failure.
6. **Adjunctive therapy.**
a. Sedation with thorazine or a benzodiazepine may facilitate pulmonary vasodilatation.
b. Muscle paralysis with pancuronium or vecuronium may facilitate hyperventilation.
c. Dopamine and/or dobutamine, 5–20 mcg/kg/min, may support cardiac output when left ventricular dysfunction is present.
d. Extracorporeal membrane oxygenators can be lifesaving in the majority of cases refractory to the above strategies. See Chapter 33 regarding patient selection.
7. **Outcome.**
a. About 75% of affected term infants survive (increases to >90% with ECMO).
b. About 75% of the survivors are developmentally and neurologically normal.
c. Onset of deafness after discharge is an occasional complication.

V. EXTRAPULMONARY AIR

Alveolar rupture, with extrapulmonary collection of air, may occur spontaneously or as a complication of ventilatory therapy in newborns. After alveolar rupture, air may accumulate in the interstitial spaces (PIE) or it may dissect along bronchovascular channels to the hilum. Rupture of mediastinal walls leads to a pneumomediastinum, pneumothorax, or both. Accumulation of air in the intrapleural space may cause minimal to severe embarrassment of pulmonary function. While spontaneous pneumothorax occurs in 1–2% of 'normal' newborns, the incidence is higher in the presence of pulmonary disease and considerably higher when ventilatory assistance is required (5–10%). Air may also dissect into the pericardium (pneumopericardium) and lead to cardiac tamponade. Dissection of gas into the peritoneum, while uncommon, is usually benign but may lead to a mistaken diagnosis of intestinal perforation.

A. PULMONARY INTERSTITIAL EMPHYSEMA.

1. **Signs.**
a. Increasing respiratory failure with signs of respiratory distress and blood gas deterioration.
b. Accentuation of breath sounds over affected lobes.
c. Hypotension and narrowing of pulse pressure if 'air block' of circulation occurs.

2. **Diagnosis.**
a. Chest radiograph shows round, oval, and linear lucencies along bronchovascular rays. May be focal, unilateral, or generalized.

3. **Management.**
a. Increased FiO$_2$.
b. Decrease in ventilator settings (inspiratory time, end-expiratory pressure and/or inspiratory pressure), if possible.
c. Positioning patient with affected lobes in dependent position.
d. High-frequency ventilation with oscillator or jet ventilator.
e. Chronic lobar PIE rarely may need to be treated by lobectomy.

4. **Outcome.**
a. May proceed to pneumothorax, which can be drained.
b. May resolve with treatment outlined above.
c. If bilateral, disseminated, and persistent, the mortality is >80%.
d. In surviving low birth weight infants, the subsequent incidence of chronic lung disease is high.

B. TENSION PNEUMOTHORAX.

1. **Signs.**
a. Sudden clinical or blood gas deterioration with signs of respiratory distress (cyanosis, tachypnea, retractions).
b. Shift of the apical cardiac impulse (most consistent finding).
c. Decreased breath sounds unilaterally, or bilaterally. (*Note:* absent breath sounds on left side or bilaterally could be due to an endotracheal tube in right mainstem bronchus or a plugged endotracheal tube.)
d. Abdominal distention with sudden descent of liver and spleen.
e. Transient increase in systolic BP followed by narrowing of pulse pressure.

2. **Diagnosis.**
a. Physical findings as above.
b. Transillumination of the chest.
c. Diagnostic and therapeutic thoracentesis.
d. Chest radiograph.

3. **Management.**
a. Asymptomatic or mildly symptomatic pneumothorax – close observation and supplemental oxygen to maintain P_aO_2 at 80–100 torr.
b. Symptomatic pneumothorax – chest tube to water seal suction ($-10cmH_2O$) or Heimlich valve.
c. Imminent demise – emergency thoracentesis used as diagnostic as well as a therapeutic maneuver.

C. PNEUMOMEDIASTINUM rarely requires treatment.

D. PNEUMOPERICARDIUM.

1. **Signs.**
a. Shock secondary to cardiac tamponade has a sudden onset.
b. On occasion, a pneumopericardium causes relatively few symptoms and disappears spontaneously.

2. **Diagnosis.**
a. Distant heart tones.
b. Narrow pulse pressure.
c. Radiographic.

3. **Treatment.**
a. Pericardial drainage via needle aspiration, placement of a pericardial drainage tube, or both is usually necessary.

VI. CHRONIC LUNG DISEASE OF PREMATURITY

CLD is a disturbing and confusing sequela of acute lung disease, prematurity, oxygen and ventilatory therapy, and possibly PDA. Some form of chronic lung disease occurs in approximately 15% of premature infants requiring mechanical ventilation for pulmonary insufficiency. However, the incidence in infants with birth weights <1kg is 30–40%. There is a significant mortality and considerable morbidity (long-term dependence on oxygen and prolonged hospitalization) from these conditions. Full recovery of lung function usually occurs in the survivors anywhere from a few months to 3 years of age. However, the most severely affected may have lifelong disability and some infants may succumb to pulmonary infection during later infancy. There is confusion because of the variety of names applied to these syndromes and whether or not they are distinct entities or on a continuum of a single disorder. Further, definitions also vary based on clinical findings of an oxygen requirement at 28 days of postnatal age or an oxygen requirement at 36 weeks postconceptual age. In general, the etiology is an abnormal healing process following an acute lung injury that is peculiar to newborn infants, especially those that are premature.

14

PULMONARY DISEASES

A. BRONCHOPULMONARY DYSPLASIA.
1. Course.
   a. Following the acute phase of RDS, failure to improve is noted. At 10–14 days of age these infants may begin to increase their oxygen requirements.
   b. Carbon dioxide retention is routinely observed.
   c. A stable oxygen requirement supervenes at 3–4 weeks of age.
   d. Resolution is slow, requiring months of oxygen dependency.
   e. These infants are predisposed to pneumonia for at least the first year of life and the respiratory syncytial virus (RSV) poses special risks in this regard.
2. **Chest radiograph** varies from a cystic, bubbly appearance in the severe forms to a streaky, fibrotic appearance in the less involved. Hyperinflation is routinely present.

B. MULTICYSTIC BRONCHOPULMONARY DYSPLASIA (WILSON–MIKITY SYNDROME).
1. Course.
   a. Was referred to as Wilson–Mikity syndrome in the past.
   b. Ureaplasma urealyteum infection appears to play a role in some (or even many) cases.
   c. This syndrome is more common in very immature infants who initially have nearly normal chest radiograph and minimal respiratory difficulty.
   d. Pulmonary insufficiency and lung cysts develop between 4 and 30 days of age.
   e. A few of these infants die in the first months of life. The survivors usually have normal chest radiograph and lung function by 1–2 years of age.
2. **Chest radiograph.** Film shows multiple cystic lesions: hyperaeration alternating with a coarse thickening of interstitial structure (honeycomb lung).

C. MILD BRONCHOPULMONARY DYSPLASIA OR CHRONIC PULMONARY INSUFFICIENCY OF PREMATURITY.
1. Course.
   a. Delayed form, with onset at 4–7 days.
   b. Infants <28 weeks gestation with less severe early lung disease.
   c. Oxygen requirements persist for 2–4 weeks. Recovery is usually complete by 60 days of age.
   d. Apneic spells and need for supplemental oxygen are early signs.
2. **Chest radiograph** seldom shows more than a diffuse haze.

D. MANAGEMENT.
1. Therapy and complications.
   a. No specific therapy exists for any of these conditions. Erythromycin treatment is indicated for ureaplasma but does not appear to prevent CLD.

b. Supportive therapy often includes oxygen and ventilatory assistance. Consider tracheostomy at 2–3 months of age if prolonged need for ventilation is anticipated.

c. Hematocrit should be maintained at 30–40%.

d. Nutritional goal is to provide sufficient calories (100–140kcal/kg/day) without excessive sodium and free water. Concentrated formula (24–30cal/oz) may be required.

e. Few of these infants tolerate normal fluid intake; fluid overload and pulmonary edema are frequently observed. Diuretics may be helpful. Aldactone and chlorothiazide are used most often. Lasix may be used for acute fluid retention but chronic use may potentiate renal calcification and osteopenia.

f. Body weight changes and serum electrolyte levels must be carefully monitored. Watch for chloride depletion, which impairs growth.

g. Consider bacterial pneumonia for any deterioration.

h. Corticosteroids, usually dexamethasone (0.125–0.25mg/kg q12h) or prednisone (2.5mg/kg q12h), may improve lung function in some infants. Dramatic improvement should occur in 2–4 days. If this is not observed, stop prednisone administration. If improvement does occur, a 10-day course is given and the dose is then tapered slowly. Some patients require chronic steroids. Prednisone given every other day is often satisfactory and is less likely to inhibit growth.

i. Theophylline has been helpful in some infants beyond 2 weeks of age with carbon dioxide retention, especially when wheezing has been noted. Monitor blood levels. Serum levels of 12–18mg/mL appear to suffice.

j. Bronchodilator therapy with nebulized β-adrenergic agonists such as albuterol, metaproterenol, or isoetherine may help to overcome bronchospasm.

k. N-Acetyl-L-cysteine nebulization for 2–3 days may be helpful in some infants with increased pulmonary secretions and/or recurrent atelectasis.

l. Prophylactic chest physiotherapy is usually prescribed once or twice a day. Frequency and intensity of physiotherapy depends on changes in P_aCO_2 and oxygen saturation and recovery time.

m. Sedation is sometimes helpful.

n. Consider bronchoscopy for diagnosis of acquired tracheobronchomalacia when severe CO_2 retention is persistent.

E. MORTALITY. 5–10% of infants with CLD die between 1 month and 1 year of age. A few die of pneumonia later, and overall mortality approaches 15%.

14

PULMONARY DISEASES

FURTHER READING

Auten RL, Notter RH, Kendig JW, Davis JM, Shapiro DL. Surfactant treatment of full-term newborns with respiratory failure. *Pediatrics* 1991; 87:101–107.

Carlo WA, Beoglos A, Chatburn RL, Walsh MC, Martin RJ. High-frequency jet ventilation in neonatal pulmonary hypertension. *Am J Dis Child* 1989; 143:233–238.

Hoekstra RE, Jackson JC, Myers TF et al. Improved neonatal survival following multiple doses of bovine surfactant in very premature neonates at risk for respiratory distress syndrome. *Pediatrics* 1991; 88:10–18.

Kinsella JP, Truog WE, Walsh W, et al. Randomized, multicenter trial of inhaled nitric oxide and high-frequency oscillatory ventilation in severe, persistent pulmonary hypertension of the newborn. *J Pediatr* 1997; 131:55–62.

Kohelet D, Perlman M, Kirpalani H, Hanna G, Koren G. High-frequency oscillation in the rescue of infants with persistent pulmonary hypertension. *Crit Care Med* 1988; 16:510–516.

Liechty EA, Donovan E, Purohit D et al. Reduction of neonatal mortality after multiple doses of bovine surfactant in low birth weight neonates with respiratory distress syndrome. *Pediatrics* 1991; 88:19–28.

NEONATAL APNEA

15

About 75% of infants weighing <1500g at birth will have at least one apneic episode during their hospital course. Associated bradycardia and hypoxemia may be life threatening. Intermittent periodic breathing is common and must be differentiated from apnea. Remember, apnea is a symptom, not a disease.

I. DEFINITIONS

A. **APNEA.** Cessation of breathing for 20 seconds or longer, or a briefer episode associated with bradycardia, cyanosis, or pallor.

B. **PERIODIC BREATHING.** Respiratory pauses of 5–10 seconds with normal respirations between episodes not associated with bradycardia, but may coincide with hypoxemia.

II. CAUSES

A. **DECREASED TISSUE OXYGEN DELIVERY.**
1. Hypoxemia.
2. Anemia.
3. Heart failure.

B. **PULMONARY DISEASE** with decreased lung compliance.
1. RDS, pneumonia, etc.
2. PDA with increased pulmonary blood flow.
3. Hypoinflation or hyperinflation of lungs.

C. **FEEDING RELATED** (vagal mediated).
1. Nasogastric tube passage.
2. Gastroesophageal reflux.
3. Gastric distention.
4. Glottic stimulation.

D. **AIRWAY OBSTRUCTION.**
1. Excessive oral secretions.
2. Anatomic obstruction.
3. Malposition.

E. **SEPSIS** – bacterial or viral.

F. **SEIZURES.**

G. **METABOLIC IMBALANCE.**
1. Hypoglycemia.
2. Electrolyte imbalance.
3. Lactic acidosis.

H. ENVIRONMENTAL TEMPERATURE FLUCTUATION. This is more common with rising environmental temperatures.
I. CNS HEMORRHAGE or abnormalities.
J. DRUG INDUCED (usually maternally administered).
K. PREMATURITY. All other causes should be considered before making this diagnosis.
1. **Respiratory drive immaturity.** Symptoms usually begin in first 2 weeks of life.
2. **Prolonged sleep** – usually during REM sleep.
a. REM sleep is more frequent in premature infants.
b. Premature infants sleep 80–90% of the time.
c. Response to hypoxia is more sustained in non-REM sleep.

III. EVALUATION

All infants who weigh <1500g at birth and larger infants at risk should have cardiorespiratory monitoring for about 10 days until mature respiratory control is documented.
A. HISTORY and physical examination.
a. Characterize frequency, duration, and temporal associations of events: e.g. feeding, reflux, sleep.
b. Characterize association with bradycardia and/or cyanosis.
B. EVALUATION OF RESPIRATORY GAS EXCHANGE.
1. ABG measurements.
2. Transcutaneous PO_2 and PCO_2 monitoring.
3. Oximetry.
C. CNS EVALUATION.
1. Cranial ultrasound and/or CT scan.
2. Brain-stem auditory evoked potentials.
3. EEG, asleep and awake.
D. CARDIAC EVALUATION.
1. ECG.
2. Echocardiography.
E. GASTROINTESTINAL TRACT.
1. Cardiorespiratory activity with feeding.
2. Radionuclide scan after feeding marker.
3. Esophageal pH with history of esophageal study.
F. PNEUMOGRAM OR POLYGRAPHIC SLEEP STUDY. Depending on ability of laboratory, many of the above studies can be incorporated into the polygraphic study.

IV. THERAPY

A. TREAT UNDERLYING CAUSE – hypoxemia, anemia, metabolic aberrations, PDA, sepsis, gastroesophageal reflux, seizure activity.

B. SYMPTOMATIC TREATMENT.
1. **Tactile stimulation** – cutaneous.
2. **Vestibular stimulation** – 'bump beds' or water beds.
3. **Environmental temperature reduction** to low neutral thermal environment.

C. PHARMACOLOGIC AGENTS for apnea of prematurity.
1. **Theophylline** – loading dose of 4mg/kg i.v. or orally, then 2mg/kg every 12 hours. Follow levels after the third to fourth dose and observe the infant for tachycardia and emesis.
2. **Caffeine citrate** – loading dose of 20mg/kg orally, then 5–10mg/kg/day in 1 or 2 daily doses. Levels not routinely available. Fewer side effects than theophylline.
3. **Doxapram** – 2.5mg/kg/h by continuous i.v. infusion may be considered when methylxanthines are ineffective.
4. **Atropine** – 0.05–0.10mg/kg every 4–6 hours p.o. or subcutaneously, may be useful when apnea follows vagally mediated bradycardia.
5. **Cisapride or metoclopramide and H$_2$ blockers** should be considered in patients with reflux-associated apnea.

V. CRITERIA FOR HOME MONITORING
Home monitoring cannot guarantee survival.

A. THE PATIENT IS READY TO BE DISCHARGED and has one of the following.
1. Documented apnea without treatable cause or with inadequate response to therapy.
2. Apparent life-threatening event requiring cardiopulmonary resuscitation (CPR).
3. Family history of a sibling with sudden infant death syndrome.
4. Potential airway obstruction or chronic hypoxemia.

B. CONSIDER FAMILY PSYCHOLOGICAL STRESS, medical/legal aspects, and use of correct monitor type.
a. All care providers should have CPR training.
b. Monitor type should be cardiorespiratory, not apnea pad.
c. Consider oximeter for infants receiving oxygen.

C. INDICATIONS FOR DISCONTINUANCE OF HOME MONITOR. The following should be considered; however, no consensus criteria exist.
a. No clinical apnea for 2 months.
b. No apnea requiring stimulation for 3 months.
c. Normal polygraphic sleep study.
d. Infant must have experienced stress of nasopharyngitis or immunizations without recurrence of symptoms.
e. Parents refuse to use, or have discontinued use of, monitor.

15 NEONATAL APNEA

FURTHER READING

Bhatt-Mehta V, Johnson CE, Donn SM, Spadoni V, Schork MA. Accuracy and reliability of dosing equations to individualize theophylline treatment of apnea of prematurity. *Pharamacotherapy* 1995; 15(2):246–250.

Kattwinkel J, Fanaroff AA, Klaus MH. Bradycardia in preterm infants: indications and hazards of atropine therapy. *Pediatrics* 1976; 58:494–499.

Miller MJ, Martin RJ. Apnea of prematurity. *Clin Perinatol* 1992; 19:789–808.

Monin P. Modification of ventilatory reflexes: an efficient therapy for apneas of prematurity? *Biol Neonate* 1994; 65(3–4):247–251.

NEUROLOGIC DISORDERS OF THE NEWBORN

I. NEONATAL SEIZURES

Neonatal seizures occur in 1.5–14 per 1000 live births, with the higher incidence in premature infants in the NICU setting. Seizures are an important prognostic indicator for later neurologic development. Bedside portable video-EEG monitoring offers a more accurate method of describing neonatal seizures by allowing correlation of the infant's abnormal movements with the brain's electrical activity. This technology has demonstrated that many forms of neonatal 'seizures' are not due to an epileptic mechanism – for example, many of the 'seizures' that are observed in severely asphyxiated newborns.

A. CLASSIFICATION OF NEONATAL SEIZURES.

This classification is based on bedside portable video-EEG correlation.

1. **Electroclinical seizures (associated with EEG seizure discharges).**
a. Focal clonic (may be unifocal, multifocal, hemiconvulsive or axial).
b. Myoclonic (generalized or focal).
c. Focal tonic (asymmetrical truncal or eye deviation).
d. Apnea (rare).
2. **Nonepileptic seizures (inconsistent or no relationship to EEG seizure discharges).**
a. Motor automatisms, or subtle seizures (e.g. oral–buccal–lingual movements, rhythmic rapid or random eye movements, pedaling, rotary arm movements, purposeless movements).
b. Generalized tonic activity (extensor, flexor, mixed).
c. Myoclonic activity unrelated to EEG seizure discharges.
3. **Electrographic seizures (EEG seizures without clinical manifestations, electroclinical dissociation).**

B. CAUSES.

1. **Hypoxemic–ischemic injury. Tonic seizures, myoclonic seizures, motor automatisms (subtle seizures) are most common.**
2. **Focal structural injury.** Focal clonic seizures are most common.
a. Unilateral infarction.
b. Intracerebral or subarachnoid hemorrhage.
3. **Metabolic.** Variable seizure types may occur.
a. Electrolyte abnormality – sodium, calcium, magnesium.
b. Hypoglycemia.
c. Pyridoxine dependence.
d. Inborn errors of metabolism – organic acidemia, hyperammonemia, aminoacidopathies.

4. **Infection** – meningitis, encephalitis.
5. **Maternal drug addiction** with subsequent withdrawal syndrome in the infant – opiates, barbiturates, propoxyphene.
6. **Toxic agents.**
a. Isoniazid.
b. Bilirubin.
c. Local anesthetic agents.
7. **Genetic/dysmorphic syndromes.**
a. Chromosomal abnormalities.
b. Tuberous sclerosis.
c. Cerebral dysgenesis.
d. Cerebral vascular anomalies.
e. Various epileptic syndromes and familial epilepsies.

C. EVALUATION.

1. **Prenatal/perinatal** and family history.
2. **Physical and neurologic examination** including serial OFC, skin and funduscopic examinations.
3. **Metabolic evaluation.**
a. Serum glucose, sodium, calcium, magnesium, bicarbonate, BUN, creatinine, bilirubin, lactate, and ammonia levels.
b. ABG.
c. Urine/serum metabolic screen for amino acids, organic acids.
4. **Lumbar puncture** to analyze CSF for protein, glucose, blood, WBCs, and bacterial/viral culture.
5. **TORCH titers** – maternal and infant.
6. **Brain imaging.**
a. MRI is preferred to evaluate for cerebral dysgenesis. CT scanning can be used to detect hemorrhagic conditions, and intracranial calcifications suspected in TORCH infections and tuberous sclerosis.
b. Angiogram may occasionally be required for complete evaluation of hemorrhage, infarction, or vascular malformation.
7. **EEG.** Maturation occurs throughout 24–40 weeks of gestational age; an EEG is most valuable within the first days of life.
a. Interictal EEG findings associated with seizure activity:
   1) Monorhythmic focal activity
   2) Focal or multifocal spikes or sharp waves
   3) Episodes of voltage attenuation
   4) Spike and wave pattern is uncommon in the neonate.
b. Video-EEG recording of clinical events provides the best information. However, this technology is not available in all NICU settings.

D. TREATMENT.

1. **Correct primary cause** if possible.
a. Correct metabolic imbalances.
   1) Glucose, 2–4mL/kg D10W i.v.
   2) Calcium, 2mL/kg of 10% calcium gluconate i.v. slowly.

3) Magnesium, 0.2mL/kg of 50% $MgSO_4$ i.m.
4) Pyridoxine, 100mg of pyridoxine hydrochloride i.v. for unexplained seizures and abnormal EEG unresponsive to anticonvulsants. In patients with pyridoxine dependence, pyridoxine treatment will stop the clinical seizures and improve the EEG, usually within minutes. To document an effect, pyridoxine should be given during continuous EEG monitoring.
5) For metabolic acidosis, give $NaHCO_3$ calculated to provide correction. If serum sodium level is high, correct slowly with i.v. glucose fluids orTHAM.
b. Remove toxins if identified.
1) Peritoneal dialysis or hemodialysis: e.g. transient hyperammonemia.
2) Exchange transfusion: e.g. kernicterus, hyperammonemia.
c. Antibiotic therapy for CSF bacterial infection.
2. **Anticonvulsant therapy.** Since many 'seizures' associated with hypoxic–ischemic injury are not due to epileptic mechanisms, aggressive anticonvulsant therapy may not be justified. Video-EEG studies may help in this decision.
a. Phenobarbital. Long half-life.
1) Loading dose, 20mg/kg i.v., followed by additional 10mg/kg doses up to total of 40–50mg/kg if seizure activity persists.
2) Maintenance, 3–5mg/kg/day i.v. or orally.
3) Therapeutic range, 15–40mg/L. Blood level usually approximates loading dose.
b. Phenytoin (diphenylhydantoin, Dilantin). Additive effects with phenobarbital. Should be used if seizures persist with phenobarbital level >40mg/L.
1) Loading dose, 20mg/kg and flush catheter with normal saline immediately (incompatible with glucose solution).
2) Maintenance dose, 5mg/kg/day i.v. twice daily, or 15–20mg/kg/day p.o.
3) Oral Phenytoin is poorly absorbed in the neonate.
4) Therapeutic range, 10–20mg/L.
c. Paraldehyde. Side effects include pulmonary edema/hemorrhage and hypotension in older children; used mainly for status epilepticus. Paraldehyde can be administered rectally 0.3mL/kg per dose, diluted 1:2 in mineral oil.
d. Lorazepam (Ativan). 0.05mg/kg i.v. over 2–5 minutes.
e. Barbiturate coma. Not often used.
3. **Continuation of anticonvulsants** after discharge is controversial. Medication can be discontinued in infants who are seizure free, have a normal neurologic exam, and have a normal EEG. Other cases need to be considered on an individual basis. The risk of later epilepsy is 5–30%.

16

NEUROLOGIC DISORDERS OF THE NEWBORN

E. PROGNOSIS.

Long-term developmental studies suggest that 40–55% of survivors of neonatal seizures have a normal outcome. However, subtle neuropsychologic abnormalities may be detected in these individuals. Death or risk of major neurologic sequelae depend on etiology (Table 16.1). Seizures due to subarachnoid hemorrhage or hydrocalcemia usually have a good outcome.

TABLE 16.1

PROGNOSES OF NEWBORNS WITH NEONATAL SEIZURES

OUTCOME BY ETIOLOGY[a]

Cause of seizure (No.)	Normal (%)	Abnormal (%)	Expired (%)
Hypoxia/trauma (180)	39	36	25
Unknown cause (139)	63	28	9
Hypocalcemia (113)	95	5	0
Infection (52)	31	35	34
Subarachnoid hemorrhage	89	0	11
Hypoglycemia (31)	49	48	3
Malformation (24)	0	29	71

OUTCOME BY SEIZURE TYPE[b]

Seizure type (No.)	Normal (%)	Abnormal (%)	Expired (%)
Clonic (14)	71	29	0
Myoclonic (12)	35	35	35
Tonic (10)	23	54	23
Automatisms (18)	27	55	18
EEG seizure only (9)	27	55	18

[a]Adapted from Bergman et al[1].
[b]Adapted from Mizrahi and Kellaway[2].

REFERENCES

1. Bergman I, Painter MJ, Hirsch RP et al. Outcome in neonates with convulsions treated in an intensive care unit. *Ann Neurol* 1983; 14:642–647.
2. Mizrahi EM, Kellaway P. Characterization and classification of neonatal seizures. *Neurology* 1987; 37:1837–1844.

FURTHER READING

Gal P. Anticonvulsant therapy after neonatal seizures – How long should it be continued? I: A case for early discontinuation of anticonvulsants. *Pharmacotherapy* 1985; 5:268–273.
Hodson A. Anticonvulsant therapy after neonatal seizures – How long should it be continued? II: A case for long-term treatment with anticonvulsants. *Pharmacotherapy* 1985; 5:274–277.

Horton EJ, Snead OC. Diagnosis of neonatal seizures. *Semin Neurol* 1993; 13:48–52.

Snead OC, Horton EJ. Treatment of neonatal seizures. *Semin Neurol* 1993; 13:53–57.

Stafstrom CE. Neonatal seizures. *Pediatr Rev* 1995; 16:248–255.

Temple CM, Dennis J, Carney R et al. Neonatal seizures: long-term outcome and cognitive development among 'normal' survivors. *Dev Med Child Neurol* 1995; 37:109–118.

Van Orman CB, Darwish HZ. Efficacy of phenobarbital in neonatal seizures. *Can J Neurol Sci* 1985; 12:95–99.

Volpe JJ. Neonatal seizures: current concepts and revised classification. *Pediatrics* 1989; 84:422–428.

II. THE FLOPPY NEWBORN

Hypotonia is a common neurologic sign in the neonate. This sign is frequently an indicator of significant neurologic, neuromuscular, or systemic disease. Specific parts of the neurologic examination aid in the differential diagnosis of hypotonia in the newborn. Characteristics of muscle strength and muscle stretch reflexes rule out certain categories of disease prior to initiating a time-consuming, expensive and, at times, invasive evaluation.

A. CLINICAL SIGNS OF THE FLOPPY INFANT.

1. **Abnormal postures** (e.g. frog leg posture of lower extremities; jug-handle posture of upper extremities).
2. **Voluntary movements** are decreased.
3. **Hypotonia.**
4. **Joint mobility** is excessive.

B. DIFFERENTIAL DIAGNOSIS.

1. **CNS** (upper motor unit) disorders.
   a. Cerebral dysgenesis (e.g. holoprosencephaly, hydrocephalus, Down syndrome).
   b. CNS or systemic infection.
   c. hypoxic–ischemic encephalopathy.
   d. Inborn errors of metabolism, including disorders of amino acid and organic acid metabolism, Leigh's encephalopathy, and peroxisomal disorders (e.g. Zellweger disease).
   e. Congenital infection (TORCH).
   f. Neonatal sepsis or meningitis.
   g. Prader–Willi Syndrome.
2. **Neuromuscular disorders** (lower motor unit).
   a. Anterior horn cell disease (e.g. spinal muscular atrophy).
   b. Neuromuscular junction disorders (e.g. myasthenia gravis).
   c. Muscle disease (e.g. congenital myotonic dystrophy, other congenital myopathies).
3. **Disorders of connective tissue** (e.g. Marfan syndrome).

16

NEUROLOGIC DISORDERS OF THE NEWBORN

C. **EXAMINATION OF MUSCLE STRENGTH** and of muscle stretch
    reflexes aids in differentiating these categories.
1. **CNS disorders.**
a. Normal muscle strength.
b. Normal or increased reflexes.
2. **Neuromuscular disorders.**
a. Decreased muscle strength or paralysis.
b. Decreased or absent reflexes.
D. **LABORATORY AND IMAGING STUDIES.**
1. **CNS disorders.**
a. MR imaging of brain (if cerebral dysgenesis is suspected).
b. EEG (if motor activity suggestive of seizures is observed).
c. Serum glucose, calcium, electrolytes, metabolic screening, karyotype
    with fluorescent in-situ hybridization (FISH) analysis for Prader–Willi
    syndrome, very long chain fatty acid for peroxisomal disorders.
d. Lumbar puncture.
2. **Neuromuscular disorders.**
a. EMG and nerve conduction studies including repetitive stimulation.
    Tensilon test is not necessary.
b. Muscle biopsy.
c. Muscle enzymes (CK).
d. Acetylcholine receptor antibody determination.
e. Molecular studies of DNA for either myotonic dystrophy or spinal
    muscular atrophy.
E. **OTHER IMPORTANT CONSIDERATIONS.**
1. **Systemic sepsis** must always be considered.
2. **Family history** must be obtained, and a neurologic examination of the
    mother can be helpful in the diagnosis of neonatal myasthenia gravis
    and congenital myotonic dystrophy.
3. **Making a diagnosis** will allow the physician to discuss the prognosis of
    the affected infant as well as to provide genetic counseling to the
    parents.

FURTHER READING

Brooke MH. *A clinician's view of neuromuscular diseases,* 2nd edition.
Baltimore: Williams & Wilkins; 1986.
Dubowitz V. *The floppy infant,* 2nd edition. Philadelphia: Lippincott;
1980.

III. BRAIN INJURY IN THE PREMATURE NEWBORN

IVH occurs in about 20% of premature infants weighing <2000g. About
15% of infants with IVH have a coexistent intraparenchymal hemorrhagic
infarction. Periventricular leukomalacia (PVL) occurs in 25–40% of VLBW

infants. These white-matter infarcts are occasionally found in more mature neonates, including full-term newborns. Both IVH and PVL may result in significant cognitive disability and motor deficits (cerebral palsy).

A. INTRAVENTRICULAR HEMORRHAGE CLASSIFICATION AND PATHOLOGY.

1. **Ultrasound/CT scan classification.**
   a. Grade I – subependymal hemorrhage (35% of lesions).
   b. Grade II – IVH without significant ventricular dilatation (40% of lesions).
   c. Grade III – IVH with ventricular dilatation (25% of lesions).
   d. Coexistent IVH and periventricular hemorrhagic infarction (older literature refers to this combination of lesions as Grade IV).

2. **Neuropathologic aspects.**
   a. Primary lesion. Bleeding from small vessels in the highly vascularized subependymal germinal matrix, most often overlying the head of the caudate nucleus.
   b. Intraventricular extension. Rupture of the germinal matrix hemorrhage through the ependyma.
   c. Intraparenchymal hemorrhagic infarction. In 80% of cases, this lesion is a consequence of a large IVH, and is due to a venous infarction of the periventricular white matter.
   d. Hydrocephalus. Acute hydrocephalus may occur with large IVH, and results from decreased CSF absorption at the arachnoid villi. Delayed or slowly progressive hydrocephalus results from an obliterative arachnoiditis at posterior fossa foramina or by blood clot obstruction of the aqueduct.

B. DIAGNOSIS.

1. **Symptoms.** Up to 50% of cases of IVH may be clinically silent. In some cases of large hemorrhages, catastrophic symptoms including shock, acidosis, anemia, pallor, acute change in requirements for ventilatory assistance, apnea, and bradycardia may accompany a rapidly progressive encephalopathy. Neurologic features may include seizures, fixed pupils, absent oculovestibular reflexes, tonic posturing, or flaccidity.

2. **Onset of IVH.** About 50% will occur within the first day of life, whereas about 90% of hemorrhages will occur within the first 3 days of life.

3. **Imaging** via bedside cranial ultrasonography is the method of choice. CT scanning is generally not required, except when neurosurgical treatment of posthemorrhagic hydrocephalus is being considered.

4. **Cranial ultrasound.** We recommend that all premature infants<1500g have a cranial ultrasound study within the first week of life.

16

NEUROLOGIC DISORDERS OF THE NEWBORN

C. PREVENTION AND TREATMENT.

1. **Prevention of premature delivery,** and/or transport of mother to a perinatal center.
2. **Appropriate neonatal resuscitation measures.**
3. **Stabilization of arterial blood pressure** and of intravascular volume.
4. **Correction of coagulation disorders.**
5. **Pharmacologic prophylaxis** using various agents such as ethamsylate, phenobarbital, indomethacin, and Vitamin E are unproven.
6. **Acute management.** Maintain adequate cerebral perfusion.
a. Maintain normal blood pressure by volume replacement and/or inotropic agents.
b. In cases with extreme increases in intracerebral pressure, lumbar puncture or ventriculostomy may be necessary.
7. **Posthemorrhagic hydrocephalus.**
a. Follow with serial ultrasound evaluation. Ventriculomegaly will occur before there is an increase in head circumference.
b. Rapidly expanding hydrocephalus should be treated with repeated lumbar or ventricular taps (often from a surgically placed ventricular reservoir) until the CSF protein is low and the infant is large enough to have placement of a ventriculoperitoneal shunt.
c. Slowly developing ventricular dilatation may resolve spontaneously or may respond to the following:
    1) Daily lumbar puncture with removal of CSF until flow stops
    2) Drugs that decrease CSF formation (e.g. furosemide, acetazolamide)
    3) Osmotic agents (e.g. glycerol) are rarely used.

D. OUTCOME.

Outcome relates to the severity of the hemorrhage and the success in stabilizing the infant's condition and maintaining cerebral perfusion following IVH. Significant neurologic morbidity (cerebral palsy, intellectual deficits) is primarily related to the amount of brain parenchymal destruction.
a. There is a 5–15% risk of major neurologic sequelae from subependymal hemorrhage or a small to moderate IVH.
b. In severe IVH, the mortality rate is about 20%, and more than 50% of survivors develop progressive ventricular dilatation.
c. Moderate to severe neurologic deficits are largely confined to infants with severe IVH. Infants who have developed IVH with intraparenchymal hemorrhagic infarction have up to an 80% mortality rate, with motor and cognitive defects occurring in >80% of the survivors.

E. PERIVENTRICULAR LEUKOMALACIA.

1. **Neuropathologic aspects.**
a. Bilateral symmetric infarctions of periventricular white matter.
b. <25% of lesions are hemorrhagic.
c. Over time, the lesions may enlarge and become cystic.

d. A variety of vascular processes may result in decreased blood flow to the periventricular white matter. In the premature newborn, this metabolically active region is at increased risk of ischemic injury.

2. **Diagnosis.**

a. Symptoms specific to PVL are uncommon during the neonatal period. Subtle weakness of the legs has been described in some affected infants.

b. Imaging of PVL lesions can be accomplished with either portable cranial ultrasonography, CT scanning, or MRI. These lesions are usually first detected by a routine bedside cranial ultrasound study as periventricular echodensities. The evolution of these lesions may be followed by serial ultrasound examinations. In certain instances, these echodensities may not represent true neuropathologic lesions and CT scanning or MR imaging may be helpful in confirming brain injury.

3. **Prevention of PVL** may be facilitated by close control of blood pressure so that systemic hypotension may be avoided. However, many cases of PVL may be due to only slight disturbances of systemic circulation, which may not be preventable.

4. **Outcome of PVL** is related, in part, to the size of the lesions. Significant motor and intellectual defects are more likely in patients with periventricular cystic changes and ventricular enlargement. There is a strong neuropathologic clinical correlation between the spastic diplegia form of cerebral palsy and PVL lesions.

FURTHER READING

Dubowitz LMS, Bydder GM, Muschin J. Developmental sequence of periventricular leukomalacia. *Arch Dis Child* 1985; 60:349–358.

Gilles FH, Leviton A, Dooling EC. *The developing human brain: growth and epidemiologic neuropathology.* Boston: Wright; 1983.

Shankaran S, Koepke T, Woldt E et al. Outcome after posthemorrhagic ventriculomegaly in comparison with mild hemorrhage without ventriculomegaly. *J Pediatr* 1989; 114:109–114.

Volpe JJ. Brain injury in the premature infant – current concepts of pathogenesis and prevention. *Biol Neonate* 1992; 62:231–242.

Volpe JJ. *Neurology of the newborn,* 3rd edition. Philadelphia: Saunders; 1995.

IV. HYPOXIC–ISCHEMIC ENCEPHALOPATHY

In the newborn, decreased blood oxygen tension (hypoxia) and decreased blood flow (ischemia) may result in a significant compromise of brain function together with chronic neurologic and developmental disability. Severe HIE should be considered as a component of a systemic disease triggered by asphyxia. Acute, severe HIE is always accompanied by a metabolic acidosis, usually with a base deficit >15–20mEq/L. hypoxic–ischemic renal, cardiac, and/or GI disease should also be apparent.

16

NEUROLOGIC DISORDERS OF THE NEWBORN

A. CLINICAL SPECTRUM.
1. Mild.
a. Irritability.
b. Jitteriness.
c. Hyperalertness.
d. Tachycardia.
2. Moderate.
a. Poor suck, swallow, abnormal cry.
b. Lethargy, poor responsiveness.
c. Hypotonia, decreased Moro reflex.
3. Severe.
a. Profound hypotonia.
b. Recurrent apnea.
c. Loss of brain-stem function (pupil responses, eye movements, gag).
d. Increased intracranial pressure due to brain swelling at 24–72 hours.
4. Seizures due to HIE usually begin at 12–24 hours. These neonatal seizures may be due to either:
a. Epileptic pathophysiology ('electroclinical seizures' – EEG discharges correlate with clinical events).
b. Nonepileptic mechanism (clinical seizures which do not correlate with the EEG).

B. DIAGNOSTIC TESTS.
1. **EEG** is an important method of assessing neurologic function. Sequential changes in the EEG may parallel the clinical encephalopathy. The development of electrographic seizures without clinical signs (electroclinical dissociation), and of a periodic EEG pattern (burst suppression), both signify a poor prognosis.
2. **Imaging studies** are of limited benefit during the acute phase of HIE. Hemorrhagic lesions may be detected by bedside cranial ultrasound, although subarachnoid and subdural hemorrhages can be missed. These lesions, as well as significant brain edema, may be demonstrated by CT scanning or MR imaging. Several days to weeks after the onset of HIE, evidence of focal and diffuse brain injury may be detected by either CT scanning or MR imaging.

C. TREATMENT.
1. **Prevention.** Fetal monitoring and scalp blood pH assessment may not prevent birth asphyxia.
2. **Maintain adequate ventilation,** oxygenation, perfusion pressure, and blood glucose.
3. **Control of epileptic seizures.**
4. **Control of brain edema.**
a. Role of brain swelling in producing brain injury is controversial.
b. Manage carefully to prevent fluid overload and recognize inappropriate ADH secretion.

c. Hyperventilation is not indicated.
d. Maintain normal to slight elevated serum sodium to decrease cellular edema.
e. Steroids are not indicated.
f. Several pharmacologic therapies are under study (calcium channel blockers, free radical scavengers, glutamate receptor antagonists).
g. Mild systemic and local cerebral hypothermia are under study.

D. OUTCOME
1. **Asphyxiated newborns** without encephalopathy do not appear to be at risk for development of long-term neurologic disabilities.
2. **Mild HIE.** Neurologic sequelae are rare.
3. **Moderate HIE.** 21% of survivors with motor or cognitive disturbances.
4. **Severe HIE.** 100% of survivors with motor or cognitive disturbances.
5. **Presence of neonatal seizures** increases the risk of sequelae.
6. **Neonatal neurologic signs** (e.g. hypotonia, poor suck) continuing after 1–2 weeks increases the risk of sequelae.
7. **Prematurity** affects the outcome. Mortality in asphyxiated premature neonates is approximately 30%, and about 10% in asphyxiated full-term newborns. The risk of neurologic sequelae in survivors is 30% in the premature group, and 20% in the full-term group.

FURTHER READING
Amiel-Tison C, Ellison, P. Birth asphyxia in the fullterm newborn: early assessment and outcome. *Dev Med Child Neurol* 1986; 28:671–682.
Low JA, Galbraith RS, Muir DW et al. The relationship between perinatal hypoxia and newborn encephalopathy. *Am J Obstet Gynecol* 1985; 152:256–260.
MacDonald HM, Mulligan JC, Allen AC et al. Neonatal asphyxia, I: Relationship of obstetric and neonatal complications to neonatal mortality in 34,405 consecutive deliveries. *J Pediatr* 1980; 96:898–902.
Mulligan JC, Painter MJ, O'Donoghue PA et al. Neonatal asphyxia, II: Neonatal mortality and long-term sequelae. *J Pediatr* 1980; 96:903–907.
Robertson C, Finer NN. Term infants with hypoxic–ischemic encephalopathy: outcome at 3.5 years. *Dev Med Child Neurol* 1985; 27:473–484.
Volpe JJ. *Neurology of the newborn*, 3rd edition. Philadelphia: Saunders; 1995.

V. INJURIES TO THE PERIPHERAL NERVOUS SYSTEM
A. BRACHIAL PLEXUS INJURY.
1. **Incidence** is 0.5–2 per 1000 live births; rarely seen in premature newborn.

16

NEUROLOGIC DISORDERS OF THE NEWBORN

2. **Pathology lesions** are usually at the nerve roots and not in the brachial plexus. Mild injury is associated with nerve root sheath edema and hemorrhage, whereas severe lesions are associated with nerve root avulsion and cord injury. The upper roots of the plexus (C5–C7) are most vulnerable to injury. Traumatic orthopedic lesions of the clavicle, shoulder, and humerus are present in about 10% of cases.

3. **Etiology.** Stretching of the brachial plexus roots due to traction on shoulder or neck during delivery; abnormal presentation, large fetal size, and fetal depression are associated with brachial plexus injury.

4. **Clinical features.**

a. Erb's palsy (C5–C7 involvement): weakness of shoulder abduction and external rotation; elbow flexion and supination; wrist and finger extension. Characteristic 'waiter's tip' posture and asymmetric Moro reflex are present. Diaphragmatic paralysis is occasionally present.

b. Total plexus palsy (C5-T1 involvement): weakness of above muscle groups as well as of intrinsic hand muscles. The grasp reflex is absent, and Horner syndrome may be present.

5. **Prognosis.** Good if onset of recovery is noted by 2 weeks of age. 92% are normal at 12 months of age. Recovery of total plexus palsy is less favorable.

6. **Management.**

a. Obstetrical prevention of traction injury.

b. Physical therapy.
   1) Support affected limb for first week of life.
   2) Passive range of motion exercises to prevent contractures should begin after a few days of life.

c. Neurosurgical exploration of the brachial plexus may be helpful in selected cases where no appreciable recovery has developed by 3 months of age.

B. FACIAL PARALYSIS.

1. **Incidence** was as high as 0.75% of term births when forceps use was more common. Facial paralysis is the most common neurologic feature of perinatal trauma.

2. **Lesion.** Usually at the point of exit of the facial nerve from the stylomastoid foramen.

3. **Etiology.** Intrauterine pressure on facial nerve by the maternal sacral promontory. Compression by forceps blade must also be considered in difficult forceps deliveries.

4. **Clinical features.**

a. Unilateral weakness of upper and lower facial muscles.

b. At rest there is a flattened nasolabial fold and widened palpebral fissure.

c. When active, the infant cannot completely close eye, wrinkle brow, or grimace on the affected side.

d. Condition must be differentiated from:
    1) 'Asymmetric crying facies' syndrome (cardiofacial syndrome) where
        there is congenital unilateral hypoplasia of the depressor anguli
        oris muscle
    2) Upper motor neuron (central) lesions causing unilateral weakness
        of lower face and ipsilateral hemiparesis
    3) Syndromes causing bilateral facial weakness (Mobius syndrome,
        congenital myotonic dystrophy, congenital myasthenia gravis).
5. **Prognosis** is excellent. Complete recovery is expected in most infants
    by 1–3 weeks.
6. **Management.** Prevention of corneal injury with artificial tears and eye
    patching.

FURTHER READING

Gordon M, Rich H, Deutschberger J et al. The immediate and long-term
    outcome of obstetric birth trauma, I: Brachial plexus paralysis. *Am J
    Obstet Gynecol* 1973; 117:51–56.
Hepner WR. Some observations on facial paresis in the newborn infant:
    etiology and incidence. *Pediatrics* 1951; 8:494–497.
Pape KE, Pickering D. Asymmetric crying facies: an index of other
    congenital anomalies. *J Pediatr* 1972; 81:21–30.

16

NEUROLOGIC DISORDERS OF THE NEWBORN

DRUG ABSTINENCE SYNDROME

17

The frequency of neonatal drug withdrawal syndromes relates primarily to the use of heroin and methadone by pregnant women. However, use of potent forms of cocaine (crack) and amphetamines may play a role. Currently, an estimated 15–20% of all newborns have been exposed to illicit drugs prior to birth. Tragically, intravenous drug use has now been further complicated with the risk of HIV as well as hepatitis for both mother and fetus. Sexually transmitted diseases also occur with increased frequency in this group of patients.

I. SCREENING

Testing the urine of all pregnant women for illicit substances is practiced on admission in some hospitals with high-risk populations.

II. PRESENTATION

Irritability, tremors, high-pitched cry, and temperature instability begin in the first few days of life. Poor feeding, emesis, and diarrhea may also be seen. Respiratory distress and seizures may occasionally be seen. There is a high incidence of IUGR in infants exposed to heroin, cocaine, or amphetamines. Cocaine has been associated with placental abruption, prematurity, and perinatal stroke. Specific side effects of different drugs are becoming more accurately described, and eventually may be helpful diagnostically.

III. DIAGNOSIS

1. **Physical examination** is often normal but may reveal increased muscle tone, fever, tachypnea, and excoriations on knees and elbows as well as IUGR and mild microcephaly.
2. **Maternal history** of, or findings of, substance abuse. Check maternal HIV status (can be done on cord blood) and tests for sexually transmitted diseases, hepatitis B, and tuberculosis.
3. **Urine toxicology.** Urine from the suspect newborns and their mothers should be tested for illicit substances. Some hospitals can also test meconium. However, their absence does not mean that the infant is not suffering from drug effects or drug withdrawal.
4. **Rule out** other causes of CNS irritability.

IV. SUBSTANCES
A. **OPIATES** (heroin, codeine, morphine, methadone).
B. **COCAINE AND AMPHETAMINES.**
C. **BARBITURATES.**
D. **ETHANOL.**
E. **TRANQUILIZERS.**

V. MANAGEMENT
A. **SUPPORTIVE** – effective for the majority of infants.
1. **Quiet, darkened environment.**
2. **Swaddling, decreased handling.**
3. **Frequent, small oral feeds.**
4. **HBIG** within 12 hours of birth if maternal hepatitis B surface antigen status is not known to be negative within 6 weeks of delivery. If positive, Hepatavax should also be given and follow-up appointments made at discharge for a subsequent two immunizations. If mother is negative, consider Heptavax for her also.
5. **Instruction of mother** or caregiver in supportive techniques prior to discharge.
B. **PHARMACOLOGIC.** Use objective measure to monitor response to treatment and weaning (e.g. Neonatal Abstinence Score). The effectiveness and long-term side effects of pharmacologic treatment for withdrawal are not known.
1. **Diazepam,** 0.3–0.5mg/kg i.m., p.o., or i.v. q8–12h.
2. **Paregoric,** 1–4 drops p.o. q6h.
3. **Morphine,** 0.1–0.2mg/kg i.m., p.o., or i.v. q4–6h
4. **Methadone,** 0.1–0.5mg/kg/day p.o. divided q8–12h.
5. **Phenobarbital,** 4–6mg/kg/day divided q12h (i.m. or p.o.).
6. **Wean doses** over 1–2 weeks.
C. **DISCHARGE PLANNING.**
a. Be cautious of discharging infants while still on medication; do not discharge on medication to substance-abusing parents.
b. Observe for recurrence of symptoms (may be delayed 4–6 weeks).
c. Frequent home visits by Public Health Nurse and/or Social Service.
d. Care by relatives of mother.
e. Foster home placement.
f. Instruct mother or caregiver in supportive techniques prior to discharge.
g. Discourage breast-feeding; contraindicated in mothers using cocaine or who are HIV+.
h. Assure adequate medical and developmental follow-up.

VI. OUTCOME
A. **GROWTH FAILURE,** microcephaly, developmental delay, hyperactivity, and learning disability may occur.

B. INCREASED RISK for child abuse, sudden infant death syndrome (SIDS), AIDS, hepatitis B, syphilis, and gonorrhea.

FURTHER READING

D'Apolito KC, McRorie TI. Pharmacologic management of neonatal abstinence syndrome. *J Perinat Newborn Nurs* 1996; 9(4):70–80.

Forest CF. The cocaine-exposed infant, part 2: Intervention and teaching. *J Pediatr Health Care* 1994; 8(1):7–11.

Kandall SR. Treatment options for drug-exposed infants. *NIDA Res Monogr* 1995; 149:78–99.

RENAL DISORDERS

I. ACUTE RENAL FAILURE IN NEONATES

A. NORMAL VALUES.

Normal values for renal function change with gestational and postnatal age (Table 18.1).

TABLE 18.1

NORMAL RENAL FUNCTION IN THE NEONATE

	Premature (<32 weeks)	Full-term	2 weeks	2 months
Glomerular filtration rate (mL/min/1.73m)	10±2	20±5	40±10	70±10
Renal blood flow (ml/min)	50±10	85±15	140±20	240±30
Maximum concentrating ability (mOsm/L)	>600	>800	>1000	>1200
Excreted fraction of filtered sodium (%)	3–8	<1	<1	<1

B. DEFINITION/DIAGNOSIS.

1. **Oliguria.**
   a. Urinary output <1mL/kg/h.
   b. Catheterize for confirmation and monitoring.
   c. Assess the state of hydration. If patient is not clinically overhydrated, give isotonic saline, 20mL/kg. If there is still no response, the patient is normovolemic and normotensive, and obstruction has been ruled out, treat the patient as having intrinsic renal failure.
2. **Urine characteristics** of renal vs prerenal failure are illustrated in Table 18.2.
3. **Elevated BUN** (>15mg/dL) or elevated serum creatinine levels (>0.7mg/dL; not applicable during the first week of life), or a delayed postpartum decline in the serum creatinine value suggest renal disease. Serum creatinine should be measured using an enzymatic method (creatinine concentrations measured using the Jaffe reaction are falsely elevated by cephalosporins, ketones, etc.).

TABLE 18.2.

RENAL VERSUS PRERENAL FAILURE IN NEWBORNS

	Prerenal	Renal
Urine osmolality (mOsm/kg of H_2O)	>400	<400
Fractional excretion of sodium ($[^U Na \times {}^S Cr]/[^S Na \times {}^U Cr] \times 100$)	<3%[a]	>3%[a]

$^U Na$, urine sodium concentration; $^S Cr$, serum creatinine concentration; $^U Cr$, urine creatinine concentration; $^S Na$, serum sodium concentration.

[a]In infants >32 weeks of gestation (not valid following the use of a diuretic).

4. **Exclude obstruction** based on clinical evaluation and, where necessary, perform abdominal ultrasound, renal scintigraphy, or i.v. pyelography.

C. ETIOLOGY OF ACUTE RENAL FAILURE.

1. **Prerenal causes** include asphyxia, dehydration, CHF, or hypotension that may occur secondary to septic or cardiogenic shock, hemorrhage, or cardiac surgery. Indomethacin may cause decreased renal blood flow.

2. **Renal causes** include congenital abnormalities (cystic dysplasia, hypoplasia, agenesis, or polycystic kidneys), inflammatory or vascular disorders (cortical necrosis, bilateral venous or arterial thrombosis or emboli, or DIC), and ATN (secondary to perinatal asphyxia, dehydration, shock, or nephrotoxins, such as aminoglycosides or indomethacin).

3. **Postrenal causes** include neurogenic bladder as well as obstruction that may occur secondary to posterior urethral valves, imperforate prepuce, urethral stricture or diverticulum, ureteropelvic or ureterovesical junction obstruction bilaterally, or extrinsic tumors compressing bladder outlet.

D. MANAGEMENT.

1. **Treat reversible or treatable cause** of acute renal failure.

a. Bladder outlet obstruction – relief of the obstruction with a catheter usually results in obligate water and electrolyte losses that require close monitoring and replacement.

b. Treat infection, reverse dehydration, and stop nephrotoxins if possible.

2. **Replace insensible water loss** as free water (full-term, 30mL/kg; premature, 50–80mL/kg) plus urinary output. Any deficit or ongoing losses such as nasogastric drainage or diarrhea should be replaced. Avoid overhydration, weigh infant 2 or 3 times daily and adjust fluid administration to maintain infant's weight.

3. **Sodium or potassium** should not be provided except to replace deficit or ongoing losses. Potassium repletion should be done carefully to avoid hyperkalemia. Hyponatremia is usually due to volume overload, not to sodium depletion; an exception is postobstructive diuresis.

4. **Hyperkalemia** may be treated with the following (use electrocardiographic monitoring).

a. Temporary measures:
   1) 10% calcium gluconate, 0.5–1.0mL/kg given slowly i.v.; monitor ECG
   2) Sodium bicarbonate, 2mEq/kg, i.v.
   3) Glucose, 0.5–1.0g/kg; insulin, i.v., one-quarter unit per gram of infused glucose; monitor blood sugar.

b. Potassium removal:
   1) Sodium polystyrene sulfonate, 1g/kg given orally or as a retention enema
   2) Furosemide if indicated
   3) Resistant hyperkalemia or acidosis should be treated with dialysis.

5. **Significant acidosis** should be corrected with sodium bicarbonate therapy to maintain a pH >7.3 (use caution if hypercarbic or hypocalcemic).

6. **Hyperphosphatemia** should be corrected with calcium carbonate ($1–2cm^3$/kg q8h if not hypercalcemic), and a low-phosphate formula (PM 60/40® or SMA®) should be used.

7. **Asymptomatic hypocalcemia** due to hyperphosphatemia should not be corrected until the serum phosphorus level is normalized, since a normal serum calcium level in the presence of hyperphosphatemia can lead to serious metastatic calcification. If the patient is clinically symptomatic, correct slowly with 10% calcium gluconate, 0.5–1.0mL/kg i.v. until symptoms disappear.

8. **Protein** may be restricted to 1.5–2.0g/kg/day.

9. **A high caloric intake,** using Polycose®, Controlyte® or medium-chain triglycerides, should be encouraged to minimize protein catabolism and generation of phosphate, sulfate, and urea.

10. **Monitor weight,** electrolyte level, intake, output, and vital signs frequently, and tabulate on flow sheets.

11. **Modify dosage of drugs** excreted by the kidneys (e.g. aminoglycosides).

12. **Hypertension** may be secondary to fluid overload (decrease fluid administration) or require therapy with propranolol or hydralazine.

II. HEMATURIA
A. CAUSES OF HEMATURIA.
1. Perinatal asphyxia.
2. Hemorrhagic disease.
3. Congenital malformations.
4. Urinary tract infection.
5. Obstructive uropathy.
6. Neoplasm.

18

RENAL DISORDERS

7. Cortical and medullary necrosis.
8. Glomerulonephritis (rare).
9. Renal vein thrombosis.
10. Hyperosmolar infusions.
11. Renal artery thrombosis.
12. Nephrocalcinosis.
13. Trauma.
14. Acute tubular necrosis.

B. EVALUATION.

1. History of predisposing factors.
a. Perinatal asphyxia: cortical or medullary necrosis.
b. Umbilical artery catheter: renal artery thrombosis with hypertension.
c. Maternal diabetes: renal vein thrombosis.
d. Furosemide usage: nephrocalcinosis.
e. Abnormal urinary stream.
2. **Abdominal mass** – renal vein thrombosis, obstructive uropathy, congenital malformation, or a renal neoplasm.
3. **Urinalysis.**
a. RBC casts suggestive of glomerulonephritis.
b. WBCs and bacteriuria suggestive of UTI (with or without urinary tract malformations). UTI should be confirmed by urine culture.
c. Crystals suggest a renal calculus: e.g. urate or calcium nephropathy.
d. Evidence of prolonged bleeding may suggest a bleeding diathesis.
e. Studies may include the following:
   1) Urine calcium/creatinine ratio
   2) Suprapubic tap for urine culture
   3) Clotting studies if bleeding diathesis is suspected
   4) Abdominal ultrasound if mass is felt or hypertensive, UTI, hematuria is persistent or nephrocalcinosis is suspected
   5) Intravenous pyelography
   6) Voiding cystourethrography
   7) Iodohippurate sodium ^{123}I or TC-diethylene triamine penta-acetic acid renal scan
   8) Renal angiography
   9) Electrolytes, calcium, phosphorus, creatinine.

III. NEONATAL HYPERTENSION

A. DEFINITION.
See Table 18.3.

1. **Vascular causes.** Renal artery thrombosis, coarctation of the aorta, renal artery stenosis, and hypoplastic aorta.
2. **Renal causes.** Renal dysplasia, renal hypoplasia, obstructive uropathy, infantile polycystic disease, renal insufficiency, renal tumors, and nephrocalcinosis.

TABLE 18.3

DEFINITION OF NEONATAL HYPERTENSION

	Newborn		4–6 weeks of age	
	Premature	Full-term	Pre-term	Term
Systolic BP (mmHg)	>80	>90	>110	>115
Diastolic BP (mmHg)	>50	>60		
Mean BP (mmHg)	>60	>70	>75	>85

3. **Other causes.** Increased intracranial pressure, fluid and electrolyte overload, ocular phenylephrine, neural crest tumor, adrenogenital syndrome, Cushing's disease (including iatrogenic), compression from closure of an abdominal wall defect, seizure, theophylline, and pneumothorax.

B. **SIGNS AND SYMPTOMS.**

1. **Cardiorespiratory.** Tachypnea, cyanosis, cardiomegaly.
2. **Neurological.** Lethargy, tremors, seizures, hemiparesis, hypertonicity, and floppiness.
3. **Other.** Nephromegaly, peripheral vascular occlusions.
4. **Asymptomatic.**

C. **EVALUATION.**

1. **Baseline diagnostic blood pressures.**
a. Four extremities.
b. Abdominal ultrasound with Doppler flow study of major vessels.
c. Urinalysis.
2. **Additional considerations.**
a. Rule out coarctation, corticosteroids, or sympathomimetic drugs, increased intracranial pressure, or fluid and electrolyte overload.
b. 24-hour urinary catecholamine, 17-hydroxysteroid, and 17-ketosteroid levels.
c. If renal artery thrombosis is suspected and a UAC is present, abdominal aortography or selective renal angiography should be done.
d. If the UAC has been withdrawn, ^{123}I or ^{131}I iodohippurate sodium renal scan, preferably with computer processing, is indicated; angiography should be done if the result of the scan is nondiagnostic.

D. **MANAGEMENT.**

1. **Correct the underlying condition** if possible (e.g. genitourinary tract obstruction, drugs, fluid overload).
2. **Treat mild hypertension** with diuretics (avoid furosemide if nephrocalcinosis is present).
3. **Severe hypertension.**
a. Diuretics.
b. Hydralazine, beginning with 1mg/kg/day and increasing the dosage up to 8mg/kg/day.

18

RENAL DISORDERS

c.   If the response is still inadequate, add captopril, beginning at
0.05mg/kg/dose and increasing gradually to 1.5mg/kg/dose q6–8h.
Captopril is contraindicated with bilateral renal artery stenosis (or
unilateral arterial stenosis in a solitary kidney), and serum creatinine
should be monitored, since severe hypotension has been reported with
captopril usage (Table 18.4).

4. **Life-threatening hypertension** may be treated with diazoxide,
3–5mg/kg/dose (which may cause severe hyperglycemia) or
nitroprusside, 1.0–5.0mcg/kg/min (with close monitoring of blood
pressure). Blood pressure should be brought down gradually, not
precipitously.

5. **Consider nephrectomy** (or partial nephrectomy) if hypertension is
caused by renal artery thrombosis and is not responding to maximal
drug therapy.

E.   **PROGNOSIS.**
1. **Initial response** to therapy is usually good.
2. **Long-term outcome** usually depends on etiology.
a.   Has improved with aggressive medical management.
b.   Re-emergence of hypertension and renal dysfunction may occur.

TABLE 18.4

AGENTS USED IN THE MANAGEMENT OF NEONATAL HYPERTENSION

Agent	Dosage range
Chlorothiazide	20–50mg/kg/24h, orally
Furosemide	1–4mg/kg/24h, i.v., orally
Hydralazine	1–8mg/kg/24h, i.v., orally
Diazoxide	3–5mg/kg/dose, i.v.
Propranolol	0.5–3.0mg/kg/24h, orally
Nitroprusside	1.0–5mcg/kg/min, i.v.
Captopril	0.05–1.5mg/kg/dose

GASTROINTESTINAL DISORDERS

I. DIARRHEA AND MALABSORPTION

Watery diarrhea indicates an osmotic, secretory, or motility disorder. Steatorrhea (fat-containing stools) may be quite variable in appearance, from loose to foul-smelling, bulky, and oily stools.

A. DIAGNOSTIC TESTS.

1. **Examine stools** for appearance and estimate their weight separate from urine.
2. **Test for blood** using the Hemoccult™ slide method.
3. **Test for white blood cells** in stool. Smear the mucousy part of the stool on a slide, and stain it with methylene blue or Wright's stain.
4. **Carbohydrate malabsorption evaluation.**
   a. Measure the pH of a fresh stool with Nitrazine™ paper (pH 4.5–7.5). If malabsorbed carbohydrates enter the colon, bacterial fermentation will lower the stool pH to <6.0. Immediate testing is necessary because bacterial breakdown of the stool continues at room temperature and the pH will quickly decrease.
   b. Test the stool for the presence of reducing substances (lactose, glucose, fructose, galactose):
      1) Mix one part stool with two parts water.
      2) Centrifuge if turbid.
      3) Transfer 15 drops of supernatant to a test tube.
      4) Add a Clinitest™ tablet to the tube and read the color change after the reaction is complete, using the Clinitest™ urine color chart.
      5) Sucrose is a nonreducing sugar. If its presence is possible, the stool must be hydrolyzed by boiling with 1N HCl prior to using the Clinitest™ method.
5. **Fat malabsorption evaluation.**
   a. Stain a stool smear with Sudan red and examine for microscopic globules of neutral fat. Fatty acids will not stain but may be apparent as refractile crystals seen under polarized light.

b. Quantitative fat determination is performed by collecting all stools in a 48 or 72 hour period, marked at the beginning and end by a colored nonabsorbable marker such as charcoal. The infant must be on at least 4g/kg/day of fat and the intake recorded. The coefficient of fat absorption is calculated by:

(g dietary fat/day − g fecal fat/day)/g dietary fat/day

If <85%, significant fat malabsorption exists.

B. INTERPRETATION OF SCREENING TESTS AND SUGGESTED FURTHER WORKUP.

1. **Mucosal injury.** A positive test for blood suggests mucosal injury. Perform a stool culture. Consider abdominal radiograph series and proctoscopy.

2. **Colitis.** The presence of white blood cells suggests colitis. Perform a stool culture and *Clostridia difficile* toxin assay. Confirm the presence of colitis with a proctosigmoidoscopy and consider a trial of protein hydrolysate-containing formula. If Hirschsprung's induced colitis is a possibility, then rectal manometry, rectal biopsy, and, when stable, a contrast enema should be obtained.

3. **Carbohydrate malabsorption.** If pH and Clinitest™ suggest carbohydrate malabsorption in a symptomatic infant, then test for Rotazyme™. When feedings are reintroduced, change to a protein hydrolysate formula, and advance the concentration as long as the stool Clinitest™ is <0.75%.

4. **Breath hydrogen.** If carbohydrate malabsorption occurs without other symptoms, then test the absorption of the individual sugars by a breath hydrogen analysis. When sugars are fermented by bacteria, hydrogen is produced and enters the blood stream where it is carried to the lungs and exhaled.

a. Give the infant nil per oram (NPO) for 4–6 hours.

b. Give the infant 2g/kg oral bolus of a 10% solution of the suspect sugar.

c. Expired air is collected by face mask into a syringe in 25mL aliquots prior to the sugar solution and at 15 or 30 minute intervals thereafter for 2–3 hours.

d. The hydrogen concentration is determined by measurement in gas chromatography. If an early peak of hydrogen is detected, then bacterial overgrowth is suspected and may be due to motility problems, a blind pouch, or partial obstruction. A later peak indicates colonic fermentation of the sugar and requires the substitution of another sugar into the diet.

5. **Fat malabsorption** may require further evaluation:

a. Sweat chloride test using pilocarpine ionophoresis to evaluate for cystic fibrosis.

b. Stool trypsin quantitation and Chymex™ test to screen for pancreatic insufficiency.

c. Liver function tests and serum bile acids to detect cholestasis.

d. Small bowel biopsy and xylose absorption test to evaluate for villus atrophy.

C. SELECTED TREATMENT PER DIAGNOSIS.

1. **Elimination diet.**

a. For cows' milk protein intolerance, substitute breast milk or a protein hydrolysate-based formula.

b. For isolated lactose intolerance, substitute a soy-based formula. Supplement premature infants with calcium and phosphorus.

c. For pancreatic insufficiency, feed Pregestimil™ and give pancreatic enzymes orally.

d. For cholestasis or bile salt deficiency, medium-chain tryglyceride (MCT) oil or Portagen™ formula should be utilized.

e. If all carbohydrates are malabsorbed or there is significant secretory diarrhea, then TPN should be initiated.

2. **Bacterial overgrowth** should be evaluated to detect any underlying anatomical reason and then treated with metronidazole.

3. **Hirschsprung's disease.** If diagnosed, a diverting colostomy or ileostomy is performed.

II. GASTROINTESTINAL TRACT BLEEDING

GI tract bleeding in the neonate may occasionally be severe, and treatment should be initiated promptly. The bleeding site should be identified if possible. With current diagnostic techniques, 90% of bleeding sites can be identified (50% anus, rectum, colon; 30% small intestine; 10% above ligament of Treitz).

A. ETIOLOGY.

1. **Stomach and esophagus.**

a. Stress (antrum most common).

b. Drugs (steroids, indomethacin, salicylates, caffeine, tolazoline).

c. Esophagitis (reflux, nasogastric tubes).

d. Coagulopathy.

e. Other (duplication cysts, Mallory–Weiss tear, AV malformation, hemangioma, milk bezoar).

2. **Small bowel** – NEC, intussusception, volvulus.

3. **Anus, rectum, and colon.**

a. Colitis (infection, cows' milk or soy protein allergy, Hirschsprung's disease).

b. Anal fissure.

19

GASTROINTESTINAL DISORDERS

B. DIAGNOSTIC TESTS.

1. **Physical examination.**

a. Hypotension, tachycardia, or both suggest at least 20% of blood volume lost.

b. Bruising or bleeding from other sites suggests coagulopathy.

c. Hepatosplenomegaly and jaundice suggest coagulopathy secondary to liver disease.

d. Abdominal distention and mass suggest duplication cyst, intussusception, or midgut volvulus.

e. Hemangioma or AV malformations on skin suggest similar lesions in GI tract.

2. **Aspiration** of gastric secretion may demonstrate upper GI tract bleeding site. No blood in the gastric aspirate indicates that bleeding has ceased or that it is beyond the pylorus.

3. **Laboratory tests.** Stool guaiac, KUB, PT, PTT, platelet count, hematocrit reading, hemoglobin values.

4. **Other diagnostic studies.**

a. Proctosigmoidoscopy will identify most lower GI bleeding sites such as colitis or anal fissures. Rectal biopsy will show colitis when it may not be apparent on proctosigmoidoscopy and will rule out Hirschsprung's disease.

b. Upper endoscopy and colonoscopy can now be performed on neonates with pediatric fiber-optic flexible scopes. More than 90% of bleeding sites can be identified with these instruments.

c. Barium enema is the diagnostic test when KUB result suggests obstruction, Hirschsprung's disease, or intussusception. Intussusception in a neonate is often associated with anatomic malformation such as duplication cyst.

d. If bleeding is massive then angiography or technetium-99m scan should be performed to identify sites. Angiography is better when the bleeding is >0.5mL/min, while the latter is more sensitive at <0.1mL/min (but less specific).

C. TREATMENT.

1. **Monitor BP and CVP.**

2. **Replace blood losses.**

3. **Correct coagulopathy** with fresh-frozen plasma, vitamin K, or platelet packs.

4. **Discontinue inappropriate drugs.**

5. **Lavage blood** from stomach with saline at room temperature.

6. **Antacids and H_2 blockers.**

7. **Antibiotics** (see Chapter 27, NEC).

8. **Surgical intervention** should be immediate for obstructive lesions such as midgut volvulus, intussusception, toxic megacolon due to Hirschsprung's disease, and for Meckel's diverticulum. If bleeding continues with blood loss >85mL/kg/24h, surgical exploration for control of bleeding is advised.

FURTHER READING

Cox KL, Ament MG. Upper gastrointestinal bleeding in children and adolescents. *Pediatrics* 1979; 63:408–413.

Sherman NJ, Clatsworthy HW Jr. Gastrointestinal bleeding in neonates: a study of 94 cases. *Surgery* 1967; 62:614.

19

GASTROINTESTINAL DISORDERS

HEMATOLOGIC PROBLEMS

I. HEMOSTATIC DISORDERS

A. NORMAL VALUES.

Normal values for routine coagulation tests are considerably different at different gestational ages and postnatal ages (Table 20.1).

TABLE 20.1

NORMAL VALUES FOR ROUTINE COAGULATION TESTS FOR TERM AND PRETERM INFANTS

Age	aPTT (s)	PT (s)	TT (s)
Child	30–40	10–12	10–15
Full-term			
(cord)	70	12–17	10–20
(48h)	60	12–20	10–16
Preterm (31 weeks)			
(cord)	105	15–22	15–20
(48h)	75	15–22	15–20

Platelet count range for all ages is 150,000–300,000/mm^3.
Clottable fibrinogen level for all ages is 150–350mg/dL.
aPTT, activated partial thromboplastin time.

B. DIAGNOSIS.

The diagnostic approach to any hemostatic problem is summarized as follows.

1. **Initially obtain:**
a. Platelet count.
b. Activated PTT (aPTT).
c. PT.
d. TT.
e. Clottable fibrinogen (Ic).
2. **If panel 'A' is abnormal,** characterize the pattern of abnormality: e.g. decreased platelet count with normal aPTT, PT, TT, Ic, or normal platelet count with prolonged aPTT, normal PT, TT Ic, etc. (Table 20.2). Order assays to delineate defect.

TABLE 20.2

PATTERNS OF LABORATORY SCREENING TESTS

	A	B	C	D	E
Platelet count	low	nl	nl	nl	nl
aPTT	nl	prolonged	nl/prolonged	prolonged	nl
PT	nl	nl	prolonged	prolonged	prolonged
TT	nl	nl	nl	prolonged	nl
lc	nl	nl	nl	nl	nl

Column headings indicate the following test procedures:

A. Work-up for thrombocytopenia includes platelet sizing, review of peripheral blood smear, maternal platelet count/sizing and platelet-associated IgG antibody, and consideration of bone marrow aspirate.

B. Work-up includes assay for factors VIII, IX, XI.

C. Work-up includes assay for factors X, V, II,VII and other liver or vitamin K-dependent factors.

D. Work-up includes assay for fibrin(ogen) degradation products, protamine neutralization.

E. Work-up includes factor VII assay in addition to other liver or vitamin K-dependent factor assays.

nl, normal.

a. A prolonged aPTT, PT, or TT should initially be assessed as to presence of inhibitor in the system by in-vitro mixing of patient's plasma and normal pooled plasma, 1:1, and repeating the screening test. If the initially prolonged test fails to correct completely to the normal range, the presence of an inhibitor should be suspected: e.g. heparin, degradation products, lupus anticoagulant, etc.

b. If clottable fibrinogen is <80mg/dL then all clotting tests (aPTT, PT, TT) will be prolonged.

3. **If all values are normal,** perform bleeding time, urea solubility, and euglobulin lysis time tests.

a. Prolonged bleeding time suggests platelet dysfunction or von Willebrand's disorder.

b. Abnormal urea solubility suggests factor XIII deficiency.

c. Abnormal euglobulin lysis time suggests excess plasmin and/or α_2 antiplasmin deficiency.

C. INHERITED DEFECTS.

1. Platelet–vessel wall disorders.

a. Von Willebrand's disorder is usually an autosomally inherited disorder characterized by a variably prolonged bleeding time and variable abnormalities of the factor VIII and von Willebrand molecules. Clinical hemorrhage is unusual in the neonate except in patients with the homozygous form. The laboratory workup includes a bleeding time and factor VIII/von Willebrand molecule assessment (factor VIII coagulant, von Willebrand factor antigen, ristocetin cofactor, mulitimer assay) for both parents and patient.

b. Severe platelet function defects are rare, although mild storage pool (aspirin-like) defects are common. Conditions to be considered are Glanzmann's thrombasthenia, Bernard–Soulier syndrome (platelet membrane glycoprotein defects), prostaglandin synthesis disorders (enzyme defects), and granule storage pool disorders.

2. **Procoagulant disorders.**

a. The hemophilias, factor VIII, IX, or XI are characterized, in the severe and moderate form, by a prolonged aPTT and otherwise normal hemostatic screening test results. Factor VIII and IX defects are inherited as sex-linked recessive traits, whereas factor XI is autosomally inherited with a high frequency to Ashkenazi Jews.

b. Isolated deficiencies of other factors are very rare.

D. ACQUIRED DEFECTS.

1. **Platelet–vessel wall disorders.**

a. The most common defect of the hemostatic system is an acquired disorder of platelet function secondary to the effects of drugs administered, either to the mother or to the neonate. Clinical bleeding is uncommon, but it may add to hemorrhage from other causes: e.g. thrombocytopenia.

2. **Procoagulant disorders.**

a. Procoagulant factor defects may occur as a result of vitamin K deficiency, secondary to inadequate intake of vitamin K, or as a result of medications that interfere with vitamin K availability (antibiotics) or that block vitamin K action (anticonvulsants, anticoagulants).

b. The most common procoagulant defect is seen in the sick neonate when an exaggerated hypocoagulable state develops owing to a combination of intravascular coagulation and decreased ability to produce adequate amounts of procoagulant proteins. The spectrum of laboratory abnormalities varies, from the case where all coagulation tests (PTT, PT, TT) are prolonged secondary to a decreased fibrinogen level (<80mg/dL) to that where only one of the tests is prolonged. The etiologies include infection, liver disease, hypoxia, or any combination of problems.

E. TREATMENT.

1. **Initial treatment.** Treatment should be instituted rapidly in the infant with clinical bleeding. If the platelet count is <50,000/mm^3, consider a platelet transfusion. A single unit of platelets administered to the neonate usually increases the platelet count by 40,000–50,000/mm^3. In addition, each platelet pack has 35–50mL of fresh plasma, and, therefore, partial correction of a prolonged procoagulant test can be accomplished simultaneously (10mL/kg of fresh plasma will increase any single procoagulant factor level by 10–15%).

2. **Hypofibrinogenemia** can best be corrected by infusion of cryoprecipitate. One unit or bag of cryoprecipitate (average volume, 10–15 mL) per 5kg of body weight will increase the fibrinogen level by 50mg/dL and provide more than adequate levels of fibrinogen for hemostasis. Cryoprecipitate also contains fibronectin, factor VIII, and factor XIII.

3. **Fresh-frozen plasma** can be used at dosages of 10mL/kg to correct most procoagulant deficiencies partially until such time as a definitive diagnosis is established. Prothrombin complex concentrates should be avoided in the neonate because of their risk for inducing thrombosis.

4. **Frequency of repeated transfusions** of any given material is determined by monitoring of hemostatic measurements and knowledge of the half-life of each deficient component.

F. **THROMBOTIC DISORDERS.** Defects leading to thrombosis in the neonate include deficiency of antithrombin (AT) III, protein C, protein S, plasminogen, prostacyclin-activated protein C (factor V Leiden mutation) and dysfibrinogenemia. Homocysteinemia should also be considered. At present, no laboratory screening tests are available for these deficiencies, but rather specific assessment is required: e.g. ATIII assay, etc. The most common etiology of neonatal thrombosis is indwelling vascular catheters.

FURTHER READING

Andrew M, Paes B, Milner R et al. Development of the human coagulation system in the healthy premature infant. *Blood* 1988; 72:1651–1657.

Andrew M, Paes B, Milner R et al. Development of the human coagulation system in the full term infant. *Blood* 1987; 70:165–172.

Lane DA et al. Inherited thrombophilias, Parts 1 and 2. *Thromb Haemost* 1996; 76:651–662, 824–834.

II. ANEMIA

Anemia may be present at birth or develop postnatally following blood loss, hemolysis, or decreased red cell production. Normal values are shown in Table 20.3.

A. **GENERAL APPROACH.** Identify and correct the cause, replacing blood as needed.

1. **The cause is often obvious** from the history and physical examination.

2. **When the cause is not apparent:**

a. Review prenatal and perinatal history for evidence of uterine trauma, perinatal blood loss, or delivery problems.

b. Obtain hematocrit and hemoglobin values (serial), reticulocyte count, and RBC smear for morphological findings.

c. Consider Coombs' test on infant blood and Kleihauer–Betke test on maternal blood.

3. **Indications for treatment.**

a. In oxygen-dependent patients with compromised oxygen-carrying capacity, it may be desirable to maintain a hematocrit >35–40%.

b. Infants requiring frequent blood sampling should be considered for packed RBC transfusions when 10% of their blood volume has been removed.

TABLE 20.3

NORMAL VALUES FOR FULL-TERM INFANTS[a]

Age	Hemoglobin Reticulocyte (g/dL)	RBCs (10^6mL)	Hematocrit (%)	MCV (mm^3)	Count (%)
Cord blood	14.6–19.6	5.4	56.6	106	3.2
Day 1	21.2(18.2)	5.6(4.7)	56.1	106(115)	3.2
Day 7	19.6(16.3)	5.3(4.4)	52.7	101(110)	0.5
Day 14	18.0(14.5)	5.1(4.1)	49.6	96(106)	0.8
Day 21	16.6(12.9)	4.9(3.70)	46.6	96(102)	0.6
Day 28	15.6(10.9)	4.7(3.2)	44.6	91(100)	0.9

[a]( )Indicates values for low birth weight infants. RBCs, red blood cells; MCV, mean corpuscular volumes. From Stockman AM, Oski F[1], used by permission.

c. Erythropoietin, 200IU/kg, begun early, and administered three times per week, may prevent late anemia in tiny preterm infants and should be given concurrently with iron 2–6mg/g/day.

d. In convalescent babies, transfusions will simply delay the normal physiologic anemia of the newborn and activation of erythropoiesis. Transfuse only in symptomatic infants with anemia when:
   1) Weight gain falls off
   2) Activity, feeding, and responsiveness decrease
   3) Baseline heart rate increases more than 40bpm
   4) Apneic episodes appear or increase in frequency.

4. **General treatment.** Give packed RBCs, 10mL/kg (maximum, 15mL/kg) i.v. over a period of 30–60 minutes. This will usually raise the hemoglobin level by 2–4g/dL.

5. **Specific conditions.**

a. Fetal–maternal transfusion. Review maternal history. Obtain Kleihauer–Betke acid elution test for fetal cells in mother's blood.

b. Identical twin–twin transfusion. Both twins may need adjustment of hematocrit.

c. Obstetric bleeding: abruption, placenta previa, torn umbilical cord, placental incision during cesarean section.
   1) Hematocrit reading at birth may be normal despite substantial blood loss.
   2) Measure central hematocrit on admission to the nursery and 4–6 hours later. Correct with volume if metabolic acidosis is present or if blood pressure is low.

d. Internal hemorrhage – covert serious bleeding may result from rupture of liver (most common) or spleen following difficult delivery. Shock, anemia, or both may be delayed with rupture of the liver capsule, which temporarily tamponades a subcapsular hemorrhage.

20

HEMOSTATIC DISORDERS

e. Hemolysis, when severe, often has RBC morphological findings which are characteristic.
    1) Spherocytes – ABO incompatibility, hereditary spherocytosis
    2) Erythroblasts – severe intrauterine hemolytic disease (usually Rh isoimmune disease)
    3) Fragmented cells, burr cells – infection DIC, metabolic disease
    4) RBC membrane defects – elliptocytosis, stomatocytosis, etc.
    5) Microcytic, hypochromic – α-thalassemias.
f. Production defects – suspect when a newborn has severe anemia and reticulocytopenia.
    1) Usually due to infection or maternal drugs
    2) Aplastic anemias (e.g. Blackfan–Diamond syndrome) are rarely apparent in the first weeks of life.
g. Delayed-onset anemia.
    1) Physiologic anemia of convalescing premature infant. Monitor hematocrit and reticulocyte count weekly when Hct <30%.
    2) Vitamin E deficiency is usually characterized by hemolytic anemia with a normal blood smear, high reticulocyte count, high platelet count, peripheral edema, and low plasma tocopherol level. Therapy is with vitamin E, 5mg/day.

REFERENCE
1. Stockman JA, Oski F. *Am J Dis Child* 1980; 134:945–946.

FURTHER READING
Lanzkowsky P. Diagnosis of anemia in the neonatal period and during childhood. In: Lanzkowsky P, ed. *Pediatric Hematology–Oncology*. New York: McGraw-Hill; 1980.

Oski FA, Naiman JL. Major problems in clinical pediatrics. In: Oski FA, Naiman JL, eds. *Hematologic problems in the newborn*, 2nd edition. Philadelphia: Saunders; 1982.

Pearson H. Anemia in the newborn: a diagnostic approach and challenge. *Semin Perinatol* 1991; 15:2–8.

Shannon KM, Keith JF 3rd, Mentzer WC et al. Recombinant human erythropoietin stimulates erythropoiesis and reduces erythrocyte transfusions in very low birth weight preterm infants. *Pediatrics* 1995; 95:1–8.

III. POLYCYTHEMIA/HYPERVISCOSITY

A. **INCIDENCE.** Hyperviscosity syndrome occurs in 2–5% of all newborns. There is a higher occurrence in IDMs, trisomies (13, 18, 21), and in cases of placental insufficiency, twin–twin transfusion, and placental transfusion at birth. It is rare in prematures born at <34 weeks gestation.

B. CLINICAL FEATURES.

1. **Polycythemia** may occur with or without accompanying signs or symptoms.
2. **Neurological:** lethargy, hypotonia or hypertonia, difficulty in arousing, irritability, tremulousness, poor sucking and feeding, and vomiting.
3. **Physical:** plethora, cyanosis when crying, tachypnea, heart failure, hepatomegaly, ileus, jaundice.
4. **Biochemical:** hypoglycemia, hypocalcemia, hyperbilirubinemia.
5. **Radiographic:** cardiomegaly, increased pulmonary vascular markings.
6. **Other:** thrombocytopenia, abnormal EEG, ECG.

C. OUTCOME.

1. **Neonatal complications.** Neonatal signs and symptoms will usually improve following partial exchange transfusion to reduce viscosity.
2. **Long-term neurological or developmental sequelae.** If the baby is symptomatic in the nursery, subsequent difficulties may arise, particularly if polycythemia is accompanied by hypoglycemia. Complications other than those resulting from major infarction include mild deficits in speech, hearing, or coordination. Serious complications include spastic diplegia and mental retardation. It is uncertain whether long-term complications can be prevented by intervention in the neonatal period.

D. DIAGNOSIS.

1. **Complications.** Diagnosis is complicated by the following relationships:
   a. Hyperviscosity is defined by a value two standard deviations above the mean for a tested population.
   b. Although hematocrit is the principal determinant of viscosity, other factors such as acidosis, hypoxia, spherocytosis, etc., which decrease RBC deformability, may increase viscosity at a given hematocrit reading.
   c. Viscosity increases more rapidly with small increases in the hematocrit reading at higher levels.
   d. Hematocrit in capillary blood obtained from heel stick (Hct_c), antecubital venous blood (Hct_v), and umbilical venous blood may differ. The Hct_c is particularly unreliable during the first 4–6 hours of life.
2. **Approach to diagnosing polycythemia.**
   a. An Hct_c should be performed on all plethoric or symptomatic babies at 4–6 hours of age.
   b. If the Hct_c is $\geq 70\%$, a Hct_v should be drawn from an antecubital vein.
   c. If the Hct_c is $>65\%$ and the infant is symptomatic, an Hct_v should also be drawn.
   d. If the Hct_v is $>65\%$, the diagnosis of polycythemia is made.

E. CRITERIA FOR TREATMENT.

1. **Symptomatic infants.** If the Hct_v is $>65\%$ and the infant has clinical

features compatible with hyperviscosity syndrome, a partial exchange transfusion should be performed.

2. **Asymptomatic infants.** Currently available evidence does not permit a recommendation regarding intervention in this group of infants. If the Hct_v is >70%, the infant should be monitored carefully for neurological and biochemical abnormalities, and treatment should be based on their appearance.

F. **TREATMENT.** Partial exchange transfusion should be performed to reduce Hct_v to about 55%.

1. **Calculation of blood volume** to be exchanged.

a. Assume blood volume (BV) of 80–90mL/kg (may be higher if polycythemia is due to placental transfusion).

b. Exchange volume = $[BV \times (Hct_v-55)]/Hct_v$.

2. **Partial exchange transfusion** may be performed through a low UVC advanced 3–5cm until there is good blood return or through a UAC.

a. Obtain a central hematocrit reading – before and after the exchange transfusion (before removing the catheter).

b. Withdraw blood (in 10mL aliquots) and replace with an equal volume of plasmanate, 5% albumin or saline. Fresh-frozen plasma is more expensive and is not usually required for this procedure.

FURTHER READING

Black VD, Lubchenco LO, Luckey DW et al. Developmental and neurologic sequelae of neonatal hyperviscosity syndrome. *Pediatrics* 1982; 69:426–431.

Ramamurthy RS, Brans VW. Neonatal polycythemia, 1: Criteria for diagnosis and treatment. *Pediatrics* 1981; 68:168–174.

JAUNDICE

I. UNCONJUGATED HYPERBILIRUBINEMIA

A. GENERAL PRINCIPLES.

1. **Physiologic jaundice.** Most newborns develop a transient elevation of unconjugated bilirubin. In the term infant, bilirubin levels usually peak on the third day. In premature infants, the bilirubin concentration may rise faster, reach maximum elevations on the 4th or 5th day, and decrease slowly thereafter. Similar patterns occur in some term Asian infants. When the bilirubin level reaches about 6mg/dL, clinical jaundice appears, increasing in a cephalocaudad progression as the serum bilirubin concentration rises.

2. **A pathological cause** for jaundice should be considered if the serum bilirubin level is >7, 9, or 11mg/dL at 24, 48, or 72 hours of age, respectively.

3. **Early discharge** of infants increases the chance of not identifying babies at risk for hyperbilirubinemia. Infants discharged before 48 hours of age should have a follow-up examination by a home nurse or physician in 2–3 days. This is particularly important if born at 36–38 weeks gestation where the risk for hyperbilirubinemia is high. In patient populations with a high follow-up failure rate, we recommend measuring a bilirubin level or screening for jaundice with a reflectometer at 24 hours of age. Newer multiwavelength reflectometers improve estimation of serum bilirubin levels. Efforts to assure follow-up are then directed toward babies with bilirubin levels >7mg/dL.

B. EVALUATING JAUNDICE. See Table 21.1.

1. **History.** Family history of recurrence is found in hemolytic disease, familial jaundice (more common in Asians), breast milk jaundice, maternal diabetes, or Gilbert's syndrome.

2. **Physical examination.** Attention should be given to the following.

a. Potential sources of bilirubin (e.g. bruising, cephalohematoma, IVH, swallowed blood).

b. Physical features of syndromes predisposing to jaundice (e.g. hypothyroid, IDM).

3. **Laboratory.**

a. Maternal prenatal testing should include ABO and Rh(D) typing and a serum screen for unusual isoimmune antibodies.

TABLE 21.1

DIFFERENTIAL DIAGNOSIS OF UNCONJUGATED HYPERBILIRUBINEMIA

Hemolytic disease	Metabolic disorders
Isoimmune hemolytic disease	Galactosemia
RH incompatibility	Crigler–Najjar disease
ABO incompatibility	Breast-milk jaundice
Minor blood group incompatibility	Familial neonatal jaundice
Inherited RBC metabolic disorders	Infants of diabetic mothers
Glucose-6-phosphate dehydrogenase	Hypothyroidism
(G6PD) deficiency	
Pyruvate kinase deficiency	
Disorders in RBC morphology	
Hereditary spherocytosis	
Infantile pyknocytosis	
Infections	**Other causes**
Bacterial sepsis	High intestinal obstruction
TORCH infections	Enclosed hemorrhage (e.g. cephalohematoma)
	Swallowed maternal blood
	Polycythemia
	Birth at high altitude

Causes of obstructive jaundice (elevated direct fraction) are not included in this table.
Elevated direct reacting bilirubin may or may not be a feature of infection or erythroblastosis fetalis

b. Blood type, Rh determination, and antibody test on mother and infant when mother has not had prenatal blood grouping or is Rh-negative.
c. Total serum bilirubin (TSB). Approximately 10% of TSB will be 'direct reacting' even when all bilirubin is unconjugated. Therefore, evaluation of jaundiced infants should be based on the TSB value.
d. Direct bilirubin should be measured in severe hemolytic disease, prolonged jaundice, dark urine, urine testing positive for bilirubin, or when there is high suspicion for hepatic disease or cholestasis.
e. Hematocrit or hemoglobin value if baby is pale or plethoric.
f. Red blood cell smear – may help identify cause of hemolysis.
   1) Rh incompatibility – nucleated RBCs, erythroblasts
   2) ABO incompatibility – microspherocytes
   3) Sepsis, G6PD deficiency-fragmented RBC
   4) Pyknocytosis – pyknocytes.
g. Other considerations in persistent, unexplained jaundice.
   1) Urine culture to rule out urinary tract infection
   2) Urine Clinitest® (galactosemia)
   3) Thyroxine (free T_4) (hypothyroidism)

4) G6PD screen if delayed hyperbilirubinemia occurs and ethnic origin suggests possibility.

C. EVALUATING RISK FOR KERNICTERUS.

1. **Interpretation of serum bilirubin levels.**

a. The serum bilirubin concentration reflects (i) the rates of bilirubin production, hepatic excretion, and intestinal reabsorption (enterohepatic shunt) and (ii) the ability of serum albumin to bind bilirubin in competition with tissue binding sites.

b. Bilirubin remains in serum because there are serum proteins which bind and hold it there. At constant bilirubin production and excretion rates, the serum bilirubin concentration is a function of the concentration and binding quality of albumin in serum. For example, if a given bilirubin load results in a serum bilirubin concentration of 24mg/dL in a baby with 4g/dL albumin, it would produce a level of about 12mg/dL in a newborn with 2g/dL albumin. The unbound bilirubin level, which is probably a better estimate of risk for encephalopathy, would be nearly identical in both babies.

c. Thus, measurement of albumin levels or, better, serum binding, may be helpful in clinical evaluation of an infant's risk for brain injury.

2. **Bilirubin monitoring frequency.**

a. Hemolytic disease. Every 4–6 hours in first day until the rate of rise is established; then every 8–12 hours until two sequential samples show decline.

b. Nonhemolytic jaundice. Every 12–24 hours in a baby whose bilirubin level is increasing and exceeds 12–15mg/dL (in term infants) and every 6–12 hours when bilirubin approaches the exchange level.

c. Post-phototherapy rebound. Bilirubin determination is not necessary unless there is suspicion of ongoing hemolysis or significantly impaired clearance.

3. **Clinical factors** which increase the susceptibility of tissue to bilirubin toxicity and/or alter the blood–brain barrier include hydrops (chronic intrauterine hypoxia-ischemia), asphyxia, sepsis, hypoglycemia, acidosis, and renal failure. Renal failure significantly impairs serum binding of bilirubin.

4. **Acidemia.** pH has little effect on binding of bilirubin to albumin, but binding of bilirubin to tissue increases in direct proportion to hydrogen ion concentration. Risk for encephalopathy is probably greater in respiratory acidosis since CO_2 readily crosses the blood–brain barrier, altering the pH of brain, and increases cerebral blood flow.

5. **Bilirubin–albumin** binding tests may improve the estimation of risk for encephalopathy.

a. Except in sick infants, serum binding (or free bilirubin levels) correlate well with the bilirubin/albumin ratio after 2–3 days of life. The quality of binding improves with advancing postnatal age.

21

JAUNDICE

b. There is good intertest agreement between the peroxidase method (apparent unbound bilirubin concentration, AUBC) and Sephadex filtration: 1+ by Sephadex agrees with AUBC ≥ 17nmol/L.

c. Binding tests do not preclude the need for clinical judgment in managing the jaundiced infant.

6. **Brain-stem auditory evoked response** (BAER). Bilirubin may produce alterations in the BAER, including prolonged II–III and I–V wave intervals or decreased amplitude of all waves before clinical manifestations of encephalopathy become apparent. These may be reversible early manifestations of toxicity. A marked alteration in the BAER may be permanent or resolve slowly over months, and it indicates a need for aggressive intervention.

7. **Clinical signs** of early kernicterus (marked lethargy, weak suck, opisthotonos, high-pitched cry, apnea) remain an absolute indication for exchange transfusion.

8. **Critical bilirubin level.** The American Academy of Pediatrics (AAP) practice parameter for phototherapy and exchange transfusion in healthy term infants is shown in Table 21.2. (These guidelines were established primarily by consensus rather than by controlled studies.)

a. We strongly advise that a serum albumin level and, when possible, a BAER be obtained in term infants whose bilirubin exceeds 20–24mg/dL. A high albumin level and normal BAER would support a clinical decision to administer intensive phototherapy rather than exchange transfusion (see Table 21.2).

b. Recommendations for intervention in sick and premature infants are shown in Table 21.3. Phototherapy should be initiated at bilirubin values about 2/3 those indicated for exchange transfusion. Intervention is based on the serum albumin level in our hospital.

D. PREVENTING/TREATING HYPERBILIRUBINEMIA.

1. **Phototherapy.**

a. Phototherapy produces structural (lumirubin) and geometric isomers

---

TABLE 21.2

MANAGEMENT OF HYPERBILIRUBINEMIA IN THE HEALTHY TERM NEWBORN[a]

Age (h)	Total serum bilirubin (mg/dL) {μmol/L}			
	Consider phototherapy	Phototherapy	Exchange Tx if intensive phototherapy fails	Exchange Tx and intensive phototherapy
[b]25–48	12 {170}	15 {260}	20 {340}	25 {430}
49–72	15 {260}	18 {310}	25 {430}	30 {510}
>72	17 {260}	20 {310}	25{430}	30 {510}

[a] AAP Practice Parameters[1].
[b] Jaundice <24h is not considered 'healthy'.
Tx, transfusion.

TABLE 21.3

ACCEPTABLE INDICATIONS FOR EXCHANGE TRANSFUSION IN PATIENTS NOT RESPONDING TO PHOTOTHERAPY[a]

Basis	>2500g	<2500g, well	<2500g, sick
TSB (mg/dL)	20–24	15–20	11–15
Albumin (g/dL)	Alb x 7.0[b]	Alb x 6.5	Alb x 5.5
AUBC[c] (nmol/L)	>20	>20	>15
Sephadex staining	1+	1+	1+
Clinical	Symptomatic	Symptomatic	Deterioration
BAER	Abnormal	Deterioration	Deterioration[d]

TSB, total serum bilirubin; AUBC, apparent unbound bilirubin concentration; BAER, brain-stem auditory evoked response.

[a] Indication for phototherapy is 2/3 level indicated for exchange.

[b] Value equals exchange level of bilirubin in mg/dL.

[c] AUBC: 1μg/dL 'free' bilirubin measured with UB analyzer® equals 18 nmol/L.

[d] Baseline BAER may be abnormal in sick or very premature infants.

21

JAUNDICE

which are water soluble and excreted by the liver without conjugation. A smaller fraction of bilirubin is excreted by kidney and liver as photo-oxidation products.

b. The efficiency of phototherapy is directly proportional to the energy output (or irradiance) of light in the blue spectrum, measured in μW/cm^2/nm. A minimum exposure of 6–8μW/cm^2 should be received by the infant. There is no maximum effective exposure.

c. Intensive phototherapy may be applied by using two or more light sources and/or adding a fiber-optic blanket. Addition of special blue fluorescent tubes (F20 T12/BB) will increase effective energy output.

d. Intensive phototherapy should lower the serum bilirubin level by 1–2mg every 4–6 hours.

e. In a healthy term infant without hemolytic disease, phototherapy may be stopped when the bilirubin level is <14mg/dL.

2. **Phenobarbital** may be administered at birth to patients with severe hemolytic disease. Antenatal treatment via the mother is more effective than treating the newborn. Phenobarbital (5 mg/kg/day) increases hepatic uptake and excretion of bilirubin and induces glucuronyl transferase and ligandin.

3. **Tin or zinc protoporphyrin** prevent jaundice by inhibiting heme oxygenase and blocking the conversion of heme to bilirubin. They are currently experimental drugs.

4. **Adequate hydration,** particularly by frequent formula feedings, is helpful in facilitating bile flow and inhibiting enterohepatic circulation of bilirubin. Excessive hydration in term infants without dehydration has not been shown to accelerate bilirubin clearance. Frequent breast-feeding, 8–10 times a day, is recommended by the AAP.

5. **Intravenous immune globulin** (IVIG) inhibits hyperbilirubinemia in hemolytic disease due to Rh sensitivity and possibly in other forms of isoimmune hemolytic disease. A dose of 500mg/kg has been used. The effect is temporary, and additional dosing may be helpful if the rise in serum bilirubin accelerates.

II. HEMOLYTIC DISEASE OF THE NEWBORN (HDN, ERYTHROBLASTOSIS FETALIS)

Erythroblastosis fetalis is usually due to sensitization of a Rh-D-negative woman by the red cells of a Rh-positive fetus, but severe hemolytic disease may be caused by maternal sensitization to many red cell antigens including c, E, Kell, and, rarely, ABO groups. Anemia, hyperbilirubinemia, or both may result in hydrops fetalis and fetal or neonatal demise.

A. **PREVENTION.** Rh immune globulin (300mg) is indicated only in nonsensitized Rh-D-negative women and given as follows.

1. **Within 72 hours of delivery and at 28 weeks gestation** (combined therapy 99% effective).

2. **After therapeutic abortion, amniocentesis, and abdominal trauma.** In the latter case, Kleihauer–Betke acid elution test for fetal cells in maternal circulation should be obtained and volume of transfusion estimated. The Rh immune globulin dose is 300mg per 30mL of fetal blood.

B. **PRENATAL MANAGEMENT.**

1. **Timing of the delivery.** Based on history of previous pregnancy outcomes, antibody titers, serial amniocentesis, ultrasound, and cordocentesis.

2. **Measure anti-D antibodies** on the first prenatal visit and periodically through pregnancy (4-week intervals during the third trimester).

a. If the titer is >1:16, perform amniocentesis at 26–28 weeks gestation to evaluate the concentration of bilirubinoid pigments in the amniotic fluid.

b. Rh genotype of the fetus can be performed from amniocytes. If the fetus is Rh negative, then no further testing is needed.

c. If the antibody titer is higher, perform initial amniocentesis at 20–24 weeks gestation.

3. **Amniocentesis.**

a. The change in optical density at 450nm provides a fair prediction of anemia or risk of fetal death, but is less accurate in predicting the postnatal course of hyperbilirubinemia (even though the ΔOD_{450} reflects the amniotic bilirubin concentration). See Figure 21.1.

b. If the initial amniocentesis indicates that the fetus is moderately affected, the procedure should be repeated at 2–3 week intervals in order to monitor ΔOD_{450} and, after 32 weeks, indices of lung maturity.

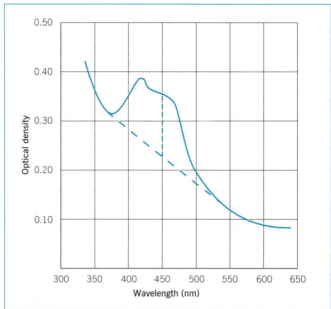

FIG. 21.1

Spectrophotometric analysis of amniotic fluid. (From Kelley[2], with permission.)

c. If the ΔOD_{450} plots in lower zone II or in zone III (Figure 21.2) or fails to decrease with advancing gestational age, we recommend the following.

   1) Perform cordocentesis to access fetal blood directly and assess antibody status and fetal hematocrit.
   2) If the fetus is <32 weeks gestation and Hct <25–30%, perform intrauterine transfusion with O Rh-negative frozen deglycerized, irradiated CMV-negative RBCs. Multiple transfusions may be necessary.
   3) If the fetus has evidence of hydrops by ultrasound and is >32 weeks gestation, administer betamethasone to the mother (if the lung profile is immature) and deliver the infant.
   4) If the fetus is severely affected (Hct <35% or zone III) and the lung profile is mature, administer phenobarbital (125mg/day) to the mother for 3–7 days before delivery to stimulate the fetal hepatic conjugating system.

4. **Severely affected fetus.** If amniocentesis indicates that the fetus is

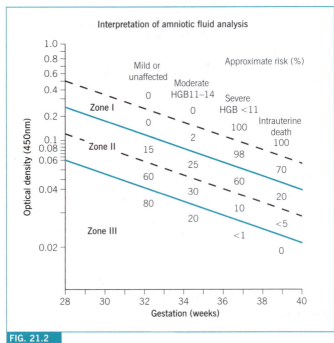

FIG. 21.2
Interpretation of amniotic fluid analysis. (From Kelley[2], with permission.)

severely affected, tightly packed type O cells compatible with the mother's blood should be available at the time of delivery. These may be later mixed with AB plasma to reconstitute as whole blood if immediate red cell exchange is not needed for neonatal distress.

C. DELIVERY ROOM MANAGEMENT OF A HYDROPIC INFANT.
1. **Assisted ventilation** with high inspiratory pressures may be required.
2. **Paracentesis** may be necessary to remove ascitic fluid, which, in combination with hepatosplenomegaly, may mechanically impair effective ventilation.
3. **Thoracentesis** is rarely needed in the delivery room.
4. **Partial exchange transfusion** with 20–40mL packed type O-negative cells may be performed in severely hydropic or pale and asphyxiated infants as the final component of the resuscitative procedure. Immediate exchange transfusion is otherwise not advised.

D. NURSERY CARE.

1. **Laboratory monitoring.**
a. The hematocrit (and occasionally bilirubin) in cord blood may be quite different from values obtained from the baby after stabilization, and should be repeated from a venipuncture or indwelling catheter at 30–60 min of age.
b. TSB concentration should be determined at 4–6 hour intervals until the concentration declines.
c. Monitor direct bilirubin periodically for development of 'inspissated bile syndrome.'
2. **Phototherapy** has little effect on the early bilirubin rise, but may be useful in decreasing the number of exchange transfusions required.
3. **Combined therapy** of phototherapy, IVIG, and antenatal phenobarbital therapy will significantly decrease the need for exchange transfusion, but will not prevent subsequent anemia.
4. **Indications for exchange transfusion** (Table 21.4) are more conservative than in nonhemolytic jaundice since the threshold for toxicity is lower in Rh hemolytic disease. A lower toxicity threshold for hyperbilirubinemia due to ABO incompatibility has not been documented.
5. **Other problems.**

21

JAUNDICE

TABLE 21.4

CRITERIA FOR EXCHANGE TRANSFUSION IN ERYTHROBLASTOSIS FETALIS

All patients
    Cord hemoglobin <8g/dL
    Cord bilirubin concentration >6mg/dL
    Rise in bilirubin concentration >0.5mg/dL/h over 12–18h

Uncomplicated HDN
    Indirect bilirubin concentration >20 mg/dL
    Indirect bilirubin concentration (mg/dL) >6.0–6.5 x albumin concentration (g/dL)
    AUBC 15–20nmol/L (if arterial pH 7.3–7.5)
    Sephadex staining 1+ (Kernlute®).

Complicated HDN (e.g. RDS, hydrops)
    Indirect bilirubin concentration (mg/dL) 5.0–5.5 x albumin
    AUBC (peroxidase) 10–15nmol/L (if pH 7.1–7.3)
    Sephadex staining 1+ (Kernlute).

Clinical deterioration:
    Irritability, lethargy, development of abnormal BAER

AUBC, apparent unbound bilirubin concentration; BAER, brain-stem auditory evoked response.

a. Hyaline membrane disease.
b. In hydropic infants, severe cardiac arrhythmias may occur.
c. Hypoglycemia (secondary to hyperinsulinemia).
d. Erythroblastotic infants may have low folate levels; consider folate supplementation.
e. Thrombocytopenia.
f. Obstructive jaundice may result from bilirubin overload to the liver (conjugated bilirubin appears) or liver bilirubin toxicity (inspissated bile syndrome).
g. Delayed anemia (at 3–4 weeks of age) is common, especially when exchange transfusion is not required.

III. CHOLESTATIC JAUNDICE

Cholestasis may result from hepatocellular disease and/or obstruction to bile flow. It is usually associated with an elevation of direct bilirubin >1.5mg/dL and should always be considered pathologic in the neonatal period, although outcomes vary with the underlying disease process.

A. CONCEPTUAL MECHANISMS OF CHOLESTASIS.

1. **Hepatocellular injury** due to infections, shock, toxins, metabolic disorders, drugs, and neonatal hepatitis.
2. **Obstruction of bile flow** due to extrahepatic and intrahepatic biliary atresia or hypoplasia, choledochal cyst, and other cholestatic syndromes.
3. **Increased bilirubin loading** due to acute hemolytic disease (ABO or Rh), multiple blood transfusions, or hemolysis related to sepsis.
4. **Congenital disorders of bilirubin excretion** (Dubin–Johnson syndrome, Rotor's syndrome).

B. DIAGNOSTIC CONSIDERATIONS.

1. **Neonatal hepatitis.**
a. Idiopathic – viral: CMV, rubella, reovirus type 3, herpesviruses, human herpesvirus type 6, adenovirus, enteroviruses, parvovirus B19, hepatitis B, hepatitis C, HIV.
b. Bacterial and parasitic: bacterial sepsis, syphilis, listeriosis, tuberculosis, toxoplasmosis.
2. **Bile duct obstruction.**
a. Cholangiopathies: extrahepatic biliary atresia, nonsyndromic paucity of intrahepatic bile ducts, choledochal cyst, neonatal sclerosing cholangitis.
b. Spontaneous perforation of common bile duct.
c. Bile duct stenosis.
d. Caroli's disease.
e. Other: inspissated bile (hemolytic disease), severe mucous plug, cholelithiasis, tumors/masses (intrinsic and extrinsic).
3. **Idiopathic cholestatic syndromes:** arteriohepatic dysplasia (Alagille's

syndrome), Byler's syndrome, hereditary cholestasis with lymphedema (Aagenaes), benign recurrent cholestasis, familial cholestasis of North American indians.

4. **Metabolic diseases.**
a. Disorders of amino acid metabolism: tyrosinemia.
b. Disorder of lipid metabolism: Niemann–Pick disease, Gaucher's disease, Wolman's disease.
c. Disorders of the urea cycle: arginase deficiency.
d. Disorders of carbohydrate metabolism: galactosemia, fructosemia, type IV glycogenosis.
e. Disorders of bile acid synthesis: peroxisomal disorders, Zellweger syndrome.
f. Disorders of oxidative phosphorylation.
g. Other: α_1-antitrypsin deficiency, cystic fibrosis, hypopituitarism (septo-optic dysplasia), hypothyroidism, neonatal hemochromatosis.

5. **Toxic.**
a. Drugs.
b. Parenteral nutrition.

6. **Miscellaneous associations.**
a. Shock/hypoperfusion.
b. Histiocytosis X.
c. Intestinal obstruction.
d. Erythrophagocytic lymphohistiocytosis.
e. Neonatal lupus erythematosus.
f. Indian childhood cirrhosis.
g. ECMO.
h. Autosomal trisomies.
i. Graft versus host disease.
j. Veno-occlusive disease.

C. CLINICAL CONSIDERATIONS.

1. **'Sick' infant.** Sudden development of direct hyperbilirubinemia may be due to hepatocellular injury from shock, sepsis (bacterial, viral, fungal), or metabolic disorders. Onset of symptoms after feeding suggests galactosemia (if fed lactose-containing formula or breast milk) or fructosemia (if fed a formula containing sucrose).

2. **Nonacutely ill infant.** Conjugated hyperbilirubinemia is common in the following conditions.
a. Idiopathic neonatal hepatitis.
b. Extrahepatic biliary atresia.
c. Intrahepatic biliary hypoplasia.
d. Choledochal cyst.
e. α_1-Antitrypsin deficiency.
f. PN-related cholestasis.
g. Hypothyroidism.
h. Congenital defects of excretion (Byler's and others).

21

JAUNDICE

i.   Cystic fibrosis.
j.   Metabolic storage diseases (Zellweger's, Niemann–Pick).
D. SCHEME OF DIAGNOSTIC EVALUATIONS.
1. The goals of any diagnostic evaluation in a neonate with cholestasis are to (i) confirm that cholestasis is present and the relative severity of hepatic dysfunction, (ii) exclude diseases which require immediate treatment (such as sepsis, endocrinopathies, and some metabolic diseases), and (iii) identify patients requiring specialized medical, nutritional, or surgical therapy. No single diagnostic study is usually sufficient to define the etiology of cholestasis in neonates, and an organized medical/surgical approach is indicated in most patients.
2. Initial investigations establish the presence of cholestasis, define the severity of the liver disease, and detect readily treatable disorders.
a.   History, physical examination (include details of family history, pregnancy, early neonatal course, presence of extrahepatic anomalies, extrahepatic disease, stool color).
b.   Fractionated serum bilirubin analysis.
c.   Serum tests for liver disease (AST, ALT, alkaline phosphatase, 5' nucleotidase or GGT).
d.   Tests of liver function to examine severity of liver impairment, (PT, PTT, coagulation factors, serum albumin, serum ammonia, cholesterol, blood glucose).
e.   Complete blood count including platelet count.
f.   Bacterial cultures of blood, urine, other if indicated.
g.   Urinalysis including reducing sugars.
h.   Paracentesis if ascites (examine for bile and infection).
3. Investigations to establish a specific diagnosis.
a.   Ultrasonography.
b. α_1-Antitrypsin level and phenotype.
c.   Serologies (HbsAg, TORCH, VDRL, Epstein–Barr virus, parvovirus, herpes virus B6, HIV, other).
d.   Sweat chloride analysis.
e.   Metabolic screen (urine and serum amino acids, urine organic acids).
f. T_4, thyroid-stimulating hormones (evaluation of hypopituitarism as indicated).
g.   Serum iron and ferritin.
h.   Urine and serum analysis of bile acids and bile precursors.
i.   RBC galactose-1-phosphate uridyl transferase.
j.   Viral cultures.
k.   Hepatobiliary scintigraphy.
l.   Radiographs of long bones, skull for congenital infection; chest for lung and cardiac disease.
m.   Bone marrow examination and skin fibroblast culture for suspected storage disease.
n.   Percutaneous or endoscopic cholangiography (rarely indicated).

o. Percutaneous liver biopsy (for light and electron microscopic examination, immunohistochemistry, viral culture and enzymology as indicated).

p. Exploratory laparotomy and intraoperative cholangiography.

E. INTERPRETATION OF SCREENING BIOCHEMICAL STUDIES.

1. **Bilirubin** concentration (total/conjugated) establishes the diagnosis of cholestasis if the direct fraction is >1.5mg/dL; direct fractions of 40–70% of the total are commonly seen.

2. **Transaminase** (AST/ALT) levels elevated >2–3 times normal suggest (but are not diagnostic of) hepatocellular injury from hepatitis.

3. **Alkaline phosphatase and** GGT values >2–3 times normal may indicate intrahepatic or extrahepatic biliary obstruction, but are not sufficient to make the diagnosis. Very high values are commonly seen in a α_1-antitrypsin disease; low or normal values are often found in patients with familial disorders of cholestasis (Byler's).

4. **Urine for reducing substances** may be positive in galactosemia, fructose intolerance, and tyrosinemia.

F. INVESTIGATIONS AIMED AT SPECIFIC DIAGNOSES.

1. **Ultrasound** of liver and biliary tract may define normal or absent extrahepatic ducts, absent gallbladder (commonly seen in biliary atresia), or presence of a choledochal cyst, but is not adequate to exclude extrahepatic obstruction.

2. **Serum α_1-antitrypsin** levels <100mg/dL are highly suggestive of α_1-antitrypsin deficiency and may eliminate the need for additional studies (confirm by protease-inhibitor phenotyping).

3. **Urine metabolic screens or qualitative urine amino acids** – while these may suggest tyrosinemia or other aminoacidurias, interpret results with caution: elevated tyrosine excretion can be seen in hepatocellular disease of various etiologies.

4. **Neonatal screening T_4, TSH, and RBC galactose-1-uridyl transferase studies** should rule out hypothyroidism or galactosemia.

5. **Biliary scans** – obtain following 3–5 days of phenobarbital (5mg/kg/day) to attempt to demonstrate patency of biliary system. (Caution: severe intrahepatic cholestasis of various etiologies may prevent isotope excretion into the GI tract, yielding false-positive results.)

6. **A percutaneous liver biopsy** may define hepatocellular disease (e.g. idiopathic neonatal hepatitis) or suggest anatomic obstruction (biliary hypoplasia, biliary atresia) in 90–95% of patients. Occasionally, serial biopsies may be required because of evolution of the characteristic histological features in extrahepatic obstruction.

7. **Surgical exploration** and an operative cholangiogram with or without

21

JAUNDICE

portoenterostomy (Kasai procedure) is indicated in selected patients when the diagnosis of biliary atresia or choledochal cyst is suspected, and should be performed prior to 6–8 weeks of age for the most optimal outcomes.

G. THERAPY.
1. **Supportive care.** Therapy for the infant with liver disease and conjugated hyperbilirubinemia is directed at supportive care, removing offending toxins, relieving anatomic obstructions, increasing bile flow, and providing adequate nutrition. Supportive care should include the following measures as required.
a. Replacement of blood loss and clotting factors with packed RBCs, fresh-frozen plasma.
b. Assisted ventilation for ascites with pulmonary compromise.
c. Early recognition/therapy of sepsis and peritonitis.
d. Careful fluid management, diuretic therapy for ascites.
e. Correction of electrolyte derangements.
f. Careful metabolic monitoring.
2. **Medical therapy.** Nutritional and drug therapy should be provided in a form which is well absorbed, even when bile flow is decreased. Offending carbohydrates or amino acids should be excluded from nutritional support in selected cases of metabolic liver disease. The management guidelines (Table 21.5) and drug therapy (Table 21.6) can be individualized as needed.

REFERENCES
1. AAP Practice Parameters. *Pediatrics* 1994; 94:558–565.
2. Kelley V (ed). *Brenneman–Kelley textbook of pediatrics.* New York: Harper & Row; 1972.

TABLE 21.5

MANAGEMENT GUIDELINES FOR CHOLESTATIC JAUNDICE

Goal	Approach
Provide adequate energy	Provide 120–130% of RDA with 20–27 cal/oz formula
	Supplemental glucose polymers (Polycose™)
	Supplement with MCT oil: 1–2mL/kg/day in 3–4 doses
Optimize fat absorption with MCT-containing formula	Pregestimil™, Alimentum™
Provide adequate levels of essential fatty acids	Oral lipid emulsions, i.v. fat emulsions
Supply adequate protein	2–3g/kg/day for infants
	0.5–1g/kg/day in hepatic encephalopathy
Supplement minerals and trace elements as needed	Calcium
	Phosphate
	Magnesium
	Zinc
	Iron
	Selenium
Avoid specific formulas in selected metabolic disease	Galactosemia: breast milk, all formulas containing lactose
	Fructose intolerance: any formula or medication containing sucrose

MCT, medium-chain triglycerides; RDA, recommended daily allowance.

21 JAUNDICE

TABLE 21.6

DRUG THERAPY AND VITAMIN SUPPLEMENTS FOR CHOLESTATIC JAUNDICE

Therapy	Use/indication(s)	Dosage/comments
Ursodeoxycholic acid (Actigall™)	Increase bile flow	10–20mg/kg/day p.o. (q12h)
Phenobarbital	Increase bile flow	3–5mg/kg/day (usual dose) i.v. or p.o.
Bile acid binding agents (cholestyramine, colestipol)	Increase bile flow	250–500mg/kg/day p.o. Constipation, metabolic acidosis, drug binding
Multivitamins (Polyvisol™, others)	Prevent/correct water-soluble vitamin deficiencies	1–2 x normal RDA p.o. or give Pediatric MVI™ i.v. (Variable absorption of fat-soluble vitamins from oral preparations related to bile flow)
Vitamin A	Prevent/correct vitamin A deficiency	5000–25,000 units/day of water-soluble vitamin A p.o. (Aquasol A™)
Vitamin D	Prevent/correct vitamin D deficiency	Vitamin D: 800–5000 units/day. 25-OHD: 3–5mg/kg/day 1,25(OH)$_2$D: 0.05–02mg/kg/day Monitor Ca, PO$_4$, Alk-phos, 25-OHD levels
Vitamin E TPGS (Nutr–E–Sol™), LiquiE™	Prevent/correct vitamin E deficiency	15–25IU/kg (as TPGS) per day p.o. (Aquasol E™ poorly absorbed in severe cholestasis.) Monitor levels
Vitamin K	Prevent/correct vitamin K deficiency, correct prolonged PT	p.o.: 2.5mg twice weekly to 1–5mg/day i.m.: 1–2mg weekly i.v.: available in Pediatric MVI™

25-OHD, 25-hydroxycholecalciferol; 1,25(OH)$_2$D, 1,25-dihydroxycholecalciferol;RDA, recommended daily allowance; TPGS, tocopherol polyethyleneglycol succinate.

ENDOCRINE PROBLEMS

I. THYROID DISORDERS

A. CONGENITAL HYPOTHYROIDISM.

Physical findings of congenital hypothyroidism are usually too subtle to detect by physical examination in the newborn. This condition has an incidence of 1 in 4000 live births. The risk of development of mental retardation in untreated infants has led all states to require newborn screening for hypothyroidism. Initiation of therapy within 4 weeks after birth is recommended to prevent abnormal brain development.

1. **Etiology.**
a. Sporadic athyreosis or ectopic thyroid gland (1:4000 births).
b. Familial goitrous hypothyroidism (1:30,000 births).
c. Hypothalamic deficiency of thyrotropin-releasing factor (TRF) and pituitary deficiency of thyrotropin (TSH) are rare (1:100,000 births).
d. Children of mothers with Graves' disease treated with propylthiouracil may have transient hypothyroidism (often followed by transient hyperthyroidism). Other infants may acquire antibodies from the mother that lead to transient hypothyroidism.
e. The condition may be idiopathic.
2. **Newborn screening.** T_4 is measured on a dried spot of blood in most states. Specimens with low T_4 concentrations also have a TSH measurement done. TSH screening alone will miss the rare cases of hypothalamic–pituitary deficiencies leading to hypothyroidism.
3. **Diagnosis.** See Figure 22.1.
a. Confirmatory testing is important, but should not delay the onset of therapy. Step b below can be carried out minutes before administration of therapy, while performance of steps c, d, and e can be done 1–2 days after therapy begins, if necessary.
b. Primary hypothyroidism is indicated by a low T_4 and an elevated TSH level. A true serum T_4 and TSH should be obtained to confirm abnormal screening results. The determination of free T_4, if available, is preferable to the determination of total T_4.
c. A low T_4 level accompanied by a normal TSH value may indicate normal thyroid status with a low concentration of TBG (common in premature infants). It is confirmed by finding a normal free T_4 level. No therapy is necessary for TBG deficiency. Alternatively, a low T_4 with a normal TSH value on screening may indicate hypopituitarism or hypothalamic deficiency, and further diagnostic measures may be

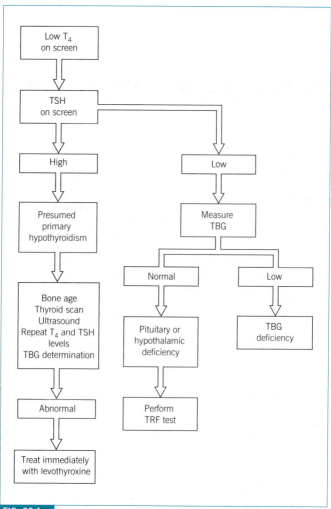

FIG. 22.1

Algorithm for diagnosis of primary hypothyroidism. T_4 indicates serum thyroxine, although free T_4 is an alternative determination (see text); TSH, thyroid-stimulating hormone; TBG, thyroid-binding globulin; TRF, thyrotropin-releasing factor.

required. Usually hypothalamic TRF deficiency or pituitary TSH deficiency is accompanied by growth hormone or adrenocorticotropin (ACTH) deficiency which may cause acute hypoglycemia; growth hormone or gonadotropin deficiency may cause microphallus and undescended testes in a male infant. Hypothalamic–pituitary deficiencies will not be detected in programs that screen only TSH.

d. An iodinated I^{124} or technetium scan of the thyroid gland is indicated, if the scanning center is experienced, to evaluate the presence of a rudimentary or ectopic thyroid gland. Maternal antibodies can suppress the newborn thyroid gland function temporarily so that there is no uptake by the thyroid gland on scan; this is a false positive. An ultrasound exam may be used to determine whether there is a normally located gland. A thyroglobulin determination will indicate the presence of functional thyroid tissue; absent thyroglobulin with no evidence of a thyroid gland on imaging studies indicates absence of thyroid tissue, while the absence of thyroglobulin in a patient with normal thyroid imaging indicates a defect in thyroglobulin synthesis which may be associated with a defect in thyroxin synthesis.

e. A bone age determination using the distal femur, proximal tibial, and cuboid epiphyses will determine the extent of prenatal hypothyroidism. The more delayed the bone age, the more likely that some loss of intellectual function has occurred.

4. Treatment.

a. Levothyroxine is administered at an initial oral dose of 10–15mcg/kg per day, if screening indicates primary hypothyroidism.

b. If the definitive test returns with normal results, re-evaluate the case. A brief period of unnecessary thyroid hormone therapy is not likely to cause ill effects.

c. Serum T_4 is measured after 5 days of therapy, and the thyroxine dosage is adjusted to keep the T_4, or free T_4, value in the upper third of the normal range for age.

d. The TSH concentration may remain elevated above 20mU/L for months after treatment because of immaturity of the feedback mechanism.

e. Monitoring growth should indicate normal progression.

f. Consultation with a pediatric endocrinologist is advised.

5. Prognosis.

a. If therapy is started within the first month after birth, the prognosis for normal intellectual function is excellent.

b. In selected cases with compliant parents and identifiable normal thyroid tissue, a 6–8 week trial of thyroxine may be tried at 3 years of age to determine whether the hypothyroidism was only transient. Serum T_4 and TSH determinations must be monitored at 2 week intervals.

22

ENDOCRINE PROBLEMS

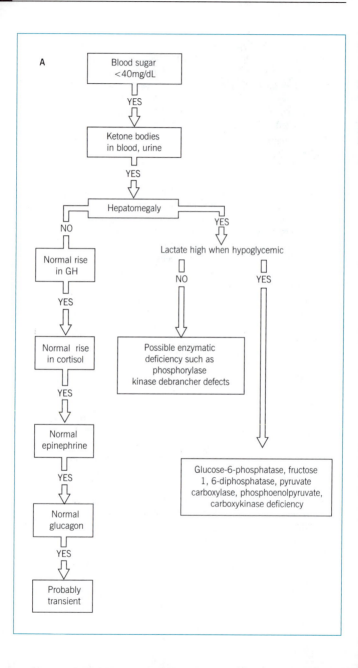

A

Blood sugar
<40mg/dL

YES

Ketone bodies
in blood, urine

YES

Hepatomegaly

NO   YES

Normal rise   Lactate high when hypoglycemic
in GH
                         NO   YES
YES

Normal rise   Possible enzymatic
in cortisol   deficiency such as
                    phosphorylase
YES   kinase debrancher defects

Normal
epinephrine

YES
                                        Glucose-6-phosphatase, fructose
Normal   1, 6-diphosphatase, pyruvate
glucagon   carboxylase, phosphoenolpyruvate,
                                        carboxykinase deficiency
YES

Probably
transient

22

ENDOCRINE PROBLEMS

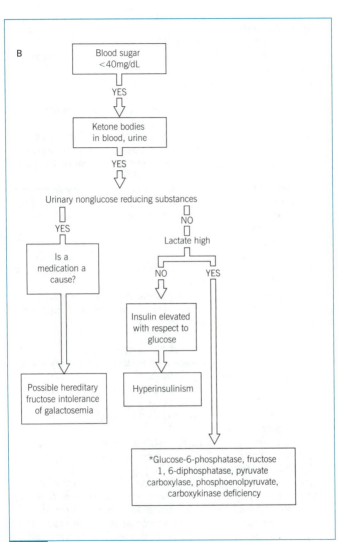

FIG. 22.2
Diagnostic schema for hypoglycemia.

B. HYPERTHYROIDISM.

Infants of mothers with hyperthyroidism may have transient hyperthyroidism. A permanent disorder can also occur sporadically, but this is extremely rare.

1. **Screening and natural history.**
a. With maternal hyperthyroidism.
    1) The T_4 values can be low, normal, or increased on the neonatal screen if the mother is receiving propylthiouracil (PTU) therapy.
    2) After 3 days or more, the maternal PTU will be eliminated, the suppressive effect will diminish, and the child will develop transient hyperthyroidism due to the persistence of maternal thyroid-stimulating immunoglobulins (TSI), usually lasting <6 weeks.
    3) Transient (≤ 6 weeks) hyperthyroidism may also occur in the infant of a mother with a history of Graves' disease treated by thyroid surgery or irradiation. TSI are still present in the mother and can cross the placenta to the infant.
b. Without maternal hyperthyroidism.
    1) Suppressed serum TSH in addition to elevated T_4 and positive TSI in the absence of maternal TSI, or history of maternal hyperthyroidism, would indicate true neonatal hyperthyroidism.
    2) Long-term therapy will usually be needed for such infants.
2. **Symptoms** include jitteriness, tachycardia, diarrhea, and hyperthermia.
3. **Treatment** depends upon whether the course is expected to be temporary or permanent.
a. Mildly affected babies may be watched prospectively.
b. Propranolol (2mg/kg/day) may be used to block the adrenergic effects of thyroxine temporarily as symptomatic therapy.
c. PTU (5–10mg/kg) is instituted (before Lugol's solution if possible) if a long course of symptoms is expected.
d. Lugol's solution of supersaturated iodine (1 drop q8h) will suppress T_4 release for several weeks.
e. Glucocorticoids have been occasionally used in severe cases.
f. Acetaminophen or a cooling blanket may be needed for hyperpyrexia.

C. THYROID HORMONE RESISTANCE.

Elevated T_4 and T_3 with elevated TSH usually indicates a form of resistance to thyroid hormone. These are rare disorders with an incidence of about 1 in 100,000 births. An autosomal dominant pattern of inheritance is usual. Those with generalized resistance to thyroid hormone (GRTH) may have developmental delay and require carefully titrated dosage of replacement thyroxine to overcome the resistance. Those with primarily pituitary resistance to thyroid hormone (PRTH) will have variable peripheral manifestations but may have signs of hyperthyroidism due to the elevated TSH driving the increased thyroid gland secretion of thyroid hormone which may encounter little to no resistance in peripheral tissues. Individual patterns of treatment are required.

II. AMBIGUOUS GENITALIA – INTERSEX PROBLEMS

The appearance of ambiguous genitalia must be considered a psychosocial emergency. The family should not be told the presumed sex of the child until the determination of sex has been firmly established. A pediatric endocrinologist experienced in such disorders should be involved in both acute and chronic care.

A. DIAGNOSIS.

1. **Variants.** The patient could be a male pseudohermaphrodite (a 46 XY individual with inadequate virilization), a female pseudohermaphrodite (a 46 XX individual with excess virilization), or a true hermaphrodite (Table 22.1).

22

ENDOCRINE PROBLEMS

TABLE 22.1

CAUSES OF AMBIGUOUS GENITALIA

I. Female pseudohermaphroditism

A. Congenital adrenal hyperplasia
1. p450c21 or 21-hydroxylase deficiency (most common)
2. 3 β-hydroxysteroid dehydrogenase deficiency
3. p450c11 or 11-hydroxylase deficiency
B. Maternal androgen administration

II. Male pseudohermaphroditism

A. Enzymatic defects affecting adrenal gland and testes
1. 20,22-desmolase deficiency
2. 3 β-hydroxysteroid dehydrogenase deficiency
3. p450c17 or 17-α-hydroxylase deficiency
B. Enzymatic defects only affecting the testes
1. 17, 20-desmolase deficiency
2. 17 β-oxidoreductase deficiency
C. End-organ resistance to testosterone
1. Syndrome of androgen resistance or testicular feminization (complete)
2. Syndrome of androgen resistance or testicular feminization (incomplete)
D. Localized enzymatic defect in sexual skin (5 α-reductase deficiency)
E. Dysgenetic testes – variants of the syndrome of gonadal dysgenesis (XO/XY) or XY gonadal dysgenesis (sometimes called pure gonadal dysgenesis)
F. Variants of the Klinefelter syndrome of seminiferous tubular dysgenesis (XXY, XXXY, etc.)

III. True hermaphroditism

2. **Examine the patient for palpable gonads.**

a. If palpable, the patient has a greater chance of being a male pseudohermaphrodite.

b. If gonads are not palpable, the infant may be a female pseudohermaphrodite or a male pseudohermaphrodite with undescended testes.

c. Ultrasound examination for cervix and uterus is useful. If the uterus is absent, the patient is most likely a male pseudohermaphrodite who is capable of making müllerian duct inhibitory substance from partially functional testes. If the uterus is present, the child could be a female pseudohermaphrodite, a male pseudohermaphrodite who has impaired testes which cannot make müllerian duct inhibitory substance, or a true hermaphrodite.

d. Perform the following laboratory tests.

   1) Plasma 17-hydroxyprogesterone, dehydroepiandrosterone, dihydrotestosterone, testosterone, androstenedione, and 11-hydroxy-cortisol to determine if an enzymatic defect is present. Request a 'rush' on the results.

   2) 24 hour urinary 17 ketosteroids, 17 hydroxy corticosteroids, and pregnanetriol excretion are difficult to collect and rarely measured now that reliable plasma measurements are available. However, some endocrine laboratories may perform detailed analysis of steroid metabolites on a spot urine to assist in diagnosis.

   3) Karyotype to determine genetic sex. This will not necessarily determine the sex of rearing but will help in diagnosis.

   4) Serum sodium and potassium levels to evaluate hyperkalemia and hypovolemia. Dehydration in adrenal insufficiency usually does not develop until the 5th to 7th day of life and can be life-threatening.

   5) No gender assignment can be made without adequate evaluation. The child should be referred to in neutral terms (e.g. 'your baby') until that time. No reference should be made to testes or ovaries or chromosomes; rather, say (e.g.) the gonads did not develop adequately. It is devastating for parents to hear a gender-related term and later hear that their child has the opposite gender.

B. MANAGEMENT OF CONGENITAL ADRENAL HYPERPLASIA.

1. **Hypoglycemia and shock** may result from absence of endogenous cortisol.

a. The normal secretion rate of cortisol is $12.5–15 mg/m^2/day$, and therapy is directed to replace this amount. In virilizing disorders, higher doses may be necessary to suppress androgen production.

b. Parenteral hydrocortisone (i.v.) at $36 mg/m^2/day$ divided into 4 doses is an appropriate beginning dose for hypoadrenal shock.

c. Intravenous preparations are immediately effective, but must be given every 4–6 hours. Intramuscular cortisone acetate is not effective until several hours after administration and, therefore, cannot be used in an emergency.

d. Intravenous glucose is important in a hypoglycemic patient.

e. Salt-losing patients will require saline infusion.

2. Parenteral and oral therapies. With early diagnosis, in absence of shock, parenteral and oral therapies are available:

a. Because intramuscular cortisone acetate lasts 3 days, one regimen is to triple the daily dose and give an injection every 3 days.

b. Oral hydrocortisone (start at 18mg/m^2/day) or cortisone acetate (start at 20–22mg/m^2/day) may be given in 3 divided doses per day.

c. While avoidance of shock is straightforward, titrating the correct dose to allow normal growth is difficult, especially in virilizing disorders: too much therapy will suppress growth and too little will allow excessive growth, virilization, and bone age advancement.

3. Mineralocorticoid therapy.

a. If salt loss has been documented, oral 9 α-hydroxy-fluorohydrocortisone (Florinef) is given at a dose of 0.05–0.10mg/day. DOCA given at 1mg/day i.m. was a classic treatment, but is not presently available.

b. Treatment with mineralocorticoids will not be effective unless sufficient sodium is administered. If the patient is NPO, normal saline may be used as the 'maintenance' intravenous fluid.

c. Salt retention and hypertension can result from excessive mineralocorticoid dosage and excessive salt administration. Blood pressure and serum electrolytes should be monitored. Plasma renin activity (PRA) is the best way to monitor salt balance and to evaluate mineralocorticoid therapy.

d. Pediatric surgeons or pediatric urologists should be consulted to plan any later reconstructive surgery.

C. MICROPENIS.

1. Definition. Micropenis is a normal-appearing penis which has a stretched length >2.5 SD less than mean. 2cm is the lower limit of length for a term infant. Measurement is made with a ruler pressed against the pubic ramus (depressing the fat completely) along the dorsum to the tip of the glans penis (eliminate the foreskin).

2. Etiology Is primary (gonadal failure), secondary (pituitary luteinizing hormone (LH) and follicle-stimulating hormone (FSH) deficiency), or tertiary (hypothalamic gonadotropin-releasing hormone deficiency) hypogonadism or partial androgen insensitivity. Growth hormone deficiency can also cause microphallus.

3. Evaluation of penile growth in response to androgen therapy is necessary to make gender assignment (without phallic growth, a male gender may prove difficult).

22

ENDOCRINE PROBLEMS

FURTHER READING

Anhalt H, Neely EK, Hintz RL. Ambiguous genitalia. *Pediatr Rev* 1966; 6:213–220.

Grumbach MM, Conte FA. Disorders of sexual differentiation. In: Williams RH, ed. *Textbook of endocrinology*. Philadelphia: Saunders; 1998.

Lee MM, Donahoe PK. The infant with ambiguous genitalia. *Curr Ther Endocrinol Metab* 1997; 6:216–223.

Styne DM. *Sexual differentiation: pediatric endocrinology for the house officer*. Boston: Williams & Wilkins; 1988: 29–45.

Styne DM. Sexual differentiation and disorders of the testes. In: Sperling MA, ed. *Pediatric endocrinology*. Philadelphia: Saunders; 1996: 423–476.

III. HYPOGLYCEMIA

A. SYMPTOMS.

1. **Subtle symptoms** such as poor feeding, apathy, lethargy, or hypotonia are most common.

2. **Serious manifestations** such as seizures, apnea, or cyanosis may occur.

3. **Onset** may be within a few hours after birth to several days of age

B. DIAGNOSIS (see Figure 22.2).

1. **Dextrostix® or other colorimetric strips** for fingerstick glucose determinations are adequate for screening, but a true blood sugar determination should be used for confirmation of hypoglycemia (blood sugar is 5mg/dL less than plasma or serum sugar, so know which test your laboratory is performing).

2. **Definition.** Previously, blood sugar <30mg/dL in a full-term infant or <20mg/dL in a premature infant was considered diagnostic of hypoglycemia; however, present practice is to maintain blood sugar >40mg/dL.

3. **In cases other than transient hypoglycemia,** it is essential to obtain serum at the time of hypoglycemia for:
   a. Glucose.
   b. Insulin.
   c. Ketones.
   d. Cortisol.
   e. Growth hormone.
   f. Lactate.
   g. Pyruvate.

4. **Extra serum** should be frozen for further specific studies.

5. **Amino acid** and/or organic acid screening is indicated if no definitive diagnosis is made from the initial test.

6. **Urinary ketone** determination should be obtained if possible.

C. PRESENTATION. Excess insulin will tend to make the glucose requirements far higher than the normal glucose production rate of 6mg/kg/min.

1. **Conditions with hyperinsulinism** (insulin level $>10^{-5}$U/mL with blood glucose ≤50mg%) are not usually associated with ketosis.

a. Transient.

    1) IDMs – hypoglycemia often occurs soon after birth following the withdrawal of the elevated maternal glucose supply

    2) Other infants experiencing the acute withdrawal of glucose: i.e. infiltration of high-rate glucose infusion

    3) Rh hemolytic disease.

b. Protracted.

    1) Beckwith–Wiedemann syndrome (with large body size, macroglossia, omphalocele)

    2) Infant giants (large head with sharp chin is characteristic)

    3) Islet cell adenomas

    4) Functional hyperinsulinism (was previously called nesidioblastosis). This condition may be autosomal recessive owing to a mutation in the high-affinity sulfonourea receptor or autosomal dominant.

1. **Conditions without hyperinsulinism.**

a. Transient hypoglycemia usually is associated with prenatal or birth complications:

    1) Intrauterine growth retardation

    2) Asphyxia or other stresses of birth

    3) Polycythemia

    4) Secondary to cardiac disease

    5) Secondary to CNS disease

    6) Sepsis

    7) Mother taking propranolol, oral hypoglycemic agents, or with narcotic addiction

    8) Secondary to other diseases.

b. Infants with protracted hypoglycemia often are born full term with no apparent complications of birth or prenatal life.

    1) Neonatal hypopituitarism including deficiencies of growth hormone (often with microphallus in males) and/or ACTH. Midline defects such as optic hypoplasia with small optic disks and nystagmus may be found (septo-optic dysplasia)

    2) Defects in carbohydrate metabolism:

    a) Glycogen storage disease Type I

    b) Glycogen synthetase deficiency

    c) Fructose 1,6-diphosphatase deficiency

    d) Fructose intolerance (onset with sucrose ingestion)

    e) Galactosemia (neonatal screening)

    f) Pyruvate carboxylase deficiency.

    3) Defects in amino acid metabolism:

a) Methylmalonic acidemia
b) Tyrosinosis
c) Propionic acidemia
d) Maple syrup urine disease.
4) Defects in organic acid metabolism.

D. THERAPY.

1. **In asymptomatic infants.**
a. Oral feedings can be tried with 10% dextrose in water or other formulas.
b. If oral feedings are not accepted, start an i.v. infusion of maintenance dextrose as below.

2. **In symptomatic infants.**
a. Give an i.v. bolus of 10% dextrose in water, 2mL/kg. (50% is too concentrated for an infant).
b. Infuse i.v. dextrose at a rate sufficient to support the blood sugar. Start with a maintenance rate of 5–7mg/kg/min. Adjust the rate upward or downward to keep blood sugar in the range 60–120mg/dL.
c. Do not abruptly decrease dextrose infusion, or rebound hypoglycemia might occur.
d. Monitor blood sugar frequently using glucose oxidase strips and confirm abnormal values with a true blood sugar.
e. When the infant is stabilized and if no persistent diagnosis is apparent, slowly decrease the dextrose infusion rate with careful monitoring of blood glucose. Aim to discontinue the infusion only if the blood glucose remains in the acceptable range.
f. After dextrose infusion is discontinued, monitor the blood sugar for at least 24 hours.

3. **Other treatment.**
a. Glucagon in doses of 300mcg/kg up to 1mg/kg by i.m. injection can be used in conditions with adequate glycogen stores such as hyperinsulinism. This is an emergency treatment.
b. Glucocorticoids are used as replacement therapy in hypoadrenal infants and can be used temporarily as pharmacologic therapy in other conditions.
c. Growth hormone is used in those infants with growth hormone deficiency.
d. Diazoxide in a dose of 5–20mg/kg/day can be used in hyperinsulinemic states and may serve as a diagnostic technique; insulinomas are far less likely to respond than functional hyperinsulinemic patients.
e. Somatostatin analogues such as octreotide are used to suppress insulin secretion. They work on different β-cell receptors than does diazoxide.
f. Pancreatectomy is reserved for intractable hypoglycemia due to

hyperinsulinism. If an isolated tumor is found, it is removed. An 85–90% pancreatectomy may be performed if a tumor is not visualized.

g. Specific diets are necessary for the metabolic diseases listed above.

E. PROGNOSIS.

1. **Asymptomatic and mild cases** usually have an excellent outcome.
2. **Symptomatic hypoglycemia** is associated with permanent CNS abnormality, so prompt therapy is essential.

FURTHER READING

Aynsley-Green A, Hawdon JM. Hypoglycemia in the neonate: current controversies. *Acta Paediatr Jpn* 1997; 39(Suppl. 1):S12–S16.

Baker L, Stanley CA. Neonatal hypoglycemia. *Curr Ther Endocrinol Metab* 1997; 6:409–413.

Cornblath M. Neonatal hypoglycemia 30 years later: does it injure the brain? Historical summary and present challenges. *Acta Paediatr Jpn* 1997; 39(Suppl. 1):S7–S11.

Halamek LP, Benaron DA, Stevenson DK. The value of neurophysiologic approaches in the anticipation and evaluation of neonatal hypoglycemia. *Acta Paediatr Jpn* 1997; 39(Suppl. 1):S33–S43.

Halamek LP, Benaron DA, Stevenson DK. Neonatal hypoglycemia, Part I: Background and definition. *Clin Pediatr* 1997; 36(12):675–680.

Sperling MA, Finefold DN. Hypoglycemia in infants. In: Sperling MA, ed. *Pediatric endocrinology*. Philadelphia: Saunders; 1996: 71–94.

Stanley CA. Hyperinsulinism in infants and children. *Pediatr Clin North Am* 1997; 44:363–374.

22

ENDOCRINE PROBLEMS

IV. ABNORMALITIES OF CALCIUM/PHOSPHORUS

Cessation of the maternal/placental supply of calcium at birth results in a prompt fall in serum total and ionized calcium to a nadir at 24–48 hours in term infants. Calcitonin in serum increases after 1–2 hours of life, peaks at 12 hours, and then falls rapidly. Parathyroid hormone (PTH) increases as serum calcium falls and serum phosphate rises. By 48–72 hours, PTH will reach adult normal or elevated values in term infants. This rise parallels the rise in serum magnesium.

A. HYPOCALCEMIA.

Hypocalcemia is defined as a serum calcium <8mg/dL in term infants and <7mg/dL in premature infants, or a serum ionized calcium <1.0mmol/L. Values >0.8mmol/L are usually tolerated in premature infants.

1. **Early neonatal hypocalcemia** in the first 3 days of life usually reflects an accentuation of the extrauterine adaptation (described above) and is usually asymptomatic and self-limiting.
a. Patients at risk.
   1) Premature infants, IDM,
   2) Asphyxiated infants are at high risk.
   3) Pre-eclampsia and postmaturity with fetal growth retardation predispose to hypocalcemia, but SGA infants as a group are not at increased risk.
   4) The use of bicarbonate, citrated blood replacement, intake of phosphate and respiratory alkalosis can all precipitate early neonatal hypocalcemia, primarily due to decreased ionized Ca (total Ca may be normal).
2. **Persistent or late hypocalcemia** after 3 days.
a. Typically occurs in term infants. With the use of modern infant formulas, the classic presentation in vitamin D-deficient populations fed cows' milk formula containing higher phosphate load is rarely encountered today. Thus, infants with late-onset hypocalcemia today more often have hypomagnesemia and/or low serum PTH and present with neurological abnormalities such as:
   1) Increased muscle tone, clonus, jitteriness
   2) Increased deep tendon reflexes
   3) Seizures.
b. Evaluation.
   1) Measure serum calcium and ionized calcium
   2) If low, measure phosphate, magnesium
   3) If persistent, measure PTH.
c. In persistent hypocalcemia, consider hypoparathyroidism with or without DiGeorge syndrome (with immune and cardiac abnormalities), abnormal renal Ca loss, and altered vitamin D metabolism. Hypoparathyroidism is heralded by low PTH, low serum Ca and high serum PO_4, while phosphate excess manifests with low serum Ca and high serum PO_4 with appropriately elevated serum PTH.
d. Pseudohypoparathyroidism is due to a PTH receptor defect as serum PTH concentrations are elevated in the face of hypocalcemia.
3. **Treatment.**
a. Treatment for asymptomatic early-onset transient hypocalcemia is controversial and may not be indicated, in view of the danger of the therapy itself. Some advocate treatment if serum Ca is <7mg/dL in term infants and <6mg/dL in premature infants or if ionized Ca is <0.85mmol/L in either.
b. Therapy for symptomatic hypocalcemia.
   1) 10% calcium gluconate, 1–2mL/kg, should be infused slowly over 5–10 minutes while monitoring the electrocardiogram for changes in QT interval and bradycardia.

2)   Make certain the i.v. line is functioning well since calcium infiltration produces tissue necrosis.

3)   *Do not* infuse concentrated calcium through an umbilical artery catheter, as severe peripheral vasospasm may ensue, producing muscle necrosis or nerve damage.

4)   *Do not* infuse through lines containing sodium bicarbonate, as calcium precipitation will occur.

c.   Seizures.

1)   Seizures in asphyxiated infants with hypocalcemia often do not respond to calcium infusion.

2)   After seizures stop in early neonatal transient hypocalcemia, 50–75mg elemental Ca/kg/day is given orally while slowly withdrawing intravenous calcium until serum Ca normalizes. See Table 22.2.

22

TABLE 22.2

CALCIUM DOSE EQUIVALENTS

1mL calcium gluconate (10%)	=	100mg calcium gluconate
1mL calcium gluconate (10%)	=	9mg elemental calcium
1mL calcium gluceptate (22%)	=	18mg elemental calcium
1mL calcium chloride (10%)	=	27mg elemental calcium
1mEq calcium	=	20mg calcium

d.   Hypomagnesemia may be associated with hypocalcemia. Magnesium levels <1.6mg/dL should be treated with 50% magnesium sulfate, at 6mg/kg or 0.12mL/kg, i.m. or i.v. Magnesium sulfate should be infused over 1 hour with careful cardiac monitoring. Correction of serum Mg will normalize PTH function and serum Ca in some cases.

e.   Chronic therapy for hypoparathyroidism. Vitamin D must be used in addition to additional calcium supplements. 1,25-dihydroxy vitamin D (calcitriol) is the usual preparation indicated in dosage of 0.03–0.08mcg/kg/day orally starting with the lower dosages. Phosphate-lowering agents may be needed as well.

B. NEONATAL RICKETS.

Premature infants may develop hypomineralization of bone or frank rickets, sometimes associated with low serum calcium. Often there is a history of severe BPD and chronic diuretic therapy with Lasix. Phosphate deficiency may predominate.

1. Evaluation.

a.   Monitor serum calcium and phosphorus twice a week in infants at risk.

b.   Alk-Phos is measured, but cannot be used as sole indicator of rickets, because of poor correlation with other biochemical and radiographic findings in this age group.

ENDOCRINE PROBLEMS

c. Evaluation of bone mineralization is necessary when biochemical abnormalities are noted. Routine radiographic screening at 6–9 weeks can be justified to identify severe osteopenia in at-risk neonates.

d. Evaluate serum PTH if bone is abnormal.

e. Severe demineralization occurs most frequently when a phosphorus deficiency is superimposed on 25-hydroxycholecalciferol (25-OHD) deficiency. Previously, human milk and infant formulas did not meet the needs of the very small premature infant, leading to a classical phosphate-deficiency rickets, but new formulas and human breast milk fortifiers have lowered the incidence.

f. With severe vitamin D deficiency, osteopenia, low normal calcium, low phosphorus, high Alk-Phos, an elevated PTH, and generalized aminoaciduria are seen. Parenteral doses of vitamin D as low as 25IU can guard against the condition.

2. Therapy for rickets.

a. Improved mineralization may be seen on a high-calcium–high-phosphorus formula.

b. Infants with rickets or severe osteopenia due to true vitamin D deficiency have been successfully treated with oral vitamin D at a dose of 1000–2000IU/day for 6–12 weeks or oral 1,25-dihydroxy-cholecalciferol ($1,25(OH)_2D$) in doses of 0.04–0.08mcg/kg/day (up to a maximum of 1–2mcg/day).

C. HYPERCALCEMIA.

Hypercalcemia occurs infrequently in neonates and is associated with several rare disorders. Signs and symptoms can be extremely serious and include weakness, anorexia, lethargy, hypertonia, seizures, polyuria, and polydipsia, leading to dehydration, hypertension, and renal failure (due to metastatic calcification in the kidney or kidney stones).

1. Neonatal hyperparathyroidism.

a. Presentation: parathyroid hyperplasia by autosomal dominant, autosomal recessive modes of inheritance or as a sporadic case is the most common cause of primary hyperparathyroidism in the neonate. Bone demineralization is common with low serum Ca, PO_4, and PTH and elevated Alk-Phos. The differential diagnosis includes maternal hypoparathyroidism leading to compensatory, transient neonatal hyperparathyroidism.

b. Therapy: subtotal parathyroidectomy is usually appropriate. Following surgery, therapy with calcium and vitamin D analogs may be required, depending upon the amount of tissue removed.

2. Maternal hypoparathyroidism with fetal parathyroid gland hyperplasia.

a. Presentation: hypercalcemia is usually transient, though skeletal lesions may be evident.

b. Therapy: both hypercalcemia and bone erosions usually return to normal without specific therapy.

3. **Idiopathic infantile hypercalcemia (IIH).**

a. Presentation: normal facial features, transient hypercalcemia, osteosclerosis, and clinical stigmata of hypercalcemia – thirst, dehydration, fever. Affected infants are alert, with normal birth weight; mild azotemia and leukocyturia with granular casts are common. There is hypercalcemia, hypercalciuria, and possibly nephrocalcinosis. High serum concentrations of $1,25(OH)_2D$ have been found.

b. Therapy: reduce intake of vitamin D and dietary calcium. Treatment with calcitonin has been effective in lowering serum calcium levels. A meat-based formula has been used successfully. Glucocorticoids will also block intestinal calcium absorption and have been used in short-term bursts.

4. **Williams' syndrome with elfin facies.**

a. Presentation: an association of hypercalcemia, cardiac lesion (commonly, supravalvular aortic stenosis), and peculiar facies, (ocular hypertelorism, depressed nasal bridge, short palpebral fissures, full prominent lips with an open mouth, malar hypoplasia, and anteverted nares). Low birth weight is common. Most patients have an ultimate IQ between 40 and 80. A gene abnormality has been found in many cases, and DNA probes are available for clinical testing.

b. Therapy: hypercalcemia is transient and only rarely requires a low-calcium, low-vitamin D diet.

5. **Fat necrosis.** These infants are either premature or SGA or have evidence of perinatal stress (hypothermia, hypoxia, birth trauma). The infants develop very high serum calcium values, 16–22mg/dL, and tender, bluish-red discolored areas of induration in the subcutaneous fat. All the consequences of hypercalcemia (azotemia, nephrocalcinosis, subcutaneous dystrophic calcification, and growth retardation) are seen. Extremely high calcium concentrations can be fatal. The hypercalcemia usually resolves in a few weeks.

6. **Severe infantile hypophosphatasia.** Rare autosomal recessive disorder characterized by hypercalcemia, severe bone demineralization, low serum Alk-Phos, elevated urinary phosphoethanolamine, and premature loss of teeth.

7. **Familial hypocalciuric hypercalcemia** is an autosomal dominant condition. While many infants have no serious morbidity, life-threatening hypercalcemia may result from homozygosity or inheritance of the gene from the father: both situations cause primary hyperparathyroidism, sometimes requiring surgery. Urinary calcium excretion is low, and nephrocalcinosis, stone formation, and azotemia are rare.

22

ENDOCRINE PROBLEMS

8. **Maternal vitamin D toxicity.** Unlikely to cause more than transient hypercalcemia.

a. A low-calcium diet with decreased vitamin D intake is the initial step for milder cases.

b. Other steps include the use of glucocorticoids (hydrocortisone 1 mg/kg body weight every 6 hours while calcium remains high, to decrease gut absorption of Ca), calcitonin (10 units/kg intravenously to decrease Ca release from the bone), and increased hydration with the use of calcium-losing diuretics.

FURTHER READING

Mimouni FB, Root AW. Disorders of calcium metabolism in the newborn. In: Sperling MA, ed. *Pediatric endocrinology.* Philadelphia: Saunders; 1996: 95–116.

Mimouni FB, Root AW. Parathyroid and vitamin D related disorders in children and adolescents. In: Sperling MA, ed. *Pediatric endocrinology.* Philadelphia: Saunders; 1996: 477–508.

NEWBORN SCREENING FOR GENETIC AND METABOLIC DISORDERS

Newborn screening programs, using blood specimens collected on filter paper and sent to regional laboratories, exist in each state of the US. Ten disorders can currently be screened for, but test panels vary from state to state.

I. PHENYLKETONURIA

A. **ETIOLOGY.** A single-gene autosomal recessive disorder resulting in decreased activity of phenylalanine hydroxylase, an enzyme which converts phenylalanine to tyrosine (located on chromosome 12q22–q24.1; 100 mutations are known).

B. **PREVALENCE.** Average for United States is 1:21,500 live births.

C. **DIAGNOSTIC SCREENING.** Phenylalanine >2–4mg/dL depending on method used.

D. **CONFIRMATION.** Amino acid panel; tetrahydrobiopterin disorders panel

E. **TREATMENT.**
1. **Low-phenylalanine diet** for life.
2. **Phenylalanine-free amino acid drink** to replace $80\pm10\%$ of daily protein intake.
3. **Monitor dietary therapy** and maintain serum phenylalanine in range 120–360μmol/L (2–6mg/dL).

F. **OUTCOME.**
1. **Normal development** in appropriately treated child.
2. **Elevated phenylalanine during period of brain growth** (<5 years of age) may lead to permanent learning disabilities.

II. HYPOTHYROIDISM
See Chapter 22, Endocrine Problems.

III. GALACTOSEMIA

A. **ETIOLOGY.** A single-gene autosomal recessive disorder involving decreased activity of galactose-1-phosphate uridyl transferase (GALT), resulting in elevated levels of galactose and galactose-1-phosphate in lactose-fed infants (located on chromosome 9p13; 13 known mutations).

B. **PREVALENCE.** Average for United States is 1:80,000 births.

C. **SCREENING.** Low enzyme activity, elevated galactose (>10mg/dL).

D. **DIAGNOSTIC CONFIRMATION.** Quantatitive assay for GALT and galactose-1-phosphate; genotyping of newborn and parents.

E. **TREATMENT.**

1. **Lactose-free diet for life.** Formula, soy, or meat based (Isomil®, Soyalac®, Prosobee®, Good Start-soy®, Nutramigen®).

2. **Monitor dietary therapy** and maintain serum galactose-1-phosphate <0.68µmoL/g Hb.

F. **OUTCOME.**

1. **Near normal development** in appropriately treated child although 50% have speech difficulties; fewer have learning disabilities.

2. **Ovarian failure** due to prenatal toxicity.

3. **Untreated** have mental retardation, cataracts, liver damage, failure to thrive, increased risk for infection.

IV. MAPLE SYRUP URINE DISEASE (MSUD) BRANCHED CHAIN KETO

A. **ETIOLOGY.** Multiple-gene autosomal recessive disorders resulting in decreased oxidation of branched-chain amino acids (located on chromosomes 19q13.1–q13.2, 1p31, 6p22–p21, 7q31–q32; known mutations 4, 4, 1, 5, respectively).

B. **PREVALENCE.** 1:200,000 births worldwide. Ten cases in US for 1992; among Mennonites of eastern Pennsylvania, classic MSUD as high as 1 in 176 births.

C. **SCREENING.** Serum leucine >4mg/dL.

D. **DIAGNOSTIC CONFIRMATION.** Quantatitive amino acid panel; keto acid decarboxylase activity.

E. **TREATMENT.**

1. **Low leucine, isoleucine, and valine diet for life.** Replace $80\pm10\%$ of daily protein intake with leucine-, isoleucine-, and valine-free amino acid drink.

2. **Evaluate thiamine responsiveness.**

3. **Monitor dietary therapy** and maintain serum leucine, isoleucine, and valine below 195µmol/L, 105µmol/L, 300µmol/L, respectively.

F. **OUTCOME.**

1. **Near-normal development** for milder forms.

2. **Intellectual impairment** despite dietary intervention if treatment is started after newborn becomes symptomatic (~10 days of age).

3. **Severe forms** are usually lethal in early infancy.

V. HOMOCYSTINURIA

A. **ETIOLOGY.** A single-gene autosomal recessive disorder with decreased activity of the cystathionine-ß-synthase in the pathway for conversion of homocysteine to cystathionine (located on chromosome 21q22.3; 9 mutations known).

B. **PREVALENCE.** 1:200,000 live births worldwide.
C. **SCREENING.** Methionine >2–4mg/dL.
D. **DIAGNOSTIC CONFIRMATION.** Quantitative amino acids; cystathionine-ß-synthase activity.
E. **TREATMENT.**
1. **Evaluate vitamin B$_6$ responsiveness;** daily pharmacologic dose.
2. **Vitamin B$_6$ nonresponders** require low-methionine diet for life. Replace 80±10% protein intake with methionine-free amino acid drink. Supplement dietary cystine. Monitor and maintain serum methionine, cystine, and homocystine levels 18–45μmol/L, 25–50μmol/L, zero to trace, respectively.
F. **OUTCOME.**
1. **Early intervention** results in near-normal development, reduced rate of lens dislocation, probably reduced seizures.
2. **Long-term study** needed to evaluate early treatments effect on thromboembolism and osteoporosis.

VI. TYROSINEMIA

A. **ETIOLOGY.** A single-gene autosomal recessive disorder with decreased activity of the fumarylacetoacetate hydrolase in the tyrosine catabolism pathway (located on chromosome 15q23–q25). Four other genetic disorders are recognized in this pathway
B. **PREVALENCE.** 1:110,000 live births worldwide; high incidence in Quebec (1:1846).
C. **SCREENING.** Tyrosine >6–12mg/dL.
D. **DIAGNOSTIC CONFIRMATION.** Quantitative amino acids, succinylacetone, fumarylacetonacetate hydrolase in selected cases.
E. **TREATMENT.**
1. **Low phenylalanine and tyrosine diet** for life.
2. **High carbohydrate diet** to reduce transcription of D-amino-levulinic acid synthase gene.
F. **OUTCOME.** Early intervention provides improved renal tubular function, but progression of cirrhosis is unchanged. Controversy regarding long-term benefits of diet therapy.

VII. SICKLE CELL ANEMIA, β-THALASSEMIA, α-THALASSEMIA

ETIOLOGY. Multiple-gene autosomal recessive genetic disorders of hemoglobin synthesis (located on chromosomes 11p15.5, 16p13.3; >400 mutations known).
B. **PREVALENCE.** Average in United States is 1:4000 live births, wide range observed due to racial/ethnic distribution of genes.
C. **SCREENING.** Hemoglobin identification.
D. **DIAGNOSTIC CONFIRMATION** by thin-layer isoelectric focusing, densiometric scanning, citrate agar electrophoresis, and/or quantitative hemoglobin.

E. **TREATMENT.** Penicillin prophylaxis in sickle cell disease and counseling.

F. **OUTCOME.** Reduction of morbidity and mortality due to infections; improved growth.

VIII. BIOTINIDASE

A. **ETIOLOGY.** Single-gene recessive disorder with decreased activity of biotinidase, necessary for biotin recycling. Biotin is a cofactor for four carboxylase enzymes involved with glucogenesis, fatty acid synthesis, and amino acid catabolism (located on chromosome 3p25; 7 known mutations).

B. **PREVALENCE.** Average for the United States is 1:60,000 births.

C. **SCREENING AND DIAGNOSTIC CONFIRMATION.** Biotinidase <30% activity.

D. **TREATMENT.** Biotin supplementation.

E. **OUTCOME.** Normal if recognized early and hypoglycemia is not severe. Untreated complications include seizures, hearing loss, optic nerve atrophy, skin rash, and hair loss.

IX. CONGENITAL ADRENAL HYPERPLASIA

A. **ETIOLOGY.** A single-gene autosomal recessive disorder resulting in decreased activity of adrenal 21-hydroxylase, necessary for conversion of 17-hydroxyprogesterone to 11-deoxycortisol in the production of cortisol and aldosterone (located on chromosome 6p21.3; 23 known mutations).

B. **PREVALENCE.** 1:12,000 live births in the United States.

C. **SCREENING.** 17-Hydroxyprogesterone >40ng/mL (borderline), >90ng/mL (strongly positive; level depends on age and birth weight at time of collection).

D. **DIAGNOSTIC CONFIRMATION.** Basal and adrenocorticotropin (ACTH)-stimulated 17-hydroxyprogesterone.

E. **TREATMENT.** Hydrocortisone. Aldosterone-deficient need mineralocorticoid and salt.

F. **OUTCOME.**

1. Reduction of mortality of males due to adrenal crisis.

2. Long-term skin pigmentation changes.

X. CYSTIC FIBROSIS

A. **ETIOLOGY.** A single-gene autosomal recessive disorder affecting apical membrane chloride ion channels (located on chromosome 7q31.2; 600 known mutations).

B. **PREVALENCE.** 1:3700 births worldwide.

C. **SCREENING.** Immunoreactive trypsin >56 units/mL.

D. **DIAGNOSTIC CONFIRMATION.** Sweat test; genetic probes.

E. **TREATMENT.** Early nutritional supplementation, pancreatic enzyme
   therapy, pulmonary care.
F. **OUTCOME.**
1. **Improved growth** with early treatment for nutritional deficiencies.
2. **Morbidity/survival** – effect of early treatments is unknown.

FURTHER READING

Applegarth DA, Dimmick JE, Toone JR. Laboratory detection of metabolic
   disease. *Pediatr Clin North Am* 1989; 36:49–65.

Burton DK. Inborn errors of metabolism: the clinical diagnosis in early
   infancy. *Pediatrics* 1987; 79:359.

Clayton PT, Thompson E. Dysmorphic syndromes with demonstrable
   biochemical abnormalities. *J Med Genet* 1988; 25:463.

Moser AB, Rasmussen M, Naidu S et al. Phenotype of patients with
   peroxisomal disorders subdivided into sixteen complementation groups.
   J Pediatr 1995; 127:13–22.

Scriver CR, Beaudet AB, William WS, Valle D, eds. *The metabolic and
   molecular bases of inherited disease*, 7th edition. New York: McGraw-
   Hill; 1995.

Ward JC. Inborn errors of metabolism of acute onset in infancy. *Pediatr
   Rev* 1990; 11:205.

23

SCREENING FOR GENETIC AND METABOLIC DISORDERS

SERIOUS INHERITED METABOLIC DISEASE

I. GENERAL CONSIDERATIONS

Individually, inherited metabolic diseases presenting in the neonate are rare, but in aggregate they are not uncommon. Most inborn errors of metabolism present as a sepsis-like syndrome but, in some, specific organ dysfunction, such as muscle weakness, seizures, or cardiomyopathy, dominates the clinical picture. Unless a previously born child is affected, a family history of unexplained neonatal deaths or morbidity is uncommon since most are rare autosomal disorders.

A. TYPICAL PRESENTATION.
1. **Unexplained deterioration** in clinical status.
2. **Differential diagnosis.** Septic shock, coma, delayed renal failure, seizures, bleeding and hemolytic disorders, jaundice, hypoglycemia, persistent metabolic acidosis.
3. **Family history.** Early unexplained neonatal deaths (uncommon, since most are autosomal recessive).

B. DIAGNOSTIC SCREENING.
1. **Serum electrolytes,** anion gap.
2. **Blood** pH, ammonia, lactate, ketones, glucose, BUN. Most life-threatening metabolic diseases presenting in the newborn are accompanied by metabolic acidosis and/or hyperammonemia.
3. **Urinalysis and metabolic screen.** Specific gravity, reducing substance, ninhydrin, $FeCl_2$, 2,4-dinitro-phenylhydrazine.
4. **Organic acid analysis in urine.** Amino acid analysis in plasma, urine.

C. TREATMENT – BASIC PRINCIPLES.
1. **Maintain maximum calories** with glucose to prevent catabolism (100–150cal/kg).
2. **Add glucose, fat, and protein** sequentially.
3. **If the patient is severely ill:**
   a. Attempt to remove toxic metabolites by exchange transfusion, peritoneal dialysis, or hemodialysis.
   b. Provide high concentrations of B vitamins and carnitine (Table 24.1).
   c. Maintain high fluid intake to increase urine output to optimize renal excretion of toxins.

D. IF THE PATIENT IS DYING.
1. **Premortem.** Save 3–5mL of heparinized blood, 3–5mL of plasma serum, and 5–10mL of urine.
   a. Separate RBCs for enzyme studies and plasma for toxins.
   b. Refrigerate RBCs.

TABLE 24.1

MEGAVITAMIN REGIMEN FOR UNDIAGNOSED SEVERE METABOLIC DISEASE[a]

Thiamine	20–50mg/day	i.v.
Hydroxycobalamine(vit B12)	1–2mg/day	i.m./i.v.
Riboflavin	100–300mg/day	i.v.
Biotin	20–40mg/day	p.o.
Carnitine	100mg/kg/day	i.v.
L-arginine-Cl$_2$[b]	4mmol/kg (800mg/kg)	i.v. bolus
	200–800mg/kg/day	i.v.
Sodium benzoate[b,c]	250mg/kg	i.v. bolus
	250–500mg/kg/day	i.v.

[a]Administer after obtaining plasma/urine for amino acid, organic acid assays.
[b]For hyperammonemia.
[c]Only for patients with low serum bilirubin and good urine output.

c. Freeze urine, plasma, and serum specimen at −20°C (−70°C preferred).

2. Postmortem. Examination must be performed immediately after death. The need for immediate examination often must be discussed with the parents before death occurs.

a. Obtain a skin biopsy for fibroblast culture.
    1) Prepare skin and use sterile technique.
    2) Place in viral culture media (nutrients plus antibiotics).
b. Obtain tissue samples, 1–5g of liver, muscle, kidney, brain.
    1) For enzyme analysis, freeze immediately in liquid nitrogen or in isopentane chilled on dry ice and stored at −70°C.
    2) For electron microscopy (EM) studies, fix fresh tissue in glutaraldehyde.

II. SPECIFIC DISORDERS PRESENTING IN THE NEWBORN PERIOD

A. TRANSIENT HYPERAMMONEMIA.

1. Usual presentation. Most cases are larger premature infants weighing 1500–2500g, who have respiratory disease. Lethargy progresses to coma, decorticate or decerebrate posturing, and seizures. Oliguria and sclerema are common. Hyperammonemia may attain >3000mg/dL, usually peaking by the 3rd to 5th day of life.

2. Diagnosis. Suspect this disorder in a newborn with a rapidly rising ammonia level in the absence of protein load. Diagnosis is confirmed by rapid resolution. Etiology is unknown.

3. Treatment. Ventilatory support is usually required. The rise in ammonia may be modified by hemodialysis. Repeated exchange transfusions and peritoneal dialysis are far less effective. Maintain low protein intake. Administer sodium benzoate, 250mg i.v. followed by a continuous infusion of 250–500mg/kg/day if the serum bilirubin concentration is low (benzoate displaces bilirubin from albumin). The disease usually resolves spontaneously by 2 weeks of age.

4. **Outcome.** Residual brain damage may be less than in other forms of hyperammonemia.

B. HYPERAMMONEMIA DUE TO UREA CYCLE ENZYME DEFICIENCIES.

1. **Usual presentation.** Periodic vomiting, lethargy, and CNS signs leading to coma, seizures, or both. May mimic transient hyperammonemia, but onset is usually more gradual and related to the quantity of protein intake. Hypoglycemia and metabolic acidosis may occur in citrullinemia.

2. **Diagnosis.** Suspect this disorder if the blood ammonia level is >300mg/dL and rises progressively with continued feeding. Obtain plasma and urine amino acid levels to identify elevations in Krebs cycle intermediates and urine orotic acid. Hyperammonemia in association with severe metabolic acidosis is usually due to organic acidemia (e.g. propionic and methylmalonic acidemias).

3. **Etiology.** Four urea cycle enzymes have been reported to produce overwhelming disease in the newborn (Figure 24.1):

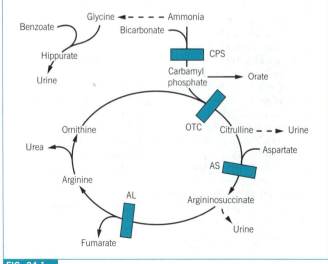

FIG. 24.1

Inborn errors in urea cycle. CPS, carbamyl phosphate synthetase; OTC, ornithine transcarbamylase; AS, argininosuccinic acid synthetase; AL, argininosuccinate lyase.

24

SERIOUS INHERITED METABOLIC DISEASE

a. Ornithine transcarbamylase: sex linked and lethal in males.
b. Carbamyl phosphate synthetase, citrullinemia (argininosuccinic acid synthetase), and argininosuccinic aciduria (friable hair) (arginosuccinate lysase) are probably autosomal recessive.
4. **Treatment.** Emergency treatment as in transient hyperammonemia. Give arginine 4mmol/kg (0.8g/kg) i.v. bolus. Maintain low protein intake. Administer a special diet. Diets with α-keto analogs of amino acids are experimental.

C. LACTIC ACIDOSIS WITH HYPOGLYCEMIA.

1. **Usual presentation.** Symptoms are related to hypoglycemia and acidosis (tachypnea).
2. **Diagnosis.** Hypoglycemia and lactic acidosis are responsive to glucose infusion. If the infant is receiving formula containing sucrose, suspect fructose intolerance. If he is taking a milk formula, suspect galactosemia (rarely a cause of severe hypoglycemia). Perform a liver biopsy for morphological findings and enzyme assay. Do a glucagon challenge test.
3. **Etiology.** Elevated lactate level is secondary to a block in gluconeogenesis (Figure 24.2). The most common causes are as follows.
a. Glycogen storage disease type I (Von Gierke's disease): glucose-6-phosphatase deficiency.
b. Fructose intolerance: aldolase B deficiency (presents only after feeding fructose).
c. Fructose-1,6-diphosphatase deficiency.
d. Phosphoenol pyruvate kinase deficiency.
4. **Treatment.** Fructose-free diet in adolase B deficiency. Continuous or frequent feedings of carbohydrate in type I storage disease.
5. **Outcome.** Variable; requires early and aggressive treatment.

D. LACTIC ACIDOSIS WITHOUT HYPOGLYCEMIA.

1. **Usual presentation.** In severe forms, patients are SGA, often with minor congenital defects, microcephalic with large ventricles, compensated severe metabolic acidosis (may become alkalotic if corrected with bicarbonate), frequently premature, and they fail to grow. Milder forms may simply have lethargy or poor coordination and are frequently asymptomatic unless stressed with a high carbohydrate load or illness.
2. **Diagnosis.** Lactic acidosis worsens on high carbohydrate load, and improves on a high-fat, low-carbohydrate diet. Specific enzyme assay on skin or liver biopsy.

3. **Etiology.** Usually involves primary or secondary blocks in either pyruvate carboxylase or the pyruvate dehydrogenase complex (Figure 24.2). Severe carboxylase deficiency may also cause hypoglycemia.
4. **Treatment.** If secondary, treat the underlying defect. If primary, a high-fat, low-carbohydrate diet may ameliorate lactic acidosis and symptoms, but will not significantly alter prognosis in infants affected prenatally. Megavitamin treatment with thiamine and biotin may be helpful.

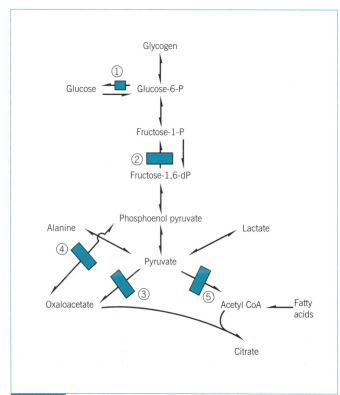

24

SERIOUS INHERITED METABOLIC DISEASE

FIG. 24.2

Inborn errors in carbohydrate metabolism, enzyme deficiencies producing lactic acidosis: (1) glucose-6-phosphatase (glycogen storage disease); (2) fructose-1,6-diphosphatase; (3) pyruvate carboxylase ($+CO_2$, biotin dependent); (4) phosphoenol carboxykinase (? decreased in SGA infants); (5) pyruvate dehydrogenase ($-CO_2$, thiamine, lipoic acid dependent). Defects in (1)–(4) are associated with hypoglycemia. Severe forms of (5) are associated with intrauterine impairment of brain development and growth.

5. **Outcome.** Microcephaly, failure to thrive, or severe mental retardation is inevitable in severe cases.

E. ORGANIC ACIDEMIAS.

1. **Maple syrup urine disease:** branched-chain aminoaciduria involving leucine, isoleucine, valine.

a. Usual presentation: apathy, hypertonia or hypotonia, and tonic seizures often in association with hypoglycemia. Death occurs without treatment. The typical maple syrup odor in urine may not be present.

b. Diagnosis: α-keto organic acids in urine are detected by 2,4-dinitro-phenylhydrazine. Branched-chain amino acid levels are elevated in plasma.

c. Etiology: defect in metabolism of branched chains and their keto acid analogs. Autosomal recessive.

d. Treatment: high-dose thiamine trial (most forms not responsive). Peritoneal dialysis. Special formulas are available.

e. Outcome: guarded prognosis for life or normal development.

2. **Disorders of propionic acid metabolism:** Propionic acidemia, ketotic hyperglycinemia, methymalonic acidemia.

a. Usual presentation: lethargy, vomiting, profound metabolic acidosis, coma. Less severe forms have mild acidosis, failure to thrive, vomiting.

b. Diagnosis: large anion gap, ketoacidosis, hyperammonemia (frequently), hyperglycinemia, elevated branched-chain amino acid levels. Elevated methylmalonic acid or propionic acid levels differentiate the three conditions. Enzyme deficiency detected in WBCs, liver, fibroblasts.

c. Treatment: restrict protein. One form of methylmalonic acidemia responds to high doses of cofactor vitamin B12. Special formulas are available.

d. Outcome: most patients do poorly and have mental retardation. Death usually occurs in the newborn period or with exacerbations.

F. PEROXISOMAL DISORDERS.

1. **Zellweger-like syndromes:** Zellweger syndrome, hyperpipecolic acidemia, infantile Refsum disease, adreno-leukodystrophy, Acyl-CoA oxidase deficiency.

a. Usual presentation: dysmorphic features, hypotonia, renal cortical cysts, epiphyseal stippling, hepatomegaly, severe retardation and early death (Zellweger). Other forms have similar but milder presentations.

b. Diagnosis: increased long-chain fatty acids, pipecolic acid in urine. The ratio of plasma very-long fatty acids (C26:0/C22:0) is an effective screening test for peroxisomal diseases. Muscle biopsy or fibroblasts have decreased or abnormal peroxisomes. Acyl-CoA oxidase deficiency is a specific peroxisomal enzyme defect with normal peroxisomes.

c. Treatment: there is no effective treatment.

G. CARNITINE DEFICIENCY. Carnitine is important in transporting long-chain fatty acids across the inner mitochondrial membrane. Carnitine deficiency in the newborn is usually secondary to increased metabolism of carnitine by acyl-CoA in organic acidemia, fatty acid ß-oxidation defects, and urea cycle defects.

1. **Usual presentation.** Decreased energy metabolism, dilated myocardiopathy.

2. **Diagnosis.** Plasma/urine carnitine, free carnitine, acylcarnitine. Plasma carnitine may be normal, but acylcarnitine will be elevated in urine and plasma.

3. **Treatment.** Supplemental carnitine may be 'lifesaving' in branched-chain organic acidemias. Supplementation in β-oxidation defects is controversial.

H. PATIENTS PRESENTING WITH SEIZURES/CNS ABNORMALITIES. (See also Chapter 16, sections I and II.)

1. **Pyridoxine-dependent seizures.**

a. Usual presentation: persistent unexplained seizures unresponsive to medication. Some forms respond to benzodiazepines.

b. Diagnosis/treatment: administer pyridoxine, 100mg i.v., while measuring EEG. Seizures usually cease immediately.

2. **Nonketotic hyperglycinemia.**

a. Usual presentation: profound neurological signs characterized by hypotonia, lethargy, poor feeding, coma, seizures, apnea.

b. Diagnosis: plasma glycine level is increased 2–20 times normal. CSF glycine should be measured.

c. Etiology: block in the glycine cleavage system to form methyl tetrahydrofolic acid. Mechanism of profound CNS signs is unknown.

d. Treatment: no effective therapy is known, although methionine and sodium benzoate may reduce the plasma glycine level.

e. Outcome: about 1/3 of the patients die in the first 2 weeks. Severe brain damage and early death usually result.

3. **Sulfite oxidase deficiency.**

a. Usual presentation: axial hypotonia and peripheral hypertonia, seizures.

b. Diagnosis: increased urinary sulfite, thiosulfate, S-sulfocysteine; decreased urinary cystine.

c. Outcome: no effective therapy is known. Microcephaly and death frequently in the first year.

24

SERIOUS INHERITED METABOLIC DISEASE

FURTHER READING

Applegarth DA, Dimmick JE, Toone JR. Laboratory detection of metabolic disease. *Pediatr Clin North Am* 1989; 36:49.

Burton DK. Inborn errors of metabolism: the clinical diagnosis in early infancy. *Pediatrics* 1987; 79:359.

Clayton PT, Thompson E. Dysmorphic syndromes with demonstrable biochemical abnormalities. *J Med Genet* 1988; 25:463.

Moser AB, Rasmussen M, Naidu S et al, eds. Phenotype of patients with peroxisomal disorders divided into sixteen complementation groups. *J Pediatr* 1995; 127:13.

Scriver CR, Stanbury JB, Wyngaarden JB et al, eds. *The metabolic and molecular bases of inherited disease,* 7th edition. New York: McGraw-Hill; 1995.

Ward JC. Inborn errors of metabolism of acute onset in infancy. *Pediatr Rev* 1990; 11:205.

TRANSIENT IMMUNOLOGIC DISORDERS

The offspring of women with certain immunologic disorders may be transiently affected during the neonatal period as a result of transplacental passage of gamma globulins, and other immunologic substances, during the third trimester.

I. IDIOPATHIC THROMBOCYTOPENIC PURPURA

A. MATERNAL.
a. ITP is the most common autoimmune disorder recognized during pregnancy.
b. Associated with premature labor, bleeding complications, and pre-eclampsia.
c. Caused by IgG antiplatelet antibodies which may cross placenta.
d. Platelet count and bleeding severity varies.
e. Treatment of mother with steroids or, preferably, intravenous gamma globulin also treats the fetus.

B. FETAL/NEONATAL.
a. About 50% of offspring of women with ITP are affected.
b. Thrombocytopenia may predispose to hemorrhage during labor and delivery, particularly intracranial or intra-adrenal.
c. Maternal antiplatelet antibodies and fetal scalp platelet counts predict neonatal platelet count better than maternal platelet count.

C. TREATMENT.
a. Prevention by maternal treatment with steroids or intravenous immunoglobulin (IVIG).
b. IVIG to neonate.
   1) 0.4g/kg/day for 5 days administered over 3–4 hours.
   2) Alternative dose: 1.0g/kg/day as 5% solution in 0.9% saline over 12 hours on two consecutive days.
   3) Appears to act by blocking Fc receptors in reticuloendothelial system.
   4) Rapid response – <24 hours.
c. Corticosteroids produce slow response – days.
d. Platelet infusions and exchange transfusion are not usually effective.
e. Infant recovers in 5–7 days.

D. ISOIMMUNE NEONATAL THROMBOCYTOPENIA.
a. Rare but often severe. Mother's platelet count is normal.
b. Mother has no platelet antigen and makes antibodies to fetal platelets, if sensitized.

c.   Transfusion of platelets from random donors will not raise platelet count.
d.   Treat by infusing maternal platelets or with IVIG as for ITP.

II. NEONATAL THYROTOXICOSIS/CONGENITAL HYPERTHYROIDISM

A. MATERNAL.
a.   Usually there is history of Graves' disease (hyperthyroidism).
b. T_4, T_3, and TSH do not cross placenta in humans.
c.   Antithyroid antibodies of IgG class do cross placenta.
d.   Antithyroid agents like propylthiouracil and iodine also cross placenta.
e.   Toxemia, prematurity, and fetal growth retardation may occur with maternal Graves' disease.
f.   Treatment of mother with PTU, 100–300mg/day, and T_4 seems preferred and also treats fetus.

B. FETAL/NEONATAL.
a.   Only 2% of offspring of women with Graves' disease are affected.
b.   Symptoms are usually delayed for a few days after birth owing to maternal treatment and the normal switch at birth from producing reverse T_3 to producing T_3.
c.   Symptoms include irritability, flushing, tachycardia, and hypertension.
d.   Arrhythmias, heart failure, and death may occur if untreated.
e.   Growth failure, craniosynostosis, and mental retardation have been reported.
f.   Maternal thyroid-stimulating immunoglobulins (TSI) of IgG class cross placenta and cause fetal and neonatal disease.
g.   Infant usually recovers by 8–12 weeks but rare cases last up to 1 year.

C. MANAGEMENT OF THE NEONATE.
a.   Measure cord blood serum T_4 and TSH (normals 6–15µg/dL and 1–20µU/mL, respectively).
b.   Repeat above studies on day 2 or 3 when they typically become elevated.
c.   Avoid early discharge.
d.   Transient hypothyroidism may occur due to maternal PTU treatment and it may require treatment.
e.   Treatment of thyrotoxicosis.
   1)   PTU, 5–10mg/kg/day is usual.
   2)   Iodine, 8mg q8h, may be added.
   3)   Propranolol, 2mg/kg/day in 3 divided doses, is useful when tachycardia is marked.

III. MYASTHENIA GRAVIS

A. MATERNAL.
a.   Affects 1 in 20,000 persons in USA.
b.   Disease worsens in 1/3 of cases during pregnancy.

c.   Prematurity rate doubled. Forceps may be required to facilitate delivery.
d. $MgSO_4$ administration will worsen the disease.
e.   Weakness of skeletal muscles is due to antibodies to the acetylcholine receptor. Smooth muscle, including uterine muscle, is not affected.
f.   Maternal treatment with pyridostigmine (Mestinon) may also treat fetus.

B. NEONATE.
a.   10–19% of offspring of women with myasthenia gravis are affected.
b.   Symptoms such as poor suck, weak cry, and hypotonia appear within the first 3 days of life.
c.   Diagnosis is made by demonstrating improvement after administration of 0.1mg neostigmine subcutaneously or 0.1mg edrophonium subcutaneously. Measurement of the antiacetylcholine receptor antibody in the serum can help differentiate this from other forms of hypotonia.
d.   Caused by transplacental transfer of antibodies against acetylcholine receptor.
e.   Recovery occurs in 1–3 months.
f.   Mortality without treatment was about 10%.

C. MANAGEMENT.
a.   Supportive care may include control of secretions, tube feeding, and mechanical ventilation.
b.   Acetylcholinesterase inhibition.
   1) Neostigmine 1–2mg p.o. q4h or pyridostigmine 4–10mg p.o. q4h.
   2) Either drug may be given i.v. at about 1/30 of the p.o. dose.
   3) Drug therapy indicated only if breathing or swallowing is affected.
   4) Either drug may increase secretions.
   5) Wean from drugs after 4–6 weeks.
c.   Breast-feeding is not contraindicated by maternal treatment with anticholinesterase agents, prednisone, or azathioprine.

IV. LUPUS ERYTHEMATOSUS
A. MATERNAL.
a.   Only about 50% of mothers have become symptomatic at time of delivery.
b.   All have autoantibodies of type Ro(SSA) or La(SSB).
c.   Autoantibodies may cross placenta and affect fetus.
d.   90–95% of affected women have HLA-DR-2 or HLA-DR-3 phenotypes.
e.   Increased fetal wastage in systemic lupus erythematosus (SLE) is not proven.
f.   Maternal treatment with steroids can decrease the severity of fetal myocarditis but does not affect established heart block.
g.   Echocardiographic evaluation of fetus recommended in second and third trimesters.

25

TRANSIENT IMMUNOLOGIC DISORDERS

B. FETAL/MATERNAL.

a. About 5% of offspring of Ro(SSA) positive mothers are affected.
   1) The majority of affected infants are born to HLA-DR-3 phenotype mothers.
   2) Infants may have any HLA phenotype.
b. Cutaneous lesions.
   1) Appear in the first month of life.
   2) More frequent in females than males (3:1).
   3) Erythematous, scaly plaques on face and scalp, but may be generalized.
   4) Sunlight or phototherapy may induce and/or worsen lesions.
   5) Resolve by 4–6 months of age.
   6) Skin atrophy, hypopigmentation, or telangiectasia are unusual residua.
   7) Not histologically similar to discoid lupus.
   8) Caused by binding of Ro(SSA) and possibly La(SSB) antibodies to epidermal antigens.
c. Heart block.
   1) Usually permanent.
   2) Males and females equally affected.
   3) Develops in utero during third trimester.
   4) May be complete or bundle-branch block.
   5) Only 6–10% have coexistent skin lesions.
   6) Maternal autoantibodies cross placenta and attach to antigens in cardiac conducting system with subsequent fibrosis.
   7) May occasionally be fatal.
d. Thrombocytopenia.
   1) Occurs in 10% of affected infants.
   2) Occasionally seen alone or with petechiae.
e. Other unusual transient findings include hemolytic anemia, leukopenia, hepatitis, and splenomegaly.
f. Diagnosis.
   1) IgG anti-Ro(SSA) in infant's serum.
   2) IgG immunofluorescence in skin lesions is helpful if present.
   3) ECG evidence of heart block.

C. MANAGEMENT.

a. Skin lesions.
   1) Avoid sunlight for first 3–6 months of life.
   2) Sun-block should be helpful.
   3) 1% hydrocortisone cream may help.
b. Heart block.
   1) Treat heart failure.
   2) Complete heart block may require pacemaker.
c. Value of plasmapheresis, IVIG, or systemic steroids unproven.
d. Long-term follow-up recommended since prognosis for developing adult SLE is unknown.

BIRTH DEFECTS AND GENETIC DISORDERS

An estimated 2–3% of all newborn infants will have a congenital birth defect, and an even higher percentage will have a genetic condition diagnosed later in life. With intensive care, more newborns with birth defects will survive. It is important therefore to develop a consistent approach to the diagnosis and care of these infants. The first step is to develop a method of classifying the type of problem seen. An understanding of the terminology used is essential.

I. CLASSIFICATION AND DEFINITION

A. **DEFORMATION.** An abnormal form, shape, or position of a part of the body caused by mechanical forces.

B. **DISRUPTION.** A morphologic defect of an organ, part of an organ, or a larger region of the body resulting from the extrinsic breakdown of, or an interference with, an originally normal developmental process.

C. **MALFORMATION.** A morphologic defect of an organ, part of an organ, or a larger region of the body resulting from an intrinsically abnormal developmental process.

D. **DYSPLASIA.** An abnormal organization of cells into tissue(s) and its morphologic result(s).

E. **SYNDROME.** A pattern of anomalies thought to be pathogenetically related and not known to represent a single sequence or a polytopic field defect.

II. CAUSATION

A. **DEFORMATION.** Uterine malformation, uterine tumor, twin gestation, large fetus, abnormal placental insertion with abnormal fetal position, abnormal fetus with poor movement or malformations which inhibit normal in-utero position.

B. **DISRUPTION.** Monozygotic twin pregnancy with twin death and twin–twin transfusion, amniotic adhesions, teratogens including viruses, drugs, radiation, or maternal diseases.

C. **MALFORMATION.** Single – polygenic, single-gene disorder, rarely chromosomal. Multiple – single-gene disorders, chromosomal abnormality.

D. **DYSPLASIA.** Single-gene disorder (metabolic or nonmetabolic), sporadic developmental abnormality.

III. DIAGNOSIS

A. PHYSICAL EXAMINATION.

1. **Placenta** – size, number of cords, size of cord, abnormalities of cord, insertion of cord, presence of fetus papyraceus, placental calcification, infarcts, tumors, evidence of infection, bogginess may suggest maternal diabetes or storage disorder.

2. **Infant/fetus** – size of infant (SGA – LGA), size of individual parts (e.g. small ears, short palpebral fissures, short digits), positional relations (hypotelorism, hypertelorism, low-set ears), minor malformations, (birthmarks, epicanthal folds, clinodactyly), major malformations (cleft lip/palate, microphthalmia, heart disease, absent limbs or digits, ambiguous genitalia), nervous system function (alertness, tone, reflexes, facial and limb movements).

B. HISTORY.

1. **Pregnancy** – maternal and paternal age, number of pregnancies, miscarriages and abnormal infants, episodes of bleeding or infections, medications, alcohol, tobacco and drug abuse (when, what, how much), diagnostic studies done, maternal diseases (PKU, myotonic dystrophy, diabetes, SLE), fetal activity, weight gain, amniotic fluid amount, delivery position, labor complications, Apgar scores, birth complications, any exposures or actions which the parents are concerned about.

2. **Family** – three generations if possible; include miscarriages, fetal demise, stillborn; ask about each family member and presence of features seen in the infant/fetus. Ethnicity and the possibility of consanguinity should be determined. Be attuned to psychosocial information such as alcoholism, depression, suicide in other family members which may give information as to the ability of the family to cope with an abnormal newborn.

C. DIAGNOSTIC STUDIES.

1. **Life-threatening problems.** Diagnose those potentially life-threatening problems which will require specific therapy.

2. **Single malformation.** The structure involved will dictate the diagnostic studies. For example, myelomeningocele is a neural tube closure abnormality and may be accompanied by midline abnormalities such as Arnold–Chiari malformation as well as secondary neurologic deficits. Imaging studies involving the brain, vertebrae, as well as the kidneys would be appropriate. Chromosome studies are indicated if there are multiple minor malformations or dysmorphic features (Table 26.1) or major CNS malformations (lissencephaly, holoprosencephaly).

3. **Multiple malformations.** Document all skeletal malformations with appropriate imaging studies and photographs. Banded chromosome studies should be done if there is not a positive family history of a similar pattern of malformation without mental retardation. If mental

TABLE 26.1

FEATURES OF COMMON DYSMORPHIC SYNDROMES

Trisomy 21 – hypotonia, brachycephaly, redundant nuchal skin, small ears, hypoplastic nasal root, Brushfield's spots, cardiac defects, mild brachydactyly, simian creases, increased fine creasing of palms and soles

Trisomy 18 – SGA, small facial features with short palpebral fissures, micrognathia, unravelled helices, short sternum, cardiac and thumb abnormalities, camptodactyly

Trisomy 13 – normal size, colobomatous microphthalmia, large nose, cleft lip/palate, cardiac defects, polycystic kidneys, postaxial polydactyly, holoprosencephaly

45 XO – redundant nuchal skin folds, pedal edema with deeply set nail beds, coarctation of the aorta

Osteogenesis imperfecta – generalized decreased mineralization of the bones, bowing or fracturing of the long bones, wormian bones of the skull, blue sclerae

Vater association – vertebral defects, vascular defects (cardiac defects, single umbilical artery), imperforate anus, trache-oesphageal fistula, esophageal atresia, radial and renal abnormalities.

Charge syndrome – conotruncal cardiac defects, hearing loss, atresia choanae, retardation (growth and mentation), genital abnormalities, ear abnormalities

Beckwith–Wiedemann syndrome – LGA, macroglossia, organomegaly, umbilical hernia or omphalocele, hypoglycemia.

Pierre Robin – micrognathia with U–shaped cleft palate. This is a diagnosis by exclusion of positive family history (Stickler syndrome) and other malformations (multiple chromosomal disorders, skeletal dysplasias) and syndromes.

retardation is present, chromosome studies are advised. If there are features of congenital infection (microcephaly, cataracts, hepatomegaly, myocardial dysfunction, etc.), obtain TORCH titers and urine for viral cultures. If a specific condition is found – e.g. lissencephaly (17p), conotruncal heart malformation with hypocalcemia (22q), cat-like cry (5p) – fluorescent in-situ hybridization (FISH) studies may be appropriate. This technique combines cytogenetics with fluorescent labelled DNA to detect small deletions. High-resolution chromosome studies should be ordered only if a specific small deletion on a specific chromosome is suspected. If the infant is not going to survive before genetic consultation can be obtained, save blood specimens in sodium heparin, obtain photographs, and obtain appropriate radiographic studies.

4. **Deformations.** Assess for neurologic abnormalities which predispose to an abnormal intrauterine position. Maternal uterine abnormalities, DES exposure, or oligohydramnios may be present.

5. **Dysplasia.** For bone dysplasias, a thorough radiographic examination is appropriate. If the metabolic abnormality or gene locus is known, more-specific blood or tissue studies are necessary for genetic counseling. These include the storage disorders, osteogenesis imperfectas, and certain other bone dysplasias. For generalized tissue dysplasias, such as Marfan syndrome, organs known to be involved, such as the heart and eye, should be examined.

D. DNA STUDIES. DNA analysis identifies a specific gene. For severely hypotonic infants thought to have spinal muscular atrophy, myotonic dystrophy, or Prader–Willi syndrome, DNA testing is diagnostic, faster, and less-invasive than neuromuscular studies. DNA mutations are now known for a number of the skeletal dysplasias, craniosynostosis syndromes, mitochondrial syndromes, and others. Information regarding test availability can be obtained from organizations such as HELIX.

E. COMMUNICATION. As the results of diagnostic studies become known, they should be discussed with the family and the primary physicians (obstetrician, pediatrician). When all studies are completed, arrange a conference with the family to discuss the diagnosis, the long-term implications, community agency support, and implications for future reproduction of the affected individual(s) and their relatives.

COMMON SURGICAL PROBLEMS

I. NECROTIZING ENTEROCOLITIS

A. **PATHOPHYSIOLOGY**: ischemia of the intestine, with bacterial invasion playing a contributory role. Feeding may place further demands on an already compromised situation.

B. **CLINICAL PRESENTATION.**

1. **Mild to fulminant,** presents anytime in first 6 weeks of life.
2. More common in premature infants.
3. **Earliest sign** is often intolerance of feedings (gastric residuals) or abdominal distention. Later findings may include blood in stools, increasing fluid requirements, abdominal tenderness, signs of shock, and sepsis.

C. **DIAGNOSIS.** Pneumatosis intestinalis is the hallmark of NEC. Portal air, pneumoperitoneum, or late strictures on contrast studies may also be seen.

D. **MANAGEMENT.**

1. **Stop feedings.**
2. **Place nasogastric tube** for GI decompression.
3. **Administer systemic antibiotics** after obtaining cultures.
4. **Take frequent abdominal radiographs** (q6–12h), including lateral decubitus to identify free air.
5. **Begin parenteral nutrition** when stable.
6. **Surgery** is indicated for perforation, progressive deterioration, or late stricture.

II. DIAPHRAGMATIC HERNIA

A. **PATHOPHYSIOLOGIC FINDINGS.** Defect (Bochdalek hernia) in posterolateral diaphragm allows abdominal contents to enter the thorax and compromise lung development bilaterally. 90% of diaphragmatic hernias occur on the left. Pulmonary hypertension frequently complicates course.

B. **CLINICAL PRESENTATION.** Respiratory distress, decreased breath sounds on the affected side, shift of heart sounds to the opposite side, and scaphoid abdomen are classic findings.

C. **DIAGNOSIS.** Chest radiograph reveals opacity or bowel in chest with lack of normal bowel gas in abdomen.

D. **MANAGEMENT.**

1. **Ventilation** by endotracheal tube. (Mask ventilation is contraindicated because of inflation of the gut.)

2. **NG tube** – place to avoid further GI tract distention.
3. **Controversial treatments:** muscle relaxants, careful ventilator management with avoidance of barotrauma, pulmonary vasodilators and alkalosis.
4. **Operative repair** following maximal decrease/stabilization of pulmonary artery pressures.
5. **Extracorporeal membrane oxygenation** if conventional therapy is unsuccessful (may precede repair).

III. INTESTINAL OBSTRUCTION

A. **PATHOPHYSIOLOGIC FINDINGS.** Intrauterine vascular accident, cystic fibrosis, meconium ileus, Hirschsprung's disease, errors in rotation or fixation.

B. **CLINICAL PRESENTATION.**
1. **Bilious vomiting.** Cause must be established without delay.
2. **Failure of passage of meconium** within 24 hours in a baby being fed or within 48 hours in a baby being kept NPO is abnormal.
3. **Abdominal distention,** visible intestinal loops, or obvious peritonitis.
4. **Delay rectal examination** until all radiographic examinations are completed.

C. **DIAGNOSIS/MANAGEMENT.**
1. **Nasogastric suction.**
2. **Chest or abdominal radiographs** should include the pelvis.
3. **Meconium obstruction** is diagnosed and usually treated by contrast enema with hypertonic water-soluble agents.
4. **Laparotomy** is usually required. Decompressive colostomy is the treatment of choice for Hirschsprung's disease.

IV. ABDOMINAL WALL DEFECT

A. **PATHOPHYSIOLOGIC FINDINGS.** Incomplete formation of the abdominal wall in the first trimester during protrusion, return, rotation, and fixation of the midgut.

B. **TYPES.**
1. **Omphalocele** is a defect with the abdominal contents covered by peritoneum and amnion.
2. **Gastroschisis** – the peritoneal membrane is absent. The cord is usually to the left of the defect.
3. **Extrophy,** a rare anomaly, occurs with lower abdominal embryogenetic defects.

C. **MANAGEMENT.**
1. **Omphalocele or hernia of the cord with intact membrane** – infants should receive nasogastric suction. The sac should be kept moist with saline-soaked gauze and plastic wrap.
2. **The herniated bowel** in gastroschisis, or ruptured omphalocele, can suffer vascular compromise if its blood supply is kinked over the edge

of the defect. The baby should be turned on his side to avoid vascular embarrassment. A nasogastric tube should be placed. Saline-moist gauze and plastic wrap or a plastic bag should be used to keep the intestine moist. Evaporative losses are large, and i.v. hydration is important. Antibiotics for systemic effect are given.

3. **Primary closure** is the ideal procedure. Temporary prosthetic pouches are used to allow slow reduction of abdominal contents only if primary closure is not possible. Antiseptic painting of the intact omphalocele sac is used if operative closure is not performed.

V. IMPERFORATE ANUS

A. **PATHOPHYSIOLOGIC FINDINGS:** a spectrum of anomalies that can be classed as either low-type (infralevator) or high-type (supralevator) depending on the location of the terminus of the colon. Fistula to the vagina is common in all types of imperforate anus in females. In males with high-type anomalies, fistula to the urinary tract (usually urethra) is common.

B. **CLINICAL PRESENTATION AND DIAGNOSIS.**

1. **Diagnosis** is not often a problem. Distinction between high- and low-type can be difficult. Radiographs can be helpful. Serial examination watching for meconium passing through a fistula or in the urine is important.

2. **An adequate-sized nasogastric tube** should be passed for decompression as well as to rule out esophageal atresia (associated in 10% of cases).

C. **MANAGEMENT.**

1. **Local peritoneal procedures** are performed in low-type imperforate anus and include dilatation, 'cut-back,' anoplasty, or anal transposition.

2. **High-type anomalies** are treated with colostomy initially. Pull-through procedures are performed after 6 months of age.

3. **Evaluation of urinary tract** with ultrasound and voiding cystourethrogram.

4. **Lumbosacral spinal MR imaging** for associated forms of caudal agenesis.

VI. TRACHEO-ESOPHAGEAL FISTULA

A. **CLINICAL PRESENTATION AND DIAGNOSIS.**

1. **Presentation** – excess oral secretions, inability to feed, gagging, respiratory distress, maternal polyhydramnios.

2. **Lateral and AP radiograph** of the thoracocervical region and abdomen with a Replogle tube in the proximal esophageal pouch usually will suffice for diagnosis, showing blind pouch and air in GI tract.

3. **Esophageal atresia without tracheo-esophageal fistula** – gas is absent from the GI tract.

B. **PRINCIPLES OF PREOPERATIVE MANAGEMENT.**

1. **Minimal disturbance of infant** to prevent reflux and aspiration of acid gastric secretions.

27

COMMON SURGICAL PROBLEMS

2. **Keep infant inclined** in a 60°, head-up prone position.
3. **Place Replogle tube** to suction in proximal esophageal pouch.
4. **Echocardiogram** to assess side of aortic arch and associated congenital heart defects
5. **Broad-spectrum antibiotics.**

C. **USUAL OPERATIVE PROCEDURE.**

1. **Division and closure of TEF,** end-to-end anastomosis of proximal and distal esophagus.
2. **Delayed anastomosis.** If the gap between esophageal segments is too long for primary anastomosis, delayed anastomosis follows stretching of the upper segment by serial bougienage.

D. **PRINCIPLES OF POSTOPERATIVE MANAGEMENT.**

1. **Suction catheters** should be inserted no further than a prescribed distance.
2. **Feeding.** If the primary anastomosis can be accomplished, feeds are begun after 1 week. Contrast study is usually performed prior to feeding.

VII. HYDRONEPHROSIS

A. **CLINICAL PRESENTATION AND DIAGNOSIS.**

1. **Presentation.** Flank mass(es), oliguria, and, rarely urinary ascites. History of oligohydramnios.
2. **Vomiting and infection** are uncommon today.
3. **Often diagnosed prenatally** during fetal ultrasound examination.

B. **LOCATION OF OBSTRUCTION.**

1. **Anatomic:** ureteropelvic junction, ureterovesicle junction or posterior urethral valves.
2. **Functional:** megaloureter syndrome with or without prune-belly syndrome.

C. **PREOPERATIVE MANAGEMENT.**

1. Monitor intake and output, body weight, and electrolytes.
2. Catheterize bladder.
3. Obtain voiding cystourethrogram and radionuclide renal scan.

D. **USUAL OPERATIVE APPROACH.**

1. **Temporary urinary diversion** (nephrostomy, ureterostomy, or vesicostomy).
2. **Repair later.** May be staged or definitive.

E. **POSTOPERATIVE MANAGEMENT.**

1. Careful fluid and electrolyte management.
2. Renal function studies serially.
3. Prophylactic antibiotics and infection surveillance.
4. Stomal dilatation.

OXYGEN THERAPY

Supplemental oxygen is an important form of therapy for many infants with cardiopulmonary disorders. Its use may be associated with the occurrence of retinopathy of prematurity and chronic lung disease. Criteria have not been established that assure minimal hazard to the patient. Therefore, we recommend that oxygen administration be regulated to maintain the P_aO_2 within the range for normal newborns: 50–100 torr.

28

I. INDICATIONS

A. **HYPOXEMIA.** Significant hypoxemia in the newborn is usually defined as P_aCO_2 <50 torr.

B. **RESUSCITATION.** Some practitioners recommend limitation of FiO_2 to 0.80 for resuscitation in the delivery room.

C. **CYANOSIS.** It is common practice to administer oxygen in a concentration just sufficient to relieve cyanosis, while awaiting the results of blood gas measurements.

II. THERAPEUTIC CONSIDERATIONS

A. **THE GOAL OF THERAPY** is to maintain P_aCO_2 in the range 50–100 torr and preferably 60–80 torr in small prematures to avoid either hypoxia or hyperoxia.

a. When cardiac output and its distribution are normal, oxygen tensions of 40–50 torr probably provide for adequate tissue oxygen delivery.

b. In premature infants, oxygen tensions <50 torr may depress respiratory effort, producing hypoventilation or apneic spells.

c. In near-term and more mature infants, oxygen tensions <50 torr may significantly increase pulmonary vascular resistance.

d. Under the best of circumstances, it may not be possible to meet your therapeutic goals consistently regarding P_aCO_2 or FiO_2.

III. MONITORING

A. **THE ARTERIAL OXYGEN TENSION.** Monitor arterial blood oxygen tension at a frequency that is determined by how rapidly the patient's pulmonary status is changing and by the availability of devices for continuous monitoring of the status of oxygenation.

a. Infants requiring >40% oxygen during the acute phase of their illness should have P_aCO_2 measurements every 4–6 hours. More frequent measurements are indicated during periods of instability.

b. Check P_aCO_2 about 30 minutes after making changes in the concentration of oxygen or ventilator settings.
c. Infants with stable chronic lung disease may require only daily or sometimes less-frequent determinations.
d. For infants requiring high oxygen concentrations, it is advisable to measure the oxygen tension periodically in the descending aorta and temporal or right radial artery simultaneously. Right-to-left ductal shunts may produce higher P_aCO_2 values above the ductus than those measured in the descending aorta (umbilical artery cather).
e. Continuous monitoring of oxygen tension with transcutaneous or intravascular oxygen electrodes improves the ability to maintain blood oxygen tensions in the desired range.

B. THE ARTERIAL OXYGEN SATURATION.
a. Oximetry (see Chapter 41) has provided a convenient method to continuously monitor oxygen saturation.
b. Adjust oxygen concentration (FiO_2) to maintain oxygen saturation of 88–95%.
c. Can be used to simultaneously monitor pre- and post-ducted oxygen saturation during right-to-left shunting.
d. May be ineffective during shock or hypoperfusion.

C. THE OXYGEN CONCENTRATION delivered to the infant should be routinely measured periodically and following changes in oxygen delivery.
a. Use a recently calibrated oxygen analyzer.
b. If the baby is in an oxygen hood, gas should be sampled near the face.

IV. OXYGEN DELIVERY

A. BLENDERS. Mixtures of oxygen and air may be delivered to an infant by a variety of means. In general, an oxygen blender should be used. However, 100% oxygen is usually administered for home care.
a. Delivered by endotracheal tube, nasal prongs, cannulae masks, funnels, and hoods.
   1) In general, use an oxygen blender and set FiO_2.
   2) Warmed, humidified oxygen should be used.
   3) The gas flow used may be dependent on the operation requirements of the mixing device, or blender.
b. Delivered by nasal cannulae for home care.
   1) In general, 100% O_2 is used and the liter flow is adjusted to achieve desired FiO_2.
   2) Humidified oxygen should be used.

B. GAS FLOW.
1. **Head hood.** A liter flow 3 times the volume of the head hood, or about 6–8L/min, is usually adequate to prevent rebreathing of exhaled carbon dioxide. Higher flows may be necessary to assure stable oxygen concentrations.

2. **INTUBATED PATIENTS.** Gas flows 1 to 2 times greater than the estimated minute ventilation are adequate in continuous-flow systems with a reservoir to provide for the peak inspiratory flow demand. Higher flows may be necessary to achieve the desired level of CPAP.

V. SPECIAL CONSIDERATIONS
A. RETINOPATHY OF PREMATURITY
a. Risk increases with decreasing gestational age (most important factor).
b. The duration and magnitude of oxygen exposure required to produce or exacerbate ROP are currently unknown.
c. Other factors, including individual susceptibility, blood transfusions, and hypercarbia, appear to be important.
d. Most cases of ROP resolve; however, a few progress to visual impairment, including blindness.
e. ROP is not totally preventable at present.
f. Laser treatment may be therapeutic.
g. Vasoconstriction of immature retinal vessels by oxygen and oxygen radical injury have been suggested as mechanisms.
h. ROP was formerly known as retrolental fibroplasia (RLF).
B. PULMONARY OXYGEN TOXICITY.
a. Often called bronchopulmonary dysplasia (BPD) or chronic lung disease of prematurity (CLD).
b. Most frequently observed in mechanically ventilated premature infants with prolonged exposure to high oxygen concentrations.
c. Other factors such as lung trauma from the ventilator, individual susceptibility, and pre-existing lung disease are probably more important.
d. Efforts to reduce incidence or severity of CLD are currently focused on limiting barotrauma and O_2 exposure. Administration of glucocorticoids may be useful.
e. Oxygen radical injury has been suggested as a mechanism.

28

OXYGEN THERAPY

ENDOTRACHEAL INTUBATION

I. INDICATIONS
A. IN THE DELIVERY ROOM.
a. Severe cardiorespiratory depression.
b. Bag and mask ventilation inadequate.
c. Upper airway obstruction (e.g. Pierre Robin).
d. Avoidance of gastrointestinal dilatation (e.g. suspected diaphragmatic hernia, abdominal wall defect).
e. When meconium aspiration is to be treated.
B. IN THE INTENSIVE CARE NURSERY.
a. Assisted ventilation (mechanical or manual).
b. Resuscitation.
c. Treatment of upper airway obstruction.
d. Tracheobronchial toilet.
e. Tracheal aspiration for microbiologic studies.

II. ROUTE
We routinely use orotracheal intubation because of the relative ease in developing and maintaining proficiency with the technique. Nasotracheal intubation may be desired on occasion or may be routine in some hospitals.

III. TUBE SELECTION AND PREPARATION
a. We use soft tubes that have markings at 1 cm intervals and a heavy black circumferential line 2.2–2.8cm from the tip.
b. Tubes may be made stiffer for intubation by using a stylet. *Be certain that the stylet does not protrude from the tip of the tube or at the side hole.* Use caution when utilizing a stylet with a 2.5mm endotracheal tube, as the stylet can be difficult to remove once the tube is inserted.
c. The tube size (see Table 29.1) should allow a small air leak around it.

IV. LARYNGOSCOPY
A. INSTRUMENT.
a. Use a Miller '0' laryngoscope blade for premature and small infants.
b. Use a Miller '1' laryngoscope blade for large, full-term infants.
c. Note: the laryngoscope is a left-handed, lifting instrument.
B. TECHNIQUE.
a. Check laryngoscope, suction setup, oxygen, and ventilatory equipment before proceeding. Empty the infant's stomach with an orogastric tube.

TABLE 29.1

ENDOTRACHEAL TUBE SIZE

Patient weight (g)	Tube size (mm)
<1000	2.5
1000–2000	3.0
2000–4000	3.5
>4000	4.0

b. Use clean technique. Wear surgical gloves.

c. If the procedure is elective, ventilate the infant with bag and mask and supplemental oxygen for 1 minute or longer before intubation. Do not bag and mask infants with meconium staining, suspected diaphragmatic hernia, or severe upper airway obstruction. Proceed directly to intubation (Figure 29.1).

d. Position the patient in 'sniff position' with the head slightly extended. Do *not* hyperextend. Suction mucus from the airway under direct vision if needed.

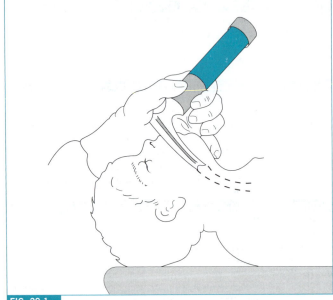

FIG. 29.1

Technique of laryngoscopy for endotracheal intubation. Note position of hand on laryngoscope handle. (From Goetzman[1], by permission.)

e. Advance the laryngoscope with the left hand, beginning at the right corner of the patient's mouth, shifting to the midline, and moving the tongue to the left. When the blade tip is in the space between the tongue and epiglottis, the epiglottis will lift, exposing the glottis and vocal cords.

f. Advance the endotracheal tube along the right side of the laryngoscope blade, but *not* within its C-shaped opening or your line of sight to the glottis will be obstructed.

g. Insert the tip of the tube into the glottis, between the vocal cords, and advance until the black line on the tube is just visible above the cords.

h. For temporary fixation, grasp the endotracheal tube near the mouth with the thumb and finger of the right hand and rest the remainder of the fingers on the infant's cheek.

i. Remove the stylet, if used, attach the ventilating device, and begin manual ventilation with oxygen-enriched gas. If intubation is successful, the following should be present:
    1) A good heart rate response
    2) Movement of the chest with positive-pressure ventilation
    3) Good breath sounds bilaterally.

j. If you cannot insert the endotracheal tube within 30 seconds, or profound bradycardia occurs, ventilate the infant using bag and mask for 2–3 minutes and try again when the heart rate is stable.

k. Premedication with atropine may be used in infants who develop immediate bradycardia with laryngoscopy.

l. Neuromuscular blockade is preferred by some operators. Can use succinylcholine, atracurium, or vecuronium.

V. TUBE FIXATION, REPLACEMENT, SUCTIONING, AND REMOVAL
A. TUBE FIXATION.

a. After successful intubation, hold the tube securely in place by resting the hand holding the tube against the baby's face. Note the number on the side of the tube at the maxillary gum margin.

b. Secure the tube with tape as follows.
    1) Apply benzoin above and below the lips, to the cheeks, and to the endotracheal tube. Allow it to dry.
    2) Three-eighths-inch white adhesive tape is cut either in 'H' or 'Y' configuration. When a 'Y' is used, the base is applied to the cheek with one arm going over the lower lip and the other arm going around the endotracheal tube positioned at the corner of the mouth. A second 'Y' is applied with the base on the cheek, one arm on the upper lip, and the other arm around the tube in the opposite direction of the first tape.
    3) Always confirm correct tube position promptly by radiograph or another technique. The tube should be approximately 1cm above the carina when the neck is in a neutral position.

29

ENDOTRACHEAL INTUBATION

B. **TUBE REPLACEMENT.** Endotracheal tubes need to be changed only if occluded by secretions, when there is accidental dislodgement, or if another diameter is deemed more appropriate.

C. **TUBE SUCTIONING.** This is a sterile procedure; use good technique and powder-free gloves. Isotonic saline, 0.5ml, should be instilled into the tube prior to suctioning. Suctioning is usually performed as needed and sometimes routinely every 4–12 hours. More- or less-frequent suctioning may be required depending on the amount of secretions and the infant's tolerance of the procedure.

D. **TUBE REMOVAL.**

a. Suction the endotracheal tube and ventilate manually for 1–2 minutes.

b. Suction the oropharynx and empty the stomach.

c. Deftly withdraw the tube during manual inflation of the lungs.

d. Place the infant in an oxygen-enriched environment 5–10% higher than that delivered via the endotracheal tube. Obtain a blood gas value in 15–30 minutes or follow O_2 saturation with oximetry.

e. If the tube was in place for 1 hour or more, maintain the infant NPO for 2–6 hours to allow return of glottic closure mechanisms.

f. We do not routinely use dexamethasone or racemic epinephrine, before and after extubation, respectively. On occasion, when extubation has not been successful, these agents are utilized. More often, we use premedication with theophylline and continue for 2–5 days after extubation.

g. Observe for postextubation stridor and chest wall retractions. Evaluate with arterial blood gas studies and chest radiograph.

VI. COMPLICATIONS

1. **Atelectasis** – deterioration in ABGs secondary to incorrect endotracheal tube placement.

2. **Laryngeal trauma,** including hematoma and perforation of hypopharynx.

3. **Vocal cord injury or paralysis.**

4. **Infection** – pneumonia or tracheitis.

5. **Subglottic stenosis** occurs in 1–5% of intubated infants. On occasion, the stenosis will be so severe as to require tracheostomy or acricoid split.

REFERENCE

1. Goetzman BW. Resuscitation of the newborn. In: Niswander KF, ed. *Manual of obstetrics*. Boston: Little, Brown; 1980: 389–397.

CONTINUOUS POSITIVE AIRWAY PRESSURE

I. INTRODUCTION

Continuous positive airway pressure (CPAP), or constant distending airway pressure (CDAP), is useful in improving oxygenation in infants whose lung disease is complicated by loss of lung volume (RDS, pulmonary edema, or diffuse atelectasis). The presumed explanation for its effectiveness is prevention of alveolar collapse during expiration. This decreases intrapulmonary shunting, improves ventilation–perfusion matching, and increases the tone in airway stretch receptors. Administration of CPAP via nasal prongs has greatly increased the number of clinical applications in which CPAP is considered as useful therapy.

II. CLINICAL APPLICATIONS

1. **RDS.**
a. Nasal CPAP early in the course may avoid endotracheal intubation.
b. Nasal CPAP may allow earlier extubation, 1–7 days, even in premature infants with BW <1kg.
2. **Atelectasis.** Postintubation nasal CPAP:
a. Postoperatively.
b. Very premature infants with soft chest walls.
3. **Airway collapse.**
a. Tracheobronchomalacia may respond to one of the forms of CPAP.
b. Pharyngeal redundancy and collapse.
4. **Apnea of prematurity.** Nasal CPAP is often effective in reducing the frequency of apneic spells.
a. Increases functional residual capacity.
b. Improves baseline oxygenation.
c. Increases central stimulation by increasing airway mechanoreceptor tone.
d. Overcomes upper-airway obstruction in phayrnx.

III. TECHNIQUES

All devices rely on a continuous flow of humidified gas with a valve that obstructs outflow. The level of CPAP is set by adjusting the outflow valve or the inflow rate. The following techniques are available.
1. **A specific CPAP device** connected to:
a. An endotracheal tube.
b. A nasopharyngeal catheter.
c. Nasal prongs.

2. **Any standard infant ventilator in CPAP mode** connected to an endotracheal or tracheostomy tube.
3. **Continuous negative pressure** (CNP) (seldom used).
   a. Body box such as Isolette® negative-pressure ventilator.
   b. Cuirass or chest jacket.
   c. CNP procedure.
      1) Place infant in chamber with head outside.
      2) Seal chamber with iris diaphragm around neck.
      3) Turn on vacuum to create negative pressure around body.
      4) Administer oxygen by head hood or nasal cannula.
      5) Increase or decrease CNP based on blood gas analysis.

IV. PROCEDURE

The nasal route is most common.
a. Connect CPAP device, with appropriate gas flow and oxygen concentration, to a properly placed endotracheal tube, nasopharyngeal tube, or nasal prongs.
b. Adjust pressure to 4–6cmH$_2$O and measure ABG in 30 minutes, or observe response on transcutaneous PO$_2$ monitor or O$_2$ saturation monitor. Adjust oxygen concentration accordingly.
c. Increase applied pressure by 1–2cmH$_2$O increments until oxygenation goal is achieved or airway obstruction is relieved. A 24–48 hour trial is necessary to determine effect on apneic spells.
d. When an applied pressure of 3–4cmH$_2$O is tolerated, and infant has improved, a trial of nasal cannula or head hood oxygen is indicated.
e. If CPAP fails, mechanical ventilation may be indicated.
f. Meticulous nursing care is necessary to maintain continuous distending pressure by nasal prongs.

V. COMPLICATIONS

1. **Pneumothorax** occurs in 5–15% of infants so treated.
2. **Decreased venous return** with decreased cardiac output, tamponade of pulmonary capillaries, and decreased ventilation have been observed at high applied pressures.
3. **Air trapping** and decreased ventilation may occur at high pressure levels.
4. **Nares skin breakdown** and nasal septal erosion may occur with nasal prongs.

FURTHER READING

Annibale DJ, Hulsey TC, Engstrom PC, Wallin LA, Ohning BL. Randomized, controlled trial nasopharyngeal continuous positive airway pressure in the extubation of very low birth weight infants. *J Pediatr* 1994; 124(3):455–460.

Gittermann MK, Fusch C, Gittermann AR, Regzzoni BM, Moessinger AC. Early nasal continuous positive airway pressure treatment reduces the need for intubation in very low birth weight infants. *Eur J Pediatr* 1997; 156(5):384–388.

Hauer AC, Rosegger H, Haas J, Haxhija EQ. Reaction of term newborns with prolonged postnatal dyspnoea to early oxygen, mask continuous positive airway pressure and volume expansion: a prospective, randomised, clinical trial. *Eur J Pediatr* 1996; 155(9):805–810.

Loftus BC, Ahn J, Haddad J Jr. Neonatal nasal deformities secondary to nasal continuous positive airway pressure. *Laryngoscope* 1994; 104(8 Pt 1):1019–1022.

30

CONTINUOUS POSITIVE AIRWAY PRESSURE

VENTILATORY ASSISTANCE

I. BAG AND MASK VENTILATION

Ventilation by bag and mask is easily learned and is usually an effective means of establishing lung expansion. Its success is usually determined by the availability of an appropriate-size mask and the experience of the operator and less often by the severity of lung disease.

A. INDICATIONS.

1. **Resuscitation** and for managing infants for short periods of time while preparing for intubation.

2. **Precautions** in the delivery room.

   a. Infants suspected of meconium aspiration should be intubated and suctioned before positive-pressure ventilation is used.

   b. Bag and mask ventilation should not be used if a diaphragmatic hernia is suspected.

   c. Very small infants and infants with micrognathia often cannot be ventilated effectively by bag and mask, and immediate intubation may be necessary. With severe micrognathia and airway obstruction (Pierre Robin anomaly), ventilation may be possible through a nasopharyngeal tube passed through the nose and past the tongue obstruction.

3. **Used intermittently** to treat or prevent postextubation atelectasis.

B. EQUIPMENT.
We usually use an anesthesia bag and mask with an attached pressure manometer. A self-inflating infant resuscitator with an accumulator attached to permit delivery of a high FiO_2 is also satisfactory.

C. TECHNIQUE.

1. **Position mask firmly** over the face with the head in neutral position and finger lifting chin. Mask should not rest on eyes.

2. **Respiratory frequency** – usually 30–50/min.

3. **Inspiratory pressure.** 20–30cmH$_2$O usually suffices. 30–60cmH$_2$O is occasionally required during initial resuscitation in the delivery room.

D. ASSESSMENT.

1. **Return of a normal heart rate and absence of central cyanosis** usually indicate adequate O_2 delivery.

2. **Chest expansion and auscultatory evidence of air entry** occur bilaterally when effective ventilation is provided.

3. **Monitoring by ABG values** is required in prolonged resuscitation.

4. **Remember** – intermittent bag and mask ventilation may worsen blood gases if the baby fights the procedure. It is necessary to evaluate each patient's response to therapy.

E. COMPLICATIONS.

1. **Pneumothorax.**

2. **Gaseous distention** of stomach may require orogastric tube or discontinuing enteral feedings.

3. **Abrasions of facial skin.**

4. **Retinal detachment.** Keep mask off eyes and do not use excessive pressure to apply mask.

II. MECHANICAL VENTILATION

The hallmark of the NICU is the ability to manage long-term assisted ventilation of sick newborns. Styles of ventilation (rapid vs slow, long vs short inspiratory times, etc.) may differ among institutions. Various styles have proven effective. A team approach (physician, nurse, respiratory therapist, radiologist, and clinical laboratory) is essential. The brand of equipment used is not critical. Success is determined by how well you use the equipment you have and by how well you assess your patients.

A. INDICATIONS. Respiratory failure may occur in infants with a wide range of disorders, including lung disease, heart disease, intrathoracic anomalies, CNS depression by drugs or disease, and in premature infants with severe apneic spells. When respiratory failure is severe and other methods for treating pulmonary insufficiency have failed, mechanical ventilation is indicated.

B. CONVENTIONAL MECHANICAL VENTILATION – pressure-limited infant ventilators for routine ventilatory and effective assistance.

1. **Principles of therapy.**

a. Oxygenation in noncompliant correlates with the FiO_2 and the mean airway pressure and thus can be improved by:

   1) Increased concentration of inspired oxygen
   2) Increased inspiratory pressure (PIP)
   3) Increased positive end-expiratory pressure (PEEP)
   4) Increased inspiratory time (IIT)
   5) Inspiratory pressure plateau (square pressure wave).

b. Ventilation (carbon dioxide removal) is related to minute ventilation and may be improved by the following:

   1) Increased tidal volume (TV)
   2) Increased rate (RR)
   3) Decreasing PEEP.

c. Ventilator settings (rate, inspiratory pressure, inspiratory pressure plateau, I:E ratio, and PEEP) will vary depending on the pathologic entity involved and on the measured response to a particular therapeutic trial.

2. **Goals.**

a. Regulate P_aO_2 in the range 50–80 torr.

b. Maintain P_aCO_2 in the range 35–55 torr.

c. Exceptions – certain conditions may require accepting P_aO_2 and P_aCO_2 limits other than those given above.

   1) In chronic lung disease, a higher P_aCO_2 may be acceptable.
   2) In cyanotic heart disease, a lower P_aO_2 may be acceptable.
   3) In pulmonary hypertension, a higher or lower P_aCO_2 may be acceptable, depending on treatment philosophy.

d. Criteria for intervention should be documented in the chart.

3. **Technique.**

a. Initial ventilator settings in RDS are typically as follows:

   1) Inspiratory pressure of 20–24cmH$_2$O
   2) PEEP of 4–6cmH$_2$O
   3) Frequency of 20–24/min (try rates l/4, l/3, or l/2 the infant's spontaneous respiratory rate)
   4) Inspiratory time of 0.3–0.4 seconds.

b. Central respiratory failure – an infant with normal lungs and decreased central respiratory drive might have initial settings as follows:

   1) Inspiratory pressure of 14–16cmH$_2$O
   2) PEEP of 3–4cmH$_2$O
   3) Rate of 15–20/min.

c. Flow and inspiratory time – controls on the ventilator may allow the pressure waveform to be altered. Useful to compensate for leak around endotracheal tube.

d. Ventilator cycling occurs automatically and is not triggered by the infant.

e. Continuous flow – fresh gas flows past the endotracheal tube when the ventilator is in the expiratory phase and allows the infant to ventilate with its own respirations, usually 2–4 times the frequency of the ventilator.

f. In-phase ventilation of the infant with the ventilator usually occurs after 5–10 minutes of cycling. Agitation may impair the effectiveness of the ventilator, and medication may be required.

   1) Benzodiazepines or morphine sulfate, 0.1mg/kg, may be used for sedation.
   2) Sometimes an infant may fight the ventilator to such an extent that muscular paralysis is indicated. Pancuronium bromide or vecuronium, 0.06–0.10mg/kg, are the recommended drugs for this purpose. Remember, a paralyzed or heavily sedated infant loses his ability to breathe and will require a higher ventilator rate and must be constantly observed for accidental extubation or mechanical failure of the ventilator. Paralyzed patients still require sedation and may require medication for pain.

31

VENTILATORY ASSISTANCE

3) Synchronous ventilation can be facilitated with several ventilators, with the patient triggering ventilator assists.

4. Assessment.

a. Trial and error methodology is required. Frequent re-evaluation by blood gas analysis is essential. Each patient is unique in his or her response to ventilator changes.

b. Physical examination.

   1) One should be able to observe chest expansion and auscultate good air entry bilaterally when effective ventilation is provided.
   2) A well-oxygenated and ventilated patient is usually well perfused, centrally acyanotic, and comfortable.

5. Complications.

a. Alveolar rupture with formation of pulmonary interstitial emphysema, pneumothorax, or pneumomediastinum is the most common complication of mechanical ventilation. This occurs in about 7–10% of RDS infants requiring mechanical ventilation in our nursery.

b. Other complications include the following:

   1) Bacterial colonization and infection
   2) Obstructed endotracheal tube or extubation
   3) Intubation of the right main-stem bronchus
   4) Pneumopericardium with cardiac tamponade
   5) Impaired venous return and decreased cardiac output
   6) Chronic lung disease
   7) Subglottic stenosis with obstruction of the trachea.

6. Withdrawal of ventilatory support.

a. Weaning, or withdrawal of ventilatory support, is a technique for testing the infant to see how well he manages without the ventilator. 'Weaning' is a misleading term because it implies that you may be able to teach the patient to get along without the ventilator.

b. Individualization – a plan for withdrawal of ventilatory support is necessary. Reduce that parameter which is considered to be most excessive and most hazardous to the patient, and reassess ABGs.

c. Nasal CPAP at 4–6cmH$_2$O can usually be tried when a rate of 14–16/min is tolerated by the infant. The inspired oxygen concentration is kept the same or raised by 5%. Arterial blood gas monitoring is necessary to assess patient response to extubation.

d. Deterioration of the infant's blood gas status during the above process may require reintubation and ventilation settings. Reassess the infant for complications of ventilatory therapy or for a new problem such as patent ductus arteriosus, low hematocrit reading, cold stress, or atelectasis.

C. HIGH-FREQUENCY VENTILATION. HFV uses a different strategy for mechanical ventilation.

1. **Small breaths** (less than the tracheal dead space) are utilized at very high rates of 7–12Hz (i.e. cycles per second).
2. **Modalities available.**
a. Jet.
   1) Inspiratory time of 0.02 seconds.
   2) Rate of 7 Hz (420 breaths per minute).
   3) Jet inspiratory pressure and PEEP are similar to those of conventional ventilator.
   4) Increase jet PIP to increase ventilation.
   5) Back-up conventional rate of 6–10/min for alveolar recruitment.
   6) Wean by decreasing jet PIP and PEEP, not rate.
b. Oscillator.
   1) Oscillates above and below PEEP at rate of 12Hz.
   2) Set PEEP at level of mean airway pressure.
   3) Mean airway pressure determines oxygenation.
   4) Change amplitude of oscillations to change ventilation.
   5) Back-up conventional rate of 6–10/min for alveolar recruitment.
   6) Wean by decreasing PEEP and amplitude not rate.
3. **Indications.**
a. Failure to respond to conventional mechanical ventilation.
b. Pulmonary air leak.
c. Pulmonary hypertension.
d. Micropremie susceptible to BPD (avoids barotrauma).

31

VENTILATORY ASSISTANCE

EXOGENOUS SURFACTANT ADMINISTRATION FOR RESPIRATORY DISTRESS SYNDROME

I. INDICATIONS

A. IN THE DELIVERY ROOM OR RESUSCITATION AREA.

1. **Infants from 24 to 29 weeks gestation** are at high risk for RDS, and some studies, but not all, have found benefit in prophylactic administration of exogenous surfactant.

2. **Immature lung profile.** Infants in whom antenatal assessment of pulmonary maturity indicates an 'immature' lung profile may also be candidates for exogenous surfactant administration.

B. IN THE NICU OR AT THE TIME OF NEONATAL TRANSPORT IN INFANTS WITH RDS

1. Infants with clinical signs and radiologic findings consistent with RDS should be treated with endotracheal administration of exogenous surfactant. Early administration, prior to 2 hours of age with the onset of respiratory distress, has been shown to be superior to waiting until an arbitary severity [e.g. arterial/alveolar oxygen $(a/AO_2) < 0.22$] had been established. Treatment at the referring site in order to stabilize an infant prior to transport is appropriate.

2. Studies have shown that exogenous surfactant may be beneficial in infants with meconium aspiration syndrome, diaphragmatic hernia, and pneumonia with ventilatory failure, although, at present, there is no specific approval by the FDA for these indications.

II. INTRATRACHEAL ADMINISTRATION

Exogenous surfactants are administrated according to their manufacturer's guidelines.

1. **Exosurf Neonatal®** is administered through a side-port adapter attached to the endotracheal tube via small boluses over 3–5 minutes through the side-port while the infant is receiving intermittent mandatory ventilation. Results of comparison trials with modified, bovine surfactants have shown more rapid improvement in respiratory function with these agents.

2. **Survanta®** is warmed to room temperature for at least 20 minutes without shaking and the single-dose vial entered once to remove sufficient Survanta to equal 100mg/kg body weight (25mg/mL) and administered according to the manufacturer's guidelines through a 5.0 end-hole feeding tube that extends to slightly beyond the end of the endotracheal tube positioned above the carina. Four positions are used during administration:

   a.   Head and body inclined 5–10∞ down. Head turned to the right.
   b.   Head and body inclined 5–10° up. Head turned to the right.
   c.   Head and body inclined 5–10° down. Head turned to the left.
   d.   Head and body inclined 5–10° up. Head turned to the left.

It is recommended that immediately preceding the initial dosing the infant should have suctioning of the endotracheal tube, the ventilator rate be adjusted to 60 breaths/min and between each dose the ventilator be adjusted to a rate of 60 breaths/min and the fractional inspiratory oxygen be 1.0. Ventilator setting need not be adjusted during the subsequent dosing procedures.

3. **Surfactant administration is a two-person procedure,** and both caregivers administering surfactant (one of whom should be a physician) should carefully position the infant while the other administers the drug intratracheally.

4. **In the prophylactic strategy,** weigh, intubate, and stabilize the infant. Administer the dose, as soon as possible after birth, preferably within 15 minutes. Position the infant appropriately, and gently inject the first quarter-dose through the catheter over 2–3 seconds. After administration of the first quarter-dose, remove the catheter from the endotracheal tube. Manually ventilate the infant with a hand-bag with sufficient oxygen to prevent cyanosis, at a rate of 60 breaths/min and sufficient positive pressure to provide adequate air exchange and chest wall excursion.

5. **In the rescue strategy,** the first dose should be given as soon as possible after the infant is placed on intermittent mandatory ventilation for management of RDS. In the clinical trials, immediately before instilling the first quarter-dose, the infant's ventilator was changed to a rate of 60 breaths/min, inspiratory time of 0.5 second, and FiO_2 of 1.0. Between each quarter-dose administration an interval of 30 seconds is allowed to permit stabilization and repositioning of the infant.

6. **Endotracheal tube suctions.** Unless clinically indicated, endotracheal tube suctions are discouraged for 1 hour after instillation of surfactant.

III. REDOSING

1. **Criteria for redosing** of each surfactant are provided by the

manufacturer.

2. **General criterion.** Generally, when an infant demonstrates an initial improvement in oxygenation, permitting a decrease in the FiO_2, additional doses are given (up to a maximum of 4 doses using Survanta) when the infant still requires an $FiO_2 \geq 0.3$ to maintain a $p_aO_2 \leq 80$ torr.

3. **Clinical experience** has documented that most infants require about 2 doses, although up to 4 doses are permitted. The frequency of dosing is every 6 hours.

4. **The technique for redosing** is identical to that for the initial dosing.

IV. COMPLICATIONS

1. **Intracranial hemorrhage.** In some studies of Survanta, there was an increased rate of intracranial hemorrhage.

2. **Pulmonary hemorrhage.** In randomized, placebo-controlled trials, there was a significant increase in pulmonary hemorrhage among infants receiving exogenous surfactant. Pulmonary hemorrhage has been attributed to several factors without a single factor, except increased left-to-right shunting through the patent ductus arteriosus, being identified.

3. **Transient oxygen desaturation, transient hypotension, and an attenuation of EEG amplitude** have been reported in some studies. Occlusion of the airway, too rapid administration of exogenous surfactant, and position of the infant with interference of the airway have all been shown to contribute to these complications.

4. **Movement of endotracheal tube.** Care must be taken not to dislodge or advance the endotracheal tube during surfactant administration.

EXOGENOUS SURFACTANT ADMINISTRATION FOR RDS

32

EXTRACORPOREAL MEMBRANE OXYGENATION

Some infants die of respiratory failure in spite of aggressive mechanical ventilation. Certain of these infants can now be saved with the short-term (<12 days) application of cardiopulmonary bypass techniques.

33

I. ECMO CENTERS

1. **Centers.** 110 centers (from four countries) are now equipped to provide ECMO as therapy for newborn infants.
2. **Transport to center** should be arranged before patient is moribund.

II. TECHNIQUE FOR VENOVENOUS AND VENOARTERIAL BYPASS

1. **Equipment.** Silicone membrane lung, small venous bladder, heat exchanger, polyvinyl chloride tubing, and roller pump.
2. **Vascular cannulation.** Right atrium via internal jugular vein using double-lumen catheter for single-site access for venovenous bypass. Alternatively, aorta via right common carotid artery and right atrium via internal jugular vein using single-lumen catheter system for venoarterial bypass. Internal jugular vein or both vessels are ligated in neck in venovenous and venoarterial bypass, respectively.
3. **Anticoagulation with heparin.**
4. **Bypass the lungs** with 80% of cardiac output for venoarterial bypass. Venovenous bypass does not decompress pulmonary circulation or support cardiac output.
5. **Personnel support** includes nurse plus an ECMO technician.
6. **Mechanical ventilation** is continued at low pressure and rate.

III. PATIENT SELECTION

1. **Potential.** Recovery within 2 weeks.
2. **Weight** >2000g.
3. **Gestational age** ≥ 35 weeks.
4. **No intracranial hemorrhage.**
5. **Severe respiratory failure** on maximum ventilatory support. Criteria should predict >80% chance for mortality. Examples follow; however, specific criteria should be established for each institution.
a. Alveolar–arterial oxygen gradient $(A–a)DO_2$ >620 torr for 8 hours and PIP >38cmH$_2$O.

$$(A–a)DO_2 = [FiO_2(p_{atm} – p_{H2O}) – P_aCO_2] – P_aO_2$$
$$= [713 – P_aCO_2] – P_aO_2 \text{ (at sea level)}$$

b. Acute deterioration (either criterion sustained for 2 consecutive hours):
   1) pH <7.15
   2) PaO2 <40 torr.
c. P_aCO_2 >50 torr and P_aO_2 <50 torr for 6 hours.
d. Oxygenation index (OI) >40 for 2 hours
   OI = mean airway pressure x FiO_2 x $100/P_aO_2$.
6. **Causes of pulmonary hypertension** include chronic vascular remodeling, meconium aspiration syndrome, sepsis, asphyxia, RDS, or diaphragmatic hernia.

IV. RESULTS

1. **Overall survival 81%.**
a. Better in aspiration syndromes (93%).
b. Worse in diaphragmatic hernia (58%).
2. **Neurological outcome.**
a. 75% normal.
b. Damage can precede ECMO.
c. Carotid ligation can interact with hypoxemia/ischemia from other causes.
d. Risk reduced with venovenous bypass and sparing of carotid artery.
3. **Chronic lung disease.**
a. 20% of survivors affected.
b. Critical injury occurs before ECMO begins.

V. FUTURE DEVELOPMENTS

1. **Single-catheter techniques** – use of smaller double-lumen catheter (12 F) may allow its use in smaller infants (1500–2000g).
2. **Improved equipment** such as pulsatile pumps.
3. **Non-thrombogenic materials** such as heparin-bonded circuitry.
4. **Perfection of techniques** to repair carotid artery.

THORACOSTOMY

I. NEEDLE THORACENTESIS

A. INDICATIONS.

1. **Evacuation of pneumothorax.**
a. Non-tension pneumothorax with ventilation/perfusion abnormalities.
b. Tension pneumothorax including sudden life-threatening deterioration in blood gas without radiographic confirmation when tension pneumothorax is suspected.
2. **Evacuation of pleural fluid.**

B. TECHNIQUE.

1. **For evacuation of air,** enter pleural space via 2nd intercostal space (ICS) midclavicular line (MCL) with neonate supine. Attach 20g (or smaller) angiocatheter or butterfly needle to a 3-way stopcock and large syringe. Use a quick, betadine preparation and insert the needle perpendicular to the chest into the intrapleural space via the second intercostal space on the midclavicular line. Avoid the areola and nipple. Remove needle stylet, if there is one, as soon as pleura is punctured and advance catheter. Attach T-connector and open stopcock to the catheter. Gently aspirate air and confirm results radiographically. Take care not to enter too far into the pleural cavity, to avoid lung perforation.

2. **For evacuation of fluid,** enter pleural space via 4th ICS (level of the nipple). Use in fluid removal from the chest cavity. Prepare as above. Using an 18-gauge butterfly or angiocath, insert the needle into the 4th ICS in the midaxillary line (MAL) and direct the needle through the pleural space toward the posterior axillary line. Aspirate fluid into the syringe as needed.

II. CHEST TUBE PLACEMENT

A. **INDICATIONS.** Satisfactory decompression of a tension pneumothorax and/or fluid collection usually requires continuous suction via a chest tube connected to an underwater seal. Aspiration with a needle and syringe usually gives only temporary relief in infants requiring assisted ventilation, but may be all that is required in infants who are breathing spontaneously.

B. **TECHNIQUES.** Chest tubes may be positioned anteriorly (for evacuation of air) or posteriorly in the pleural cavity (for fluid drainage).

1. **Anterior placement of chest tube.**

a. Prepare with betadine and alcohol, drape area, wear sterile gloves, and pass instruments in a sterile fashion.

b. The site of insertion may be in the 2nd–4th intercostal space just lateral to the midclavicular line (risk of injury to internal mammary vessels) or in the 4th–6th intercostal space in the anterior axillary line (AAL).

c. Argyle trocar catheters (size 12 F) may cause pulmonary lacerations and are preferably used without trocar.

d. Position the infant with the affected side elevated 60°. Anesthetize the area of skin incision (6th–7th ICS MAL) with 1% lidocaine. Make 1/2 cm skin incision with a No. 15 scalpel blade. Make a tract with a closed, curved Kelly forceps tunneling to the 4th ICS puncturing the pleural space in the 4th ICS over the top of the 5th rib, allowing air to leak. Gently spread the forceps to open the space. Either grasp the tube between the blades of the forceps or place the closed tip of the forceps into the tip of the catheter via the first side hole. Advance the catheter along the tract into the pleural space, directing the catheter across the anterior thorax. Remove the forceps and advance the catheter 1–2cm past the last side-hole.

e. Connect the chest tube to a chest-tube suction apparatus at 10cmH$_2$O or to a Heimlich valve (when transport of infant is anticipated).

f. Anchor chest tubes securely with a purse-string suture (4-O silk) and a high-tie. Cover site with bacitracin ointment, or vaseline gauze, and a small dressing.

g. Obtain an ABG value, BP measurement, and chest radiograph immediately after placing the tube to assess the effectiveness of the tube and its position.

2. **Posterior placement of chest tube.**

a. Prepare as above. Position the infant supine without elevating the affected hemithorax.

b. Incise the skin at the level of the 6th ICS AAL. With a curved hemostat, tunnel into the subcutaneous tissue posteriorly along the 6th ICS to the MAL. Puncture the pleural space at the level of the MAL and spread the hemostat gently to open the pleura. Advance the chest tube posteriorly to desired length while removing the hemostat. Connect chest tube to suction apparatus and suture and secure as with anteriorly placed chest tubes. Confirm placement with radiograph.

c. A simple percutaneous device referred to as a pigtail catheter for pleural drainage in newborns is available. The area is prepped and draped. An introducer needle is inserted as in chest tube placements and a guide wire is threaded. The needle is withdrawn taking care to leave the guide wire at the desired area, and a dilator is threaded through the wire to help open the skin area. Once that is accomplished, the dilator is withdrawn and the pigtail catheter is placed making sure that all six holes are inside the pleural space. The guide wire is then pulled out and the catheter is connected by a Luer lock to a closed drainage system. A suture is tied around the catheter to secure it.

C. COMPLICATIONS.

1. **Inappropriate placement** either from misdiagnosis or placement too far into the cavity with entry into the mediastinum; side-hole outside pleural space

2. **Trauma:** lung laceration or perforation; perforation of a major vessel with hemorrhage or chylothorax; residual scarring; damage to breast tissue.

3. **Nerve damage:** diaphragmatic paralysis or eventration from phrenic nerve injury, or Horner's syndrome from pressure of right-sided posterior chest tube.

4. **Infection.**

5. **Subcutaneous emphysema** with leak of pneumothorax.

III. CHEST TUBE REMOVAL

A. INDICATIONS.

1. **Pulmonary air leak has sealed,** as indicated by cessation of bubbling from the chest tube for a period of 24 hours.

2. **Pneumothorax has disappeared on radiograph.**

3. **Pneumothorax does not reappear** after 4 hours clamping of the chest tube or cessation of bubbling for at least 4–6 hours on water seal.

B. TECHNIQUE.

1. **Removal of tube.** Remove the dressing and wipe area with antiseptic solution. Cut the suture to the chest tube. Cover the insertion site with petroleum gauze. At the end of the inspiration phase of respiration or positive pressure ventilation, rapidly remove the tube while applying pressure with the gauze over the site to produce an airtight seal.

2. **Wound closure.** The wound may then be closed with a 4-0 silk suture or small strips of tape.

3. **Monitoring.** Follow the infant's vital signs closely and obtain a follow-up chest radiograph.

34

THORACOSTOMY

PERICARDIOCENTESIS FOR PNEUMOPERICARDIUM

35

I. INDICATIONS

1. **Pericardial air,** on chest radiograph, causing cardiovascular compromise.
2. **Sudden, life-threatening deterioration** in blood gases and circulation without radiographic confirmation when cardiac tamponade is suspected; transillumination may be helpful in locating air collection.
3. **Tamponade** secondary to fluid or blood collection.

II. TECHNIQUE

1. **Instruments.** A 20-gauge angiocatheter or a 19–22-gauge intracatheter, T-tube connector, 3-way stopcock, and sterile syringe are needed.
2. **Preparation.** The subxiphoid area is prepped with betadine.
3. **Procedure.** The angiocatheter is advanced from the subxiphoid position toward the left midclavicle at about a 30° angle with the chest wall. Once a 'pop' is sensed, negative pressure is applied to the syringe to aspirate air or other contents. The catheter is then advanced and sewn in place with the T-tube connector attached to an underwater seal at $-10cmH_2O$ pressure.
4. **Alternative procedure.** An intracatheter with 1 or 2 additional side-holes is used. An ECG lead in the precordial position is connected to the needle. A tracing is present when the skin is contacted, disappears when the needle is advanced subcutaneously, and reappears when the pericardium is entered. The catheter is then advanced, secured, and attached as above.

ADJUNCTS TO MECHANICAL VENTILATION

A. PURPOSE.

a. To improve ventilation and to reduce incidence of atelectasis.

b. To improve the clearance of mucus and debris from the airways.

B. INDICATIONS.

For patients with excess or thickened pulmonary secretions, atelectasis, and prophylactically in patients with chronic lung disease and impaired respiratory mechanics (e.g. paralyzed infants).

C. EQUIPMENT.

a. Percussion tools:
   1) Newborn percussor
   2) Infant or premature mask
   3) Nipple attached to syringe holder
   4) Battery-operated toothbrush with padding or mechanical percussor.

b. Suction equipment.

c. Blanket roll (optional to aid in positioning infant).

D. TECHNIQUE.

a. The combination of suctioning, chest percussion, and vibration (PVS) can be considered as a treatment unit.

b. Steps:
   1) Auscultate lungs and/or view recent radiographs to determine areas of greatest need for treatment.
   2) Place infant in position which promotes maximal drainage of involved lobes.
   3) Percussion: tap the infant's chest to loosen bronchial secretions, in sets lasting approximately 1 minute, in desired position as tolerated, as an aid to suctioning.
   4) Vibration: rapidly produce an even vibratory motion. Usually we follow one set of percussions with 1 minute of vibration. Vibrate areas of greatest need for 2 minutes.
   5) Suctioning upon completion of procedure, and if necessary during procedure.
   6) Auscultate to evaluate effectiveness and need for further suctioning.

c. PVS should be interrupted immediately if the neonate's color or clinical condition deteriorates.

d. Care must be exercised to avoid tender areas, including sites of trauma or surgery.

e.   These techniques are often fatiguing to the infant and time-consuming for nursery personnel and therefore should be used judiciously.

E.   FREQUENCY.

Frequency depends on productivity of secretions, therapeutic goals, and tolerance. General guidelines for PVS orders are as follows.

1.   RDS. The acute phase (first 48 hours) is not accompanied by significant tracheobronchial secretions, and PVS is usually not needed. Routine endotracheal suctioning should suffice. At about 48 hours of age, an exudative phase begins, and PVS every 4–8 hours (usually scheduled before feedings) is helpful. As RDS resolves, the frequency of PVS can be decreased.

2.   **Meconium aspiration.** PVS every 2–4 hours may be helpful during the first 8–12 hours of life. Subsequently a lesser frequency should suffice.

3.   **Pneumonia.** PVS is usually of benefit only when there are increased secretions.

4.   **Atelectasis of isolated lobes.** PVS should be concentrated on those areas.

5.   **Paralyzed and comatose infants and infants with chronic lung disease** probably benefit from routine PVS every 12–24 hours whether or not secretions are evident. The addition of a nebulized or metered-dose inhaler (MDI) bronchodilator, such as albuterol, may be helpful in infants with chronic lung disease. Such therapy must be re-evaluated periodically.

F.   ASSESSMENT.

PVS orders must be individualized, not ritualized, and frequently reassessed.

a.   Personnel providing PVS therapy are often the best judges of effectiveness and patient tolerance.

b.   Auscultate lungs and/or view recent radiographs to determine areas of greatest need for treatment

c.   Tolerance of PVS therapy should be evaluated initially and periodically using a transcutaneous CO_2 monitor and pulse oximetry.

G.   RELATIVE CONTRAINDICATIONS AND PRECAUTIONS.

1.   **Relative contraindications.**

a.   Bronchopulmonary fistula.

b.   Bronchospasm.

c.   Coagulopathy.

d.   Large pleural effusions.

e.   Anoxic spells in premature neonates.

f.   Pulmonary edema with CHF.

g.   Pneumothorax.

h.   Airway risk of aspiration.

i.   Rib fractures.

j.   Recent pulmonary embolus prior to adequate anticoagulation.
2.   **Precautions.** If an infant does not tolerate PVS, blood gases may deteriorate for the subsequent 30 minutes or even longer.
a.   Infants who have cardiorespiratory instability (e.g. persistent pulmonary hypertension, uncontrolled systemic hypertension, unstable arrhythmias) are the most likely to deteriorate during PVS.
b.   The Trendelenberg (head down) position is *not* recommended during care of the premature neonate since it may contribute to increased intracranial pressure and intraventricular hemorrhage.

II. INHALATION ADJUNCTS
See Table 36.1.

TABLE 36.1
INHALATION ADJUNCTS

Drug/Route[a]	Action	Indication	Dosage	Comments	Adverse Rxn
Albuterol (Ventolin), salbutamol (Proventil)/ ET, naso-oral, or MDI	Stimulates β1 (minor) β2 (strong), duration 4–6h	Bronchoconstriction	0.05–0.2 mL in 2mL NS, or MDI: 2 puffs q2–6h	Use 0.5% soln. If 0.083%, do not dilute. Increase dose if given orally (2–5mg q6h). May titrate dose to weight, desired effect or side effects. Consider continuous aerosol option	Slight CV, slight CNS (see footnote[b]). Interactions: propranolol (β-blockers)
Terbutaline sulfate (Breathine, Bricanyl)/ET or naso-oral	Selective β₂ agonist	Severe broncho-constriction/BPD	0.2–0.5mL/kg in 2mL NS	No approved FDA or manufacturer dose published for inhalation. Use the injectable form, 1mg/ml	See footnote[b]
Cromolyn sodium (Intal)/ ET, naso-oral, or MDI	Prevents degranulation of sensitized mast cells, duration 2–6h	Bronchoconstriction	1mL(10mg), or MDI: 1-2 puffs q5h	Desired effect in 4 weeks or less. Compatible with all other bronchodilators	Bronchospasm, cough, local irritation, vertigo
Racemic epinephrine (Micronefrin, Vaponefrin)/ naso-oral	Stimulates: (mild) β₁ (medium) β₂ (short) duration 1–2h	Tracheobronchial inflammation, bronchoconstriction	0.1–0.2mL in 2mL NS	For postextubation stridor, ET bypasses affected desired area. Titrate dose to weight, desired effect, or side effects. May repeat up to 3 times	See footnote[b]

Ipratropium bromide (Atrovent) / MDI	Anticholinergic, potentiates β_2 stimulation	Bronchoconstriction	MDI: 1–2 puffs q6h (10–80mg)	Can be administered via ET with adaptors. Major effect is on larger airways	Few side effects, epistaxis, dry mouth or throat, nasal congestion or dryness
Glycopyrrolate (Robinol)/ ET or naso-oral	Anticholinergic muscarinic	Excess salivation and respiratory secretions	0.8mg in 2mL NS	No approved FDA or manufacturer dose published for inhalation. Recommended to add albuterol in conjunction	Atropine-like effect: bronchospasm, glaucoma, tachycardia, urinary retention, ileus, colitis, or liver disease
N-Acetylcysteine (Mucomyst) 10% (Do not use 20%)/ ET or naso-oral: aerosol or direct instillation	Breaks mucous disulfide bonds, decreases mucous viscosity	Thick secretions	0.5–1.5mL in 2mL NS up to q2h	Recommend adding broncho-dilator (i.e. albuterol) due to possibility of bronchospasm associated with administration. May increase secretions if used too long or too often	Allergic sensitivity, incompatible with some antibiotics; stomatitis, rhinitis, nausea, bad odor/ taste

MDI, metered dose inhaler (need to be bagged into infants as they rarely have enough negative inspiratory force); ET, endotracheal tube; NS, normal saline.

[a]Aerosolized agents administered during inhalation via endotracheal tube or naso-oral breathing.

[b]Adverse reactions with sympathomimetic bronchodilators:

Pulmonary – bronchial irritation and edema;

CNS – restlessness, nervousness, headache, weakness, anxiety, tremor, fear, irritability, insomnia, vertigo.

Cardiovascular – increased BP, increased heart rate, palpitations, anginal pain, coronary insufficiency, peripheral vasoconstriction.

Other – vomiting/nausea, urinary retention, hypersensitivity, tachyphylaxis.

ADJUNCTS TO MECHANICAL VENTILATION

36

ANALGESICS, SEDATIVES, AND MUSCLE RELAXANTS

37

Analgesia and sedation should be administered for humanitarian reasons since pain is associated with certain necessary medical and surgical procedures. Remember, pain can still be appreciated during pharmacologic paralysis. In addition, infants with pain or discomfort may exhibit agitated behavior and struggle against mechanical ventilation. Under such circumstances, sedation and analgesia not only improve ventilation, they may hasten recovery and may decrease complications such as pneumothorax and intraventricular hemorrhage.

I. ANALGESIA

A. MORPHINE.

a. Opium alkaloid (stimulates opiate receptors in the CNS).
b. Produces sedation, analgesia, and respiratory depression.
c. Decreases gut motility, increases anal and urinary sphincter tone.
d. Well absorbed by all routes.
e. Onset of action peaks at about 1 hour after injection.
f. Duration of action in neonates about 2–4 hours.
g. Detoxified by hepatic conjugation with glucuronide, which is then excreted in the urine and bile.
h. Usual individual dose is 0.1–0.15mg/kg of the sulfate. May be repeated every 2–6 hours.
i. May be given by continuous i.v. infusion at 0.05–0.1mg/kg/h after an initial loading dose of 0.10mg/kg.
j. With prolonged administration, some degree of tolerance, requiring an increasing dosage, can be expected.
k. A weaning regimen, reducing the dose by 10–20% per day, is recommended.
l. Morphine effects may be reversed by administering naloxone, 0.1mg/kg.

B. FENTANYL.

a. Synthetic opioid 80 times more potent than morphine.
b. Lacks sedative properties of morphine.
c. In high doses, it can cause chest wall rigidity and hypotension.
d. Fewer other side effects than morphine.
e. Onset of action is minutes but duration of action only 1–2 hours.
f. Can be given by intravenous bolus, 1–2mcg/kg, when short-term analgesia is desired.

g. For longer-term effects, infusion is begun at 1–2mcg/kg/h and increased according to symptom relief.

h. Tolerance occurs more readily than with morphine, and a weaning regimen is recommended.

i. Effects can be reversed by naloxone.

C. NALBUPHINE (NUBAIN).

a. Synthetic narcotic agonist.

b. As potent as morphine.

c. Respiratory depression also similar to morphine.

d. May precipitate withdrawal in infants dependent on other narcotics.

e. Onset of action 2–3 minutes after i.v. dose.

f. Dose is 0.1– 0.2mg/kg q4–6 hours as needed.

D. ACETAMINOPHEN.

a. Analgesia produced by raising pain threshold.

b. Antipyretic activity on hypothalamus.

c. Hepatic toxicity rare except with massive overdosage.

d. Rare blood dyscrasias.

e. Contraindicated in glucose-6-phosphate dehodrogenase (G6PD) deficiency.

f. Dose is 10–15mg/kg q6h orally or 20–30mg/kg q6h rectally.

II. SEDATION

A. DIAZEPAM.

a. Characteristic benzodiazepine.

b. Has anxiolytic, hypnotic, anticonvulsant, muscle relaxant, and amnesic effects.

c. Benzodiazepines have no analgesic properties.

d. Long-acting sedative

e. Elimination half-life 75 hours in premature infants and 30 hours in full-term infants.

f. Metabolized in the liver.

g. May help infants to 'settle' on the ventilator.

h. Dose is 0.10–0.25mg/kg q6h i.v.

B. MIDAZOLAM (VERSED).

a. A benzodiazepine.

b. Onset of action, 5–6 minutes.

c. Twice as potent as diazepam but shorter duration of action.

d. Metabolized in the liver and excreted in the urine.

e. Not clear what impact it would have on development.

f. Dose is 0.1mg/kg i.v. q2–4h as needed.

g. Toxicity unusual and may present as excessive somnolence.

h. Can be obtained without benzoyl alcohol as a preservative.

C. LORAZEPAM (ATIVAN).

a. A benzodiazepine with potent anticonvulsant activity.

b. Onset of action 5–6 minutes.

c. Duration of action 3–24 hours.

d. Conjugated in the liver.

e. Low incidence of toxicity. Apnea, somnolence, and movement disorders might be anticipated.

f. Dose is 0.10mg/kg i.v. q4–12h depending on effect.

g. May be given in conjunction with morphine or fentanyl.

D. THORAZINE.

a. A phenothiazine.

b. Limited information in infants.

c. Dose is 0.5–1.0mg/kg i.v. q4–6h.

d. May also produce pulmonary vasodilatation.

E. CHLORAL HYDRATE.

a. A hypnosedative with actions similar to the barbiturates.

b. Does not significantly depress respiratory drive.

c. No analgesic properties, and it is a gastrointestinal irritant.

d. Converted to trichloroethanol by the liver.

e. With repeated and prolonged use, trichloroethanol can accumulate to toxic levels and cause paradoxical CNS stimulation and cardiac arrhythmias.

f. Dosage of 50mg/kg for one-time sedation appears to be well tolerated.

III. MUSCLE RELAXANTS

While muscle relaxants are not routinely used during mechanical ventilation of neonates, they may be useful in selected infants whose own respiratory efforts interfere with ventilation and in severely hypoxemic infants with persistent pulmonary hypertension. The paralyzed neonate is dependent on mechanical ventilation, and careful monitoring is required. Paralysis also obscures the detection of seizures and pain. Their effects on the incidence of pneumothorax and intraventricular hemorrhage and the magnitude of cardiac output in preterm infants are unclear. Paralysis for more than a few days has been associated with a decrease in dynamic lung compliance and an increase in total pulmonary resistance. Some infants suffer subsequent hypotonia and skeletal muscle growth failure.

Muscle relaxants are usually administered as a therapeutic trial and continued if ABG values improve, if nursing care is greatly simplified, or if patient comfort is obvious.

A. PANCURONIUM.

a. Long-acting, competitive neuromuscular blocking agent.

b. Has vagolytic effect, and an increase in heart rate is commonly observed.

c. Maximum paralysis within 2–4 minutes.

d. Variable duration in neonates from one to several hours.

e. Primarily renal excretion.

f.   Dosage in neonates varies in the range 0.06–0.10mg/kg q2–4h.
g.   Continuous infusion best avoided in neonates because of potential for accumulation.
h.   Effects can be rapidly reversed with neostigmine, 0.08mg/kg i.v. preceded by glycopyrrolate, 0.01mg/kg, to block the muscarinic side effects.

B. VECURONIUM.

a.   A short-acting nondepolarizing muscle relaxant.
b.   Onset of action 1.5–2.0 minutes after i.v. bolus.
c.   Duration only 30–60 minutes.
d.   Few cardiovascular side effects.
e.   Cleared rapidly by biliary excretion.
f.   Safer than pancuronium in the presence of renal failure.
g.   Dose by continuous infusion is 0.1mg/kg/h after an initial bolus dose of 0.1mg/kg/h.
h.   Intermittent bolus dosing impractical for long-term paralysis.
i.   Can be reversed by neostigmine as described above.

FURTHER READING

Costarino AT, Polin RA. Neuromuscular relaxants in the neonate. *Perinatal Pharmacol* 1987; 14:965.

Fitzpatrick KTJ, Black GW, Crean PM, Mirakhur RK. Continuous vecuronium infusion for prolonged muscle relaxation in children. *Can J Anaesth* 1990; 38:169.

Hartley S, Franck LS, Lundergan F. Maintenance sedation of agitated infants in the neonatal intensive care unit with chloral hydrate: new concerns. *J Perinatol* 1989; 9:162.

Jacqz-Aigrain E, Wood C, Robieux I. Pharmacokinetics of midazolam in critically ill neonates. *Eur J Clin Pharmacol* 1990; 39:191.

Levene MI, Quinn MW. Use of sedatives and muscle relaxants in newborn babies receiving mechanical ventilation. *Arch Dis Child* 1992; 67:870.

McDermott CA, Kowalczyk AL, Schnitzler ER, et al. Clinical and laboratory observations: pharmacokinetics of lorazepam in critically ill neonates with seizures. *J Pediatr* 1992; 120:479.

FLEXIBLE FIBER-OPTIC BRONCHOSCOPY

Flexible fiber-optic bronchoscopy and laryngoscopy permits direct visualization of the dynamic anatomy of the upper and lower airway during spontaneous breathing. This is particularly advantageous in neonates, where the small airway is susceptible to dynamic collapse – a frequent cause for extubation failures, obstructive apneas, and feeding difficulties. Flexible bronchoscopy is also useful for identifying congenital anomalies of the airway, for obtaining lower airway secretions for cytologic and microbial analysis, and for the removal of mucus plugs contributing to atelectasis.

I. INDICATIONS FOR BRONCHOSCOPY

1. **Intubated patients.**
a. Unexplained CO_2 retention.
b. Unexplained extubation failure.
c. Atelectasis causing significant respiratory embarrassment.
d. Intubation of a difficult airway.
2. **Nonintubated patients.**
a. Stridor (inspiratory wheezing).
b. Lower-airway (expiratory) wheezing.
c. Evaluation of obstructive apnea.
d. Poor feeding, especially when associated with hypoxia.
e. Recurrent focal lobar atelectasis or pneumonia.

II. COMMON BRONCHOSCOPIC DIAGNOSES

a. Laryngomalacia (up to 85%).
b. Subglottic stenosis.
c. Vocal cord paralysis.
d. Vascular rings and slings.
e. Tracheal or bronchial stenosis.
f. Tracheomalacia and bronchomalacia.
g. Laryngeal cleft.
h. Mass lesions (granulation tissue, papillomatosis, cystic hygroma, hemangiomas).

III. ALTERNATIVES TO FLEXIBLE BRONCHOSCOPY

Direct examination of the upper airway with a laryngoscope can identify structural abnormalities of the larynx and pharynx. However, this procedure distorts normal anatomic relationships, making it difficult to establish the functional importance of a particular lesion. A limited evaluation of the upper airway with either a flexible bronchoscope or laryngoscope can be performed, but associated lower-airway anomalies (e.g. tracheomalacia) will be missed by this procedure. Rigid bronchoscopy is not effective for evaluating dynamic lesions that are best observed during spontaneous respiration. Rigid bronchoscopy is the procedure of choice when surgical intervention is anticipated (e.g. removal of granulation tissue). The flexible bronchoscope can also be used to examine the lower airway in an intubated, mechanically ventilated patient. Table 38.1 gives a comparison of the techniques.

TABLE 38.1
COMPARISON OF TECHNIQUES

	Flexible bronchoscopy	Direct laryngoscopy	Rigid bronchoscopy
Sedation	Conscious sedation. Procedure performed in ICU or monitored setting	Sedation not required	General anesthesia. Procedure performed in OR
Anatomic relationships	Normal dynamic anatomic relationships maintained	Anatomic relationships may be distorted by laryngoscope blade	Some distortion of anatomic relationships and no spontaneous airway movement
Risks	Small with skilled bronchoscopist. Sedation is principal risk	Minimal	Risks related to anesthesia and postop airway management
Image quality	Good, documented on videotape and print film	Depends on the skill of the operator	Excellent, documented on print film
Airway management	No control of airway in nonintubated infants but can be performed in intubated infants with sufficient endotracheal tube size	Some control of airway	Complete control of airway by anesthesiologist

IV. PROCEDURE
1. **Patient preparation.**
a. Reliable i.v. access.
b. NPO for 4 hours prior.
c. Hemodynamic and respiratory stability.

d.   Control of hemostasis abnormalities, stable acid/base, and electrolyte status.
2.   **Monitoring.** Bronchoscopy should be performed in a setting with sufficient equipment and skilled personnel to administer sedation safely and manage the airway. Monitoring includes continuous pulse oximetry and ECG. Transcutaneous CO_2 monitoring is useful for prolonged procedures. Blow-by oxygen is delivered during the procedure.
3.   **Sedation and anesthesia.** Narcotic analgesics that can be reversed with naloxone are the preferred means for managing sedation. Anesthesia is delivered topically by applying lidocaine to the nasopharynx, larynx, and lower airway through the bronchoscope suction channel.

V. RISKS/COMPLICATIONS
1.   **Common.**
a.   Sedation-related airway obstruction.
2.   **Uncommon.**
a.   Bleeding.
b.   Swelling/trauma.
c.   Laryngospasm.
d.   Infection.
e.   Aspiration.
f.   Pneumothorax.

VI. PEDIATRIC BRONCHOSCOPES
Examples of typical pediatric bronchoscopes are given in Table 38.2.

TABLE 38.2

TYPICAL PEDIATRIC BRONCHOSCOPES

Name	Overall diameter (mm)	Tip diameter (mm)	Minimum ET size (mm)	Suction channel (mm)
Olympus BF3C10	3.7	3.5	4.5	1.2
Pentax FB10X	3.5	3.4	4.5	1.2
Pentax FI-7P	2.5	2.4	3.0	none
Olympus BFN20	2.2	1.8	3.0	none

38

FLEXIBLE FIBER-OPTIC BRONCHOSCOPY

BLOOD-SAMPLING TECHNIQUES

I. CAPILLARY BLOOD SAMPLING (HEEL STICK)

1. **Purpose.** To obtain small amounts (1mL or less) of blood for capillary blood gas determinations, hematology, and blood chemistry measurements
2. **Equipment.**
   a. Lancet.
   b. Chemical warmer.
   c. Alcohol, cotton ball or gauze.
3. **Technique.** The large lancets are used for larger premature and term infants. The small lancets are used exclusively for small premature infants. A 25-gauge needle may also be used as a lancet in very small premature infants (<500g) requiring frequent heel sticks.
   a. Warm extremity.
   b. Clean with alcohol.
   c. Insert the lancet in the posterior lateral instep.
   d. Collect blood sample in a large heparinized capillary tube or specially designed microtainer tube.

II. ARTERIAL PUNCTURE

1. **Purpose.** To obtain blood for arterial blood gas analysis, as well as hematology, coagulation studies, blood chemistry, cultures, etc. Radial, temporal, and posterior tibial arteries are the most accessible and are safest for percutaneous arterial sampling. Brachial and femoral arterial puncture should be avoided. Radial artery puncture is described in detail.
2. **Equipment.** The same equipment is used for each site and is of individual preference. Heparin is not used if sample is to be sent for coagulation studies.
   a. Heparinized tuberculin syringe with a 25-gauge needle, or
   b. Scalp vein needle, 23- or 25-gauge preflushed with heparin and connected to a syringe by assistant after blood flow has been established.
3. **Technique.**
   a. Immobilize extremity with armboard and tape, or enlist the help of an assistant.
   b. Cleanse area thoroughly with alcohol (and povidone-iodine if blood culture is being obtained).

c. After identifying arterial pulsation, insert needle bevel up at a 45° angle to skin, aiming proximally; advance until blood appears in hub or tubing. Occasionally blood will be obtained while needle is being withdrawn rather than advanced.

d. Once blood flow is evident, have assistant attach syringe to tubing if using scalp needle and gently withdraw until desired sample is obtained.

e. Remove needle and apply direct pressure to entry site for 5–10 minutes to minimize hematoma formation.

III. UMBILICAL CATHETERS

1. **Purpose.** To obtain blood for blood gas analysis, hematology, chemistry, culture, etc.; generally not acceptable for coagulation studies, because of heparin contamination; glucose measurement may also reflect contamination if glucose-containing solution is being infused through line.

2. **Equipment.** (For catheter insertion, see Chapter 40.)

a. Sampling syringes.

b. Flush syringes (saline or infusate).

3. **Procedure.**

a. Place the stopcock and tubing on a sterile pad.

b. Clean the stopcock with an alcohol swab.

c. For ABG and usual laboratory studies, clear the line by withdrawing 2–3mL of blood. For coagulation studies, attempt to clear the line by withdrawing 4mL of blood and note the source of the sample for the laboratory.

d. Disconnect the syringe, letting one drop of blood overflow. For arterial blood gas, draw 0.3mL of blood into heparinized syringe, expel air, attach stopper, and place on ice (0.6mL if electrolyte and ionized calcium panel is requested).

e. Reinfuse the 2–4mL of blood previously withdrawn and clear the line with 0.5mL flush solution.

f. Record volumes of blood removed and flush infused in appropriate section of nursing notes.

IV. PERIPHERAL VENOUS BLOOD SAMPLING

1. **Purpose.** To obtain blood for blood gas analysis and routine hematology, coagulation, chemistry, blood glucose; generally not acceptable for metabolic studies (lactate, pyruvate, ammonia) which require free-flowing blood.

2. **Equipment.**

a. Scalp vein needle or straight needle (user's preference). Size will be dictated by vessel location and caliber.

b. Tourniquet.

c. Alcohol; povidone-iodine if for culture.

3. **Select vein.** Suitable veins include scalp, posterior auricular, external jugular, dorsal arch (hand or foot), basilic, cephalic, cubital, and saphenous veins

3. **Technique.** In general, limb is tourniqueted, vessel identified visually or by palpation, area prepped appropriately, and vessel entered with needle bevel up at approximately 15–30° degree angle to skin. Once blood is seen in needle hub, gentle withdrawal into collecting syringe is necessary.

4. **Alternative technique.** The vena comitans of the brachial artery, or deep basilic vein, lies deep in the antecubital fossa lateral to the artery with little variation between individuals. Blood may be obtained safely by inserting a larger (18–21 gauge) straight needle at a 45° angle 1–1.5cm distal and perpendicular to a line connecting medial and lateral condyles with the arm fully extended. The path of the needle bisects the line and extends until periosteum is felt. Then withdraw gently with a 3–10mL syringe while withdrawing the needle until blood is obtained. Pressure should be applied to the site for at least 5 minutes following the procedure. Tourniqueting the extremity prior to blood draw may be helpful, but is not always necessary.

39

BLOOD-SAMPLING TECHNIQUES

PLACEMENT AND MANAGEMENT OF INTRAVASCULAR CATHETERS

I. UMBILICAL ARTERIAL CATHETER

A. INDICATIONS.
1. ABG monitoring.
2. Continuous BP monitoring.
3. Angiography.

B. PERMISSIBLE USES (NOT INDICATIONS).
1. Obtaining blood specimens.
2. Blood transfusion and blood product infusion if other site is not available.
3. Alkali therapy.
4. Exchange transfusion (for blood withdrawal only).
5. Infusion of maintenance solutions. All infusates should contain heparin, 0.5–1.0 units/mL.

C. PROHIBITED SUBSTANCES (EXCEPT IN RESUSCITATION).
1. Concentrated calcium solutions of 400–600mg/dL.
2. Tolazoline (bolus infusion).
3. PN solutions (except with attending physician's approval).
4. Hypertonic glucose solutions in excess of 12.5%, excluding TPN.
5. Vasotoxic drugs.

D. INDICATIONS FOR REMOVAL.
1. When alternative for monitoring becomes available.
2. When FiO_2 is low and frequent ABGs no longer needed.
3. Thromboembolic complications.
4. Sepsis with positive culture drawn.

E. CONTRAINDICATIONS. Should not be used in presence of the following.
1. Omphalitis.
2. Peritonitis.
3. NEC.
4. Omphalocele.
5. Evidence of local vascular compromise in lower extremities.

F. EQUIPMENT REQUIRED.
1. Umbilical artery catheterization tray supplemented with the following.
a. Polyvinyl chloride or silastic UAC, No. 3.5 F for infants with birth weight <1500g, No. 5 F for larger infants.
b. Three-way stopcock attached to a blunt needle if not attached to UAC.
c. Umbilical tape.

d. Scalpel blade.
e. 4-0 silk suture.

G. TECHNIQUES.

1. Insertion of UAC.

a. Attach the infant to a cardiac monitor. Sterile gloves, clean gown, mask, and cap must be worn by the operator. Prepare the cord and surrounding skin thoroughly with betadine while an assistant holds the cord off the abdomen.

b. Place umbilical tape loosely around the base of the umbilical cord (for control of bleeding). Cut the umbilical cord 1–2cm from skin with a scalpel (not scissors). Drape the infant, but allow for observation.

c. Grasp cord with thumb forceps and hold upright. When the cut surface is blotted, the umbilical vessels can be identified: the single, large, thin-walled oval vein can readily be distinguished from the two smaller, thick-walled, round arteries.

d. The closed tips of the small curved iris forceps should be gently inserted into the lumen of one artery until the cut end of the artery is at the bend in the forceps; the spring of the forceps is allowed to spread the tips apart, thus dilating the artery. Repeatedly dilate the lumen until the orifice appears large enough to accommodate the catheter.

e. Grasp the catheter about 1cm from the tip between the thumb and forefinger or with forceps, and, while the cord stump is held upright, insert the catheter into the lumen of the dilated artery. An assistant may grasp the arterial wall with forceps to facilitate insertion of the catheter.

f. One of two positions for the tip of the catheter may be chosen. The calculation of the length of the catheter for placement is done by measuring shoulder-to-umbilicus length or by using birth weight in kilograms.

   1) High UAC at level of T6–9 (110% of shoulder-to-umbilical length plus length of stump): catheter tip is above the celiac axis and below the ductus arteriosus. Associated with fewer episodes of blanching of lower extremities but may be associated with increased incidence of IVH and hypertension.

   2) Low UAC at level of L3–4 (60% of shoulder-to-umbilical length plus length of stump): catheter tip is below major aortic branches (renal/mesenteric).

2. Troubleshooting.

The catheter may encounter obstruction at the level of the anterior abdominal wall or the bladder. Obstruction can usually be bypassed by gentle, steady pressure for 30–60 seconds. Do not attempt to force the catheter. As a last resort, remove the catheter, empty the saline, partially fill with 2% xylocaine without epinephrine, fill with normal saline so that xylocaine now fills tip of catheter, reinsert catheter, and infuse 0.1–0.2mL of xylocaine. Wait 1–2 minutes until the drug has relaxed the vasospasm, then advance the catheter. If false tracks are encountered, leave catheter in same vessel (this technique assumes that the first catheter will occupy the false track and the new catheter will advance within the arterial lumen). Remove first catheter after second catheter is successfully placed. If unsuccessful, catheterization of the other artery should be attempted. If difficulty is encountered, consult fellow or attending physician.

3. **Stabilization of catheter.**
a. When the catheter has been inserted to the desired length, ensure that there is free flow of blood before the catheter is stabilized.
b. Flush the catheter. Observe both legs for evidence of blanching, cyanosis, or mottling.
c. Place a purse-string suture in the interior wall of the cord around the catheter. Tie the suture snugly, but not so tightly that you kink the catheter. Leave the ends of the suture long. Wrap these around the catheter about 0.5cm from the end of the cord, using a clove hitch, and then tie with a square knot.
d. Paint the abdomen with tincture of benzoin and allow to dry. Secure catheter to a tape bridge.
e. Apply antibiotic ointment to umbilicus stump.
f. Attach catheter and stopcock to i.v. tubing, making sure all bubbles have been removed from the system. Begin infusion to prevent blood from clotting in the catheter.

4. **Removal of catheter.**
a. Cut and remove sutures holding catheter in place.
b. Gently loosen adhesive tape from skin.
c. Withdraw catheter slowly, then apply several centimeters at a time over 3–5 minutes, and then apply pressure directly to umbilicus with 2x2 sponges. Maintenance of pressure for up to 5 minutes is usually adequate to stop bleeding. If persistent or brisk bleeding occurs, control can be obtained by pinching the lower abdominal wall just inferior to the umbilicus for several minutes. Insertion of a purse-string suture may be necessary if bleeding continues.
d. Apply antibiotic ointment to the umbilicus.
e. Observe umbilicus for bleeding.

H. COMPLICATIONS.
1. **Vasospasm causing blanching of a leg or buttocks.** May resolve by warming of the opposite leg. Remove catheter if there is no improvement within the hour.
2. **Vessel perforation.**
3. **Thrombosis and embolism.**
4. **Hemorrhage** from accidental dislodgement, disconnection of the catheter, breaks in the catheter, or vessel perforation.

40

PLACEMENT/MANAGEMENT OF INTRAVASCULAR CATHETERS

5. Infection.
6. **Hypertension,** especially if tip is located close to the origin of the renal arteries.
7. **Rare complications:** peritoneal perforation, false aneurysm, air embolism, transection of an omphalocele, sciatic nerve palsy.

II. RADIAL ARTERY CATHETERS
A. INDICATIONS.
1. ABG monitoring.
2. Arterial BP monitoring.
3. When UAC placement is not possible, a UAC thromboembolic complication has occurred, or surgery requires ABG and BP monitoring.
B. PERMISSIBLE USES (NOT INDICATIONS).
1. Fluid administration.
2. **Sodium administration** (0.45 normal sodium chloride containing 0.5–1.0 units of heparin per milliliter of infusate to maintain catheter patency).
3. Drawing blood specimens.
C. PROHIBITED SUBSTANCES: known vasotoxic substances.
D. CONTRAINDICATIONS.
1 Inadequate collateral blood flow.
2. Extremity ischemia.
3. Local skin infection.
4. Bleeding disorder.
E. COMPLICATIONS.
1. Infection.
2. Thrombus formation/thromboembolism.
3. **Air embolism** leading to tissue ischemia which may result in limb shortening or amputation.
F. EQUIPMENT.
1. **Angiocatheter,** 22 or 24 gauge.
2. Short extension tubing, T-connector.
G. TECHNIQUE.
1. Percutaneous radial artery puncture.
a. Occlude radial artery by compression for 30 seconds to ensure adequate collateral circulation to the hand (modified Allen test).
b. Fix arm to armboard with wrist in slight extension. Avoid hyperextension. Do not obstruct view of fingers to check for color changes.
c. Clean area with betadine, allow to dry, and re-prep with alcohol. Allow site to dry.
d. Using sterile gloves, identify radial artery pulse. A transilluminator placed under or lateral to the wrist may aid in the identification of the radial artery.

e. Insert angiocatheter at an angle of 30–40° from forearm for a distance of 0.5–1.0cm.

f. Remove stylet and slowly withdraw catheter until blood returns. Then angle catheter slightly and advance until resistance is met. If no blood appears as the stylet is withdrawn, do not reinsert stylet as this may sheer the cannula tip off into the artery. Instead, slowly pull back the catheter until blood flows. Remove the catheter if there is still no blood return and retry.

g. Attach extension tubing, withdraw arterial blood gas sample, and slowly flush with heparinized saline.

h. Fix the catheter in place with suture or tape and secure extension tubing.

2. Cutdown on radial artery.

a. If unsuccessful with percutaneous catheter, let vessel recover for 1 hour (if possible) before proceeding.

b. Identify location of radial artery pulse and surgically prepare area. Use sterile surgical technique.

c. Anesthetize locally with 1% plain lidocaine and make superficial 0.5–1.0cm skin incision across wrist medial to the radial styloid process (at or just above the proximal wrist crease).

d. Carefully blunt dissect tissue, identifying the radial artery (it may not pulsate visibly).

e. Puncture the vessel, inserting the Medicut® (or similar catheter) at a 30° angle (from the wrist–forearm) through the artery.

f. Remove the needle and gently remove the catheter until the tip is in the lumen. Blood flow usually returns unless the artery is in spasm. Then advance the catheter until resistance is met.

g. *Do not* ligate the radial artery or tie suture around the vessel and catheter. The vessel will recanalize following removal.

h. When blood returns, attach the extension tubing and flush the catheter slowly with heparinized saline.

i. Stabilize the catheter with tape and sutures used in wound closure.

3. Removal.

a. Compress over insertion site and slowly withdraw.

b. Maintain compression for 5 minutes

4. Posterior tibial artery. If radial artery cannot be catheterized, posterior tibial artery is an alternative.

III. UMBILICAL VENOUS CATHETER
A. INDICATIONS.

1. Central venous pressure monitoring.
2. Exchange transfusion.
3. Emergency vascular access during resuscitation.
4. Balloon atrial septostomy.

40

PLACEMENT/MANAGEMENT OF INTRAVASCULAR CATHETERS

B. PERMISSIBLE USES (NOT INDICATIONS).

1. Infusion of:
a. Fluid, glucose, and electrolyte administration.
b. All resuscitation drugs.
c. Antibiotic.
d. Blood product or albumin infusions.
e. Cardiotonic agents (if advanced thorough ductus venous into vena cava).

2. **Drawing blood specimens.**

C. PROHIBITED SUBSTANCES. See Section I.

D. INDICATIONS FOR REMOVAL. Duration should not generally exceed 48–72 hours unless critically needed as in venous access for VLBW infants.

E. CONTRAINDICATIONS.

1. **Omphalitis.**
2. **Omphalocele.**
3. **Peritonitis.**
4. **NEC.**

F. COMPLICATIONS.

1. **Infections.**
2. **Thromboembolism.**
3. **Malpositioned in heart,** causing arrhythmias, endocarditis, effusion, cardiac tamponade.
4. **Catheter malpositioned in portal system,** causing hepatic necrosis.

G. TECHNIQUES.

1. **Insertion.**
a. The preparation is the same as for UAC placement. Cut umbilical stump 1–2cm from skin.
b. Grasp umbilicus with thumb forceps and gently probe vein lumen. Since the vein extends cephalad from the umbilicus, the entering probe may be held almost parallel to the abdomen below the umbilicus. Remove any visible clots with forceps.
c. Ensure that the catheter is filled with heparinized saline and attached to a syringe when it is introduced. *Extreme care* must be taken that the catheter is not open to the atmosphere, since air embolus can occur if the infant takes a deep inspiration producing negative pressure in the thoracic inferior vena cava.
d. The calculation of the length of the catheter for placement is done by measuring shoulder-to-umbilicus length or by using birth weight in kilograms. For UVC at level of T8–11 or just above the diaphragm (66% of shoulder-to-umbilical length plus length of stump), verify location of the catheter tip by radiograph or venous pressure tracing. If the tip is in the liver, slowly remove the catheter until blood can no longer be withdrawn and then advance 0.5cm. This will prevent

infusing hypertonic or toxic substances directly into the lower hepatic circulation.

2. **Troubleshooting.**
a. If resistance is met at 2–3cm, the cord is pulled caudally to 'straighten' a tortuous vein.
b. If the catheter 'bounces back' before the measured length, it is most likely in the portal vein. The catheter is withdrawn, rotated and reinserted in an attempt to pass through the ductus venosus. Do not use force in inserting catheter.
c. If there is no blood on drawback at 2–3cm length, there may be a clot. Remove the clot by applying gentle suction as the catheter is being withdrawn. Then reinsert catheter.
3. **Removal.** Same as with UAC.
4. **In emergency** situations and for exchange transfusion, the catheter is inserted just far enough to get a blood return (approximately 4–5cm length).

IV. DEEP VENOUS CATHETER

A. INDICATIONS AND USES. Intravenous access for:
1. Parenteral nutrition.
2. Fluids, glucose and electrolytes.

B. INDICATIONS FOR REMOVAL.
1. Sepsis.
2. Occlusion of catheter.
3. Vascular complications.
4. Indication has resolved.

C. EQUIPMENT. Sterile materials needed:
a. Silastic radiopaque medical grade tubing 0.7mm o.d., 0.3mm i.d. in 30cm and 40cm lengths.
b. 27 gauge blunt needle.
c. 19 gauge scalp vein needle.
d. Fine forceps.
e. Scalpel.

D. PLACEMENT.
1. Percutaneous placement.
a. An antecubital, external jugular, or scalp vein can be selected for use.
b. For an antecubital vein placement, the extremity is taped on an armboard. A soft rubber band acts as a tourniquet.
c. The skin is cleansed with betadine and draped with sterile towels.
d. The silastic catheter is flushed with heparinized saline.
e. A 19 gauge needle is introduced a short distance into the vein and, using fine forceps, the catheter is threaded into the needle. The catheter is advanced 1 or 2 mm at a time, until it is thought to be in the superior vena cava. When an arm vein is used, the catheter

40

PLACEMENT AND MANAGEMENT OF INTRAVASCULAR CATHETERS

occasionally will meet resistance at the shoulder. Manipulation of the arm often makes it possible to pass this resistance.

f.   The needle is then withdrawn, the catheter removed from the connector, and the needle discarded.

g.   Position of the catheter tip in the superior vena cava should be confirmed by radiograph. Collodion is then applied at the catheter insertion site to prevent slippage.

h.   The site is covered with dry gauze or Op-Site®. The connector of the silastic catheter is attached to the i.v. tubing. A strip of pH paper placed beneath the blunt needle and catheter will identify any leakage of solution.

2. **Cutdown.**

a.   The basilic vein in the antecubital fossa is most commonly used.

b.   Following preparation of the extremity (as above), the area is infiltrated with 1% lidocaine, and a small incision is made in the medial antecubital fossa.

c.   The basilic vein is located by blunt dissection, a ligature placed beneath it, and the vessel nicked with a scalpel or veniotomy scissors if available. The silastic catheter, flushed with heparinized saline, is inserted with the fine forceps and advanced into the superior vena cava.

d.   Tunneling of catheter through 19 gauge butterfly needle.

e.   The position is confirmed by radiograph, the wound is sutured, and the site is covered with a dry, sterile gauze or Op-Site®.

CONTINUOUS MONITORING OF OXYGENATION AND VENTILATION

Oxygen saturations can be monitored continuously using pulse oximetry. Continuous monitoring of transcutaneous PO_2 and PCO_2 may be accomplished with a heated skin electrode.

I. PULSE OXIMETRY

A. PRINCIPLE.

a. Utilizes two diodes in a single probe emitting light at 660nm and 940nm that are absorbed differently by saturated and unsaturated hemoglobin.

b. Measurements are made of the change in light transmittance through an extremity or digit during arterial pulses of blood, and an algorithm calculates the oxygen saturation (SaO_2).

B. SPECIAL CONSIDERATIONS.

a. Pulse rate measured by oximeter must match monitored heart rate to assure accuracy ($\pm 2\%$). Inaccurate sensing of arterial pulsations will result in invalid (falsely low) SaO_2 readings. Causes of inaccurate sensing include movement, restriction of blood flow, edema, cardiovascular collapse, and environmental light interference, such as phototherapy light.

b. Carboxyhemoglobin absorbs light in the same wavelength as oxyhemoglobin; thus the sensor will not differentiate between the two and will give falsely high SaO_2 readings when COHb levels are high ($>3\%$).

c. Differences in HbF, bilirubin, and skin pigmentation do not cause clinically significant changes in saturations determined by pulse oximeter.

d. It is important to note that in general the saturation as determined by pulse oximetry reflects a true measure of the actual hemoglobin saturation in the infant. Simultaneous blood gas sample results may give a lower saturation value because it is determined from an HbA oxygen-saturation curve using only the measured P_aO_2 in the sample and assuming a Hgb of 15g%.

II. TRANSCUTANEOUS PO_2

A. PRINCIPLE.

a. The skin is maintained at a preset temperature by a heated electrode (term infant 44–45°C, preterm 43–44°C) while an electrochemical skin sensor measures the skin surface partial pressure of oxygen.

b. The response time for detection of acute changes in transcutaneous pO_2 ($TcpO_2$) is about 15–20 seconds.

c. In general, the monitor must be calibrated every 4 hours and skin site rotated every 2–4 hours.

B. SPECIAL CONSIDERATIONS.

a. $TcpO_2$ is not identical to directly measured $p_a O_2$, and the relationship must be established for each patient. Correlation coefficients should be 0.92 or better if properly used.

b. Causes of poor correlation include:
   1) Altered skin perfusion at the sensor site (i.e. local ischemia when skin is stretched taut over rib or other bony prominence as electrode is applied)
   2) Shock or hypoperfusion
   3) Edema.

c. If the infant is crying while blood is sampled by arterial puncture, a decrease in $P_a O_2$ may occur which may not be reflected in the cutaneous $TcpO_2$ for another 20–30 seconds.

d. Right-to-left shunting through the ductus arteriosus will produce a higher $TcpO_2$ in the right upper chest than over the abdomen.

C. COMPLICATIONS.

a. Local irritation and skin abrasion, due to adhesive on sensor, is difficult to avoid.

b. Burns:
   1) First degree – erythema may last several days
   2) Second degree – blister formation may also occur. This can be minimized by changing site more frequently and usually precludes use in infants <1000g.

III. TRANSCUTANEOUS PCO_2

A. PRINCIPLE.

a. Similar to $TcpO_2$ above, but heating the skin to 41.5°C will suffice.

b. Site must be changed and monitor recalibrated every 4 hours.

B. SPECIAL CONSIDERATIONS.

a. Complications related to heating are fewer and accuracy is high, making $TcpCO_2$ the current measure of choice.

b. See II.B above.

c. Correlates better with changes in $P_a CO_2$ than with the actual $P_a CO_2$.

IV. END-TIDAL CO$_2$ MONITORING

Common in the pediatric and adult ICU setting but not yet practical in the neonate. Problems include excess weight and dead space (in-line sensors) and mechanical/circuit difficulties (side-stream sensors and slow response time). Currently only of use in larger term infants. In smaller newborns, end-tidal CO$_2$ is not a direct measure of P$_a$CO$_2$, because of high anatomic dead space to tidal volume ratio and changing physiologic dead space with varying degrees of lung disease, and it should therefore be standardized by correlating with blood gas measurements.

41

CONTINUOUS MONITORING OF OXYGENATION AND VENTILATION

OBTAINING SPINAL FLUID

42

The four procedures available for collection of CSF are lumbar, subdural, cisternal, and ventricular punctures.

I. LUMBAR PUNCTURE

Lumbar puncture is most frequently used for obtaining CSF for diagnostic purposes.

1. **Positioning of infant.** Lumbar puncture may be performed in either the lateral recumbent or sitting position. In sick premature infants being ventilated, or with chest tubes present, the procedure is more easily done in the lateral recumbent position. The surface on which the infant is placed should be firm and flat. The infant is restrained with hips, knees, and neck flexed. Make sure that the cardiorespiratory status is not compromised with positioning.

2. **Skin preparation.** Prepare the skin over the lumbar area with betadine as for a surgical procedure.

3. **Pertinent landmarks** are the spinous processes and iliac crests. The line joining the tops of the iliac crests passes through the 4th spinous process. The space between L3 and L4 or between L4 and L5 is the site of choice for puncture.

4. **Spinal needle with stylet** (to prevent epidermoid tumor from being introduced into epithelial tissue) is inserted into the chosen intravertebral space in the exact midline and perpendicular to the plane of the body, aiming cephalad. When the dura mater is pierced, remove the stylet and examine the needle hub for the appearance of fluid. In premature infants, one may not feel a 'pop' as the dura is entered.

5. **When the fluid is obtained,** collect samples in tubes 1, 2, and 3 for the following studies: protein and sugar; cell counts with differential, culture and sensitivity; and Gram stain. Concurrent blood glucose level should be obtained for comparison. 'Dry' taps and bloody taps are more frequent in neonates. However, the presence of blood may be a pathological finding indicating subarachnoid or intraventricular hemorrhage.

II. CISTERNAL, SUBDURAL, AND VENTRICULAR PUNCTURES

These are usually performed by the neurosurgical service.

SUPRAPUBIC BLADDER ASPIRATION

43

I. TECHNIQUE

1. EQUIPMENT.

a. Antiseptic solution: e.g. betadine.
b. 3mL or 6mL sterile syringe.
c. 22 gauge 1in or 1.5in needle.

2. PROCEDURE.

a. Ensure that the patient has not just voided.
b. The infant is placed on a flat surface.
c. An assistant stands opposite the operator and immobilizes the infant by grasping the lower thorax with one hand, and the thighs and hips with the other (frog-leg position). Occlusion of the urethra in the male or anterior rectal pressure in females will prevent reflex voiding during cleansing and needle insertion.
d. Operator locates the symphysis pubis with one finger and inserts the needle 1–2cm above the symphysis in the midline and perpendicular to the flat surface.
e. With a single steady motion, the needle is inserted until a perceptible change in resistance is felt as the needle enters the bladder. Light suction is applied to aspirate the urine specimen. It may be necessary to rotate the needle if the bevel is against the bladder wall.

II. COMPLICATIONS

Essentially a benign procedure, the most frequent complication has been transient hematuria. Entering the bowel may occur, and, in a dehydrated patient, resultant fistula formation has been reported.

ADMINISTRATION OF BLOOD AND BLOOD COMPONENTS

44

I. BLOOD SUPPLY

Since newborns require small volumes of blood (except for exchange transfusions), a single-donor unit of RBCs can provide multiple transfusions, provided that the unit has attached satellite bags. The blood components are from donors negative for hepatitis B surface antigen, syphilis testing and antibodies to HIV and hepatitis C. RBC, WBC and platelet components should be from donors negative for antibodies to CMV. Fresh-frozen plasma, frozen-thawed deglycerolized RBCs and cryoprecipitate need not be tested for antibody to CMV since freezing destroys the WBCs in which the virus is located.

II. USE OF BLOOD COMPONENTS

1. **Infants <1200g in birth weight** should receive irradiated RBC, WBC, and platelet components to prevent graft-versus-host disease. Irradiation destroys the mitotic spindle, making the donor lymphocytes incapable of division. However, other functions such as oxygen-carrying capacity of RBCs or phagocytosis by WBCs are not impaired by irradiation.
2. **Infants with acidosis** should receive RBC and platelet components <3 days old since the pH drops to 7.0 after several days of storage.
3. **Infants who are premature** and need replacement blood only because of frequent blood drawing or from chronic anemia due to prematurity can be transfused with RBCs that are up to 21 days old. 2,3-glucose 6-phosphate dehydrogenase is restored in vivo within 24 hours.
4. **Anticoagulant.** All infants should receive blood components collected in citrate-phosphate-dextrose (CPD) anticoagulant. Adsol® contains too much adenine, which may be harmful to the immature kidney and also contains 100mL of normal saline added to 250mL of RBCs, so this component is not recommended.
5. **Cross-matching.** Since infants are unable to mount an immune response to foreign RBC antigens until 4 months after term delivery, it is necessary to cross-match the infant only once. In addition, the mother's serum is cross-matched at this time since her antibodies might be of higher titer than the infant's. Thereafter, ABO Rh compatible RBCs with no cross-match are given.
6. **All infants** can receive O Rh negative RBCs (universal donor red cells) if convenient.

7. **Multiple infants.** A whole or part of a Pedi-Pack® set can be cross-matched with multiple infants. Three or more infants may be cross-matched with and receive aliquots of a single part if transfused concurrently. Mixing plasma and packed cells at a 1:1 ratio will yield a hematocrit reading of about 45%. Test the hematocrit value after adding plasma.

8. **Pedi-Packs® with three bags** are usually set up to minimize exposure to multiple donors. Three Pedi-Packs, each with approximately 80mL volume, can be made from one adult unit of packed RBCs.

9. **Platelets, cryoprecipitates, and fresh frozen plasma** are usually needed to combat DIC due to sepsis. Septic infants are prone to undergo T-antigen activation of their red blood cells. (The bacterial enzymes digest the infant's blood group antigens to a primitive antigen called T.) Since all adult plasma contains antibodies to T, hemolysis of the infant's cells would develop if T activation had occurred. A plant lectin test for T antigen can be done within 10 minutes in the laboratory on a drop of RBCs. It should be done within 6 hours of anticipated transfusion. If T activation has occurred, platelets are washed and resuspended in 5% albumin. If fresh-frozen plasma is needed, the least incompatible of five units is given after a minor cross-match has been done.

10. **Granulocyte transfusion** may be needed in septic conditions. Irradiation of the component does not interfere with the phagocytotic ability of the granulocytes.

11. **Pediatric fresh-frozen plasma is usually of AB blood type** since that is the universal plasma. Three Pedi-Packs® are made from one adult unit each containing about 60mL.

12. **Filtering.** All blood components should be filtered.

EXCHANGE TRANSFUSION

I. SELECTION OF BLOOD

Use fresh blood <48 hours old. Blood stored in citrate-phosphate-dextrose longer than 48–72 hours may have an unacceptable serum potassium concentration, increased acid load, and decreased 2,3-diphosphoglycerate content.

1. **For Rh hemolytic disease,** select blood as follows.
   a. If the baby's ABO group is unknown, suspend group O, Rh-negative packed cells in AB fresh-frozen plasma.
   b. If the baby's blood group is known, prepare blood as shown in Table 45.1.
2. **ABO hemolytic disease** is not very common, because α and β antigens are poorly expressed at birth. Use group O, Rh-specific, packed cells cross-matched with both mother and infant serum specimens, accompanied by group-specific fresh-frozen plasma.
3. **Hyperbilirubinemia** with negative direct Coombs test result, or exchange transfusion for sepsis or hyperammonemia – use group-specific, Rh-specific, whole blood.

TABLE 45.1
BLOOD PREPARATIONS FOR BABIES WITH KNOWN BLOOD TYPE

Types		
Mother's	Baby's	Give baby
A	A	A Rh negative whole blood
O	O	O Rh negative whole blood
O	A	O Rh negative cells in A or AB plasma
O	B	O Rh negative cells in B or AB plasma
AB	A	A Rh negative whole blood
AB	B	B Rh negative whole blood

Use red cell products as fresh as possible.

II. TECHNIQUE

1. **Exchange transfusion** may be performed through a UVC, via an inferior vena cava catheter placed from a peripheral vein, or by simultaneous infusion through a UVC and withdrawal from an UAC.
2. **General conditions.**

a. Evacuate gastric contents and restrain the infant under a radiant warmer. Place the infant on cardiorespiratory monitor.
b. Use aseptic technique in placing catheters and throughout the procedure.
c. Nurse should monitor and record heart rate, respiratory rate, temperature, behavior, volume of blood infused, and volume removed through the exchange.

3. Catheter placement.

a. Catheter should ideally be placed through the ductus venosus into the inferior vena cava with the tip at the level of the diaphragm. It should not lie in the pulmonary, hepatic, or portal veins, as pressure from infusion or injection of calcium may cause damage.
b. Location of the tip of the catheter should be verified radiographically before exchange transfusion; if it is technically impossible to pass the catheter through the ductus venosus, exchange transfusion should be performed with the catheter removed as far as possible and still obtaining blood return.

4. Preparation of blood.

a. When exchange transfusion is performed with reconstituted whole blood, calculate the amount of plasma (V_{plasma}) to add to packed cells (V_{RBC}) as follows:

$$V_{plasma} = V_{RBC} (Hct_{RBC} / Hct_{desired} - 1)$$

b. Since the Hct of citrate-phosphate-dextrose packed cells is usually about 80% and the desired Hct of the exchange blood is 40–50%, it is usually satisfactory to add 60–100mL plasma per 100mL packed RBCs. Note that packed cells containing additive have Hcts of 60–65% and lower serum proteins.
c. Practical considerations in determining desired Hct:
   1) Patient's bilirubin level (plasma volume more important)
   2) Patient's Hct and oxygen requirement (RBC volume more important)
   3) Size of infant and exchange volume desired. CPDA packed cell units are about 240mL. Do not sacrifice exchange volume in order to achieve a higher Hct.
d. Blood should be warmed to 37.5°C in blood warmer. Mix blood periodically during the procedure to prevent settling.

5. Procedure.

a. Normally, a double-volume exchange transfusion is performed (one volume = 80mL/kg for term infants and 90–100mL/kg for preterm infants).
b. Exchange increments (syringe size) vary from 5mL in the smallest unstable infant to 20mL in a term infant.
c. Initially, withdraw the first increment and save for laboratory tests (Hct,

total/direct bilirubin, calcium, etc.). Then transfuse with an equal amount.

d. Do not leave infant with a deficit unless there is evidence of CHF (enlarged liver, high CVP).

e. Calcium gluconate 10%, 0.5–1.0mL, may be given slowly after every 100–150mL of blood if the infant is jittery or has a low pre-exchange calcium level.

f. Velocity of replacement is important. A slow (1–2 hour) procedure is probably more efficient in removing bilirubin from tissue stores and is safer.

g. As an alternative to venous exchange, blood may be simultaneously infused into the venous catheter and removed from a UAC using 30–50mL syringes and two operators.

h. Infusion through the umbilical artery should be avoided since spinal injuries due to microemboli may occur. A high UAC may perfuse the brain circulation directly with acidic exchange blood.

i. Postexchange specimen:
   1) Send to blood bank for cross-match with new blood donor for subsequent exchange transfusion.
   2) Send to laboratory for Hct, total/direct bilirubin, binding tests, platelets, calcium, sodium, potassium, and glucose analysis.

j. Volume deficit – except for severely hydropic infants, erythroblastotic infants have near-normal blood volumes, and high CVPs are usually the result of acid–base imbalance. However, donor blood has a high plasma protein concentration compared with that of premature or erythroblastotic infants. This may result in fluid shifts and volume overload that may not be apparent until after the procedure is over. Careful monitoring of CVP, limited exchange transfusion with packed cells, and appropriate adjustment of vascular volume by leaving a volume deficit may be required in severely affected newborns.

III. EFFICIENCY

1. **A two-volume exchange transfusion** will remove about 90% of the circulating fetal RBCs.

2. **Postexchange bilirubin concentration** will usually be about one-half the pre-exchange value and will typically rebound to about two-thirds the initial concentration. If the postexchange bilirubin concentration is higher than two-thirds the pre-exchange level, a large extravascular reservoir of bilirubin probably exists, and an additional exchange will usually be required within hours.

IV. POSTPROCEDURAL CARE

1. **Observation.** Observe the infant for evidence of heart failure, enlarging liver, tachycardia, arrhythmias, tachypnea, and abnormal distention.

45

EXCHANGE TRANSFUSION

2. **Feeding.** If the condition is stable, feed the baby 2–4 hours after the procedure.
3. **Blood glucose.** Monitor the blood glucose level (Dextrostix) after the exchange.
4. **Bilirubin.** Check bilirubin concentration for postexchange rebound 4 hours after the exchange. This value should provide a baseline for evaluating the subsequent rate of rise of serum bilirubin.

V. COMPLICATIONS

Complications are infrequent, but include the following.

1. **Cardiac arrest** due to hyperkalemia, hypocalcemia, citrate toxicity, air embolization, volume overload, and arrhythmias.
2. **Vascular complications** due to air or clot embolization, thrombosis, phlebitis, tissue necrosis from calcium infusion, and NEC (colonic perforation).
3. **Electrolyte imbalance** from hyperkalemia, hypernatremia, hypocalcemia, and acidosis.
4. **Hemorrhage** from heparin, thrombocytopenia, and vessel perforation.
5. **Infection** from hepatitis, CMV, or bacteria.
6. **Miscellaneous complications** from mechanical injury to donor cells, transfusion reaction, graft-vs-host syndrome, and reactive hypoglycemia.

PERITONEAL DIALYSIS

46

I. INDICATIONS
1. **Renal failure** in association with the following.
a. Severe hyperkalemia (serum potassium level >7.5mEq/L, presence of ECG abnormalities, or both).
b. Severe acidosis (serum bicarbonate level <12mEq/L) and azotemia (BUN level >75mg/dL).
c. Volume overload with congestive failure, hypertension, or massive edema.
2. **Other.**
a. Hyperammonemia.
b. Drug overdosage.

II. SELECTION AND PREPARATION OF DIALYSIS SOLUTIONS
1. **Peritoneal dialysis** is performed with commercially available dialysate solutions warmed to body temperature prior to usage. Patients with significant lactic acidosis, which may occur in the presence of liver disease and hypoxia/hypoperfusion and which is initially identified by an elevated anion gap, should not be dialyzed with solutions containing lactate. A bicarbonate dialysis solution may be used with the necessary calcium provided parenterally.
a. Heparin, 1 unit/mL, should be used initially.
b. A 1.5% glucose solution should be used initially.
c. Higher glucose concentrations can be used if fluid removal has been inadequate with lower concentrations. Severe hyperglycemia may occur with high dextrose-containing dialysate solutions.
2. **Potassium.** Normokalemic patients should have potassium (3.5mEq/L) added to dialysate solution, while hyperkalemic patients should be initially treated without added potassium until serum values return to normal.

III. PROCEDURE
1. **Catheter placement.**
a. A 14 gauge intravascular catheter with three side-holes added, or a pediatric dialysis trocar catheter shortened if necessary by cutting the tip to ensure that side-holes remain in the peritoneum, is used.
b. If long-term dialysis is anticipated, a Tenckhoff catheter is preferred.
c. Place the catheter through the surgically prepared area in the left lower or right lower quadrant.

d. Connect the catheter to an extension tube, a 'Y' connector, and to a clamped tube leading to the dialysate and evacuation bottles. Maintain a closed system and change tubing and bottle every 12 hours. A commercially available peritoneal dialysis kit is usually used to supply the needed tubing and connectors.

2. **Dialysate** is infused by gravity, using a dwell time of 30–45 minutes. Fluid is then removed by gravity.

3. **Small exchange volume** should be used in the range 20–30mL/kg, since large volumes can compromise ventilation.

4. **Weighing.** The infant should be weighed 2–4 times daily. Strict recording of the patient's weight, intake, and output must be maintained.

5. **Monitoring.** Serum sodium, potassium, and glucose values should be monitored every 2–6 hours, and routine chemistry studies performed every 24 hours. Calcium should be monitored closely if a bicarbonate dialysis solution is used.

6. **Antibiotics** may be provided in the dialysate at the first sign of peritonitis or to maintain levels in infants who are already receiving antibiotics.

IV. COMPLICATIONS

1. **Infections.** Gram stain and culture solutions every 12–24 hours.

2. **Fluid overload.** Increase the amount of glucose in the dialysate to 2.59g/dL and monitor the blood glucose level carefully. Occasionally 4.25g/dL glucose is required.

3. **Hyperglycemia** may require insulin, 0.1–0.3 units every 4 hours, or as needed, to maintain normal glucose levels.

4. **Hypokalemia.** Increase the amount of potassium in the dialysate.

INFANT TRANSPORT

47

I. REGIONALIZATION OF NEONATAL CARE

1. **Rural (primary) and community (secondary) facilities** may need to transfer sick infants to regional (tertiary) centers for special care. (Maternal transport is generally preferred but not always feasible.) Ground transportation is used for most transports within 100 miles. Air transport (fixed wing) is more efficient for longer distances. Occasionally, helicopter transport is utilized for shorter distances when patient's medical condition warrants more rapid team arrival for stabilization and transport.

2. **Consultation.** Following initial resuscitation of a sick infant, referring physicians are encouraged to contact their tertiary center and the attending neonatologist, or other specialists, for consultation or patient referral. A 24-hour 'hotline' is often available for this service.

II. STABILIZATION FOR TRANSPORT

Steps taken by the referring physician and the transport team to stabilize infants for and during transport may differ from those normally taken in the care of an inborn infant, but the goals are similar.

1. **Initial history and physical examination** should provide the major diagnosis or diagnoses.

2. **Circulation.** Pretransport assessment should include BP determination, assessment of capillary filling, blood volume, and an Hct reading. Therapy for hypoperfusion should be initiated before transport.

3. **Oxygenation and ventilation.**

a. The goal is to maintain the arterial oxygen tension in the range 50–80 torr and the arterial carbon dioxide tensions in the range 35–55 torr during transport.

b. If available, transcutaneous oxygen and carbon dioxide monitors and/or pulse oximeters should be used.

c. Team members may have to rely on their clinical assessment and provide enough oxygen to relieve central cyanosis.

d. Criteria for ventilatory assistance during transport are more lenient than in the NICU in order to ensure a safer transport and should be individualized in consultation with the neonatologist responsible.

4. **Glucose homeostasis.**

a. Parenteral glucose infusion at ≥ 4–6mg/kg/min is indicated if the patient is normoglycemic, and at 8mg/kg/min if the patient has been hypoglycemic.

b. During transport, Dextrostix monitoring should be continued and the GIR adjusted to maintain an estimated glucose concentration of 40–120mg/dL.

5. **Sepsis/meningitis.** If infection is suspected, evaluation and initiation of treatment should normally be begun before transporting the infant.

6. **Thermal protection.**

a. Prewarm the transport module and pad.

b. You may also place an inner heat shield in the transport module or wrap the infant in thin plastic blankets.

c. Minimize the time outside the warmer or incubator. Manipulate the infant through the entry portals only.

d. If the infant is already hypothermic, rewarming is accomplished by setting the module air temperature a maximum of 1.5°C above the abdominal skin temperature. Gooseneck lamps should not be used. Warm water bottles (surgical gloves filled with warm water) or preferably chemical (sodium thiosulfate, dextrose, and water) warming mattresses may be used, provided that direct skin contact is avoided.

e. If the infant is hypothermic, measure an initial rectal temperature and follow as necessary. Assisted ventilation may be required if apnea develops during rewarming.

7. **Gastrointestinal decompression.** Infants with vomiting or abdominal distention or who are at risk for aspiration should have a nasogastric tube placed for intestinal decompression prior to transport.

8. **Specific stabilization procedures.** See appropriate sections.

9. **Parental contact.** Talk to the parents and show them the infant before leaving the referring hospital. Make sure all consent forms are signed and properly witnessed.

48 NEONATAL DRUG FORMULARY

DRUG	ROUTE	DOSAGE	COMMENTS
Acetaminophen	p.o., p.r.	10mg/kg/dose q6–8h p.o.; 20mg/kg/dose q6–8h p.r.	Analgesic and antipyretic.
Acetylcysteine	ET, p.o., p.r.	Nebulize 2–5mL of 5–10% solution q4–12h	May induce bronchospasm in larger infants.
Acetylcysteine		10mL of 10% solution p.o. or p.r. q6h x 3 for meconium ileus	Surgery if not relieved.
Acyclovir	i.v.	10mg/kg q8h for 10 days	Increase dosing interval to 24 hours if renal function is <25% of normal.
Adenosine	i.v. push	0.1–0.3mg/kg. Dilute 1:10 prior to giving with NS	Do not allow to mix with blood in syringe. For diagnosis and therapy of supraventricular tachycardia.
Albumin 25%	i.v.	1.0g/kg (4mL/kg).	Repeat as necessary, monitoring BP. Usually diluted 1:4 with saline.
Albuterol	Neb	0.1–0.5mg/kg/dose q2–6h	Selective β_2 agonist. May cause tachycardia.
Aminophylline	i.v.	5mg/kg loading dose; 5mg/kg/day divided q12 h	Monitor serum levels. Maintain theophylline level 6–13mcg/mL. Do not use with erythromycin.

48   NEONATAL DRUG FORMULARY

DRUG	ROUTE	DOSAGE	COMMENTS
Amoxicillin	p.o.	20–40mg/kg/day q8h dosing	Adjust dose for renal impairment.
Amphotericin B	i.v.	0.25mg/kg/day in single dose over 6h (dilute in D5W. Concentration not to exceed 0.1mg/mL). Increase daily as tolerated to 1mg/kg/day	See manufacturer's package insert. Renal and hematologic toxicity. Test dose not necessary in neonates.
Ampicillin	i.v.	*Initial dosage:* <1 week, 100mg/kg/day divided q12h; >1 wk, 150mg/kg/day divided q8h. *Continuing dosage:* Sepsis <1 week, 50mg/kg/day q12h; >1 wk, 100mg/kg/day q8h. Meningitis: continue initial dosage	
Atropine	s.c./i.v./i.m.	0.01–0.03mg/kg/dose	May also be given intratracheally.
Bethanechol	p.o.	0.6mg/kg/day divided q6–8h	Give 30–60min before feeding.
Caffeine citrate	p.o.	20mg/kg loading dose; 5mg/kg/day maintenance in 1 or 2 doses	Maintain blood levels 8–25 mcg/mL.
Calcium chloride (10%)	i.v.	Severe hypocalcemia or cardiac dysfunction, 20–30mg/kg/dose.	Give slowly. 27mg elemental calcium/mL (1.36 mEq/mL).

		Maintenance dose: 1mg/kg elemental calcium/kg/h	Avoid extravasation – severe tissue damage.
Calcium gluceptate (22%)	i.v.	Cardiac arrest/severe hypocalcemia: 10–20mg/kg/dose (1–2mL/kg/dose); Maintenance dose: 1mg elemental calcium/kg/h	Infuse no faster than 20mg Ca^{2+}/kg/min. 18mg elemental calcium/mL (0.9mEq/mL). Avoid extravasation – severe tissue damage.
Calcium gluconate (10%)	i.v.	Cardiac arrest/severe hypocalcemia: 10–20mg/kg/dose (1–2mL/kg/dose); Maintenance dose: 1mg elemental calcium/kg/h	Infuse no faster than 20mg Ca^{2+}/kg/min. 9.3mg elemental calcium/mL (0.46mEq/mL). Avoid extravasation – severe tissue damage.
Captopril	p.o.	Initial: 0.05mg/kg.	Give on an empty stomach.
Captopril	p.o.	Maintenance: 0.1–1.5mg/kg q6–12h	Contraindicated in bilateral renal artery thrombosis. Observe for neutropenia.
Cefazolin	i.v./i.m./p.o.	20mg/kg every 8–12h	Half-life 3–4.5h. Modify dosing interval for renal function below 50% of normal.
Ceftazidime	i.v./i.m.	50mg/kg/dose q12h, until 7 days of age, then q8h	Monitoring level not necessary. Synergistic with aminoglycosides. Third-generation cephalosporin.

48 NEONATAL DRUG FORMULARY

DRUG	ROUTE	DOSAGE	COMMENTS
Cefotaxime	i.v./i.m.	50mg/kg/dose q12h. >1 wk, 50mg/kg/dose q8h	
Ceftriaxone	i.v./i.m.	50mg/kg q24h for sepsis. 50mg/kg q12h for meningitis	Long half-life, third-generation cephalosporin.
Chloral hydrate	p.o./p.r.	25–50mg/kg/dose	Use for sedation. Gastric and mucous membrane irritant. Use with caution in renal and hepatic disease. Half life 37h. Requires 15min for sedation, 40min for sleep. Not analgesic. Check trichloroethanol levels if paradoxic agitation occurs.
Chloramphenicol	i.v./p.o.	<1 week, 25mg/kg/day; >1 week, 50mg/kg/day divided q12h	Monitor blood levels. Peak: 15–25mcg/mL; trough: 5–10mcg/mL.
Chlorothiazide	p.o.	10–20mg/kg q12h	Monitor electrolytes. May cause hypokalemia, hyperbilirubinemia, alkalosis, hyperglycemia.
Cholestyramine	p.o.	80mg/kg/dose q8h with feeds	Not absorbed; complexes with bile acids in intestine.
Cimetidine	p.o./i.v.	20mg/kg/day. Divided q6h or added to TPN	Histamine-receptor blocker. Contraindicated with cisapride because of potential for arrhythmias.
Cisapride	p.o.	0.8–2mg/kg/day divided q6h	Contraindicated with cimetidine or with GI bleeding or obstruction

Clindamycin	p.o.	10mg/kg q8h	Pseudomembranous colitis, rare in children. Do not use for meningitis.
Clonidine	p.o.	3–4mcg/kg/day divided q6h	For drug withdrawal.
Cortisone acetate	i.m./p.o.	Physiological replacement, 0.7mg/kg/day p.o. divided q8h. Pharmacologic dose, 2.5–10mg/kg/day divided q8h	
DDAVP	Intranasal	5–30mcg/day divided q12–24h	Titrate to effect. Use with caution in patients with predisposition to thrombus formation.
Desoxycortisone acetate (DOCA)	i.m.	1–5mg q24h	Adjust according to electrolyte level.
Dexamethasone	i.v./i.m./p.o.	0.1–1.0mg/kg/day divided q6–8h	Higher dose for short-term trial in brain edema or chronic lung disease.
Diazepam	i.v./i.m./p.o.	0.1–0.4mg/kg/dose. May repeat up to maximum total of 1mg/kg for status epilepticus	Titrate carefully to control seizures. Risk for circulatory and respiratory depression. Tolerance may develop. Long half-life.

48

FORMULARY

48 NEONATAL DRUG FORMULARY

DRUG	ROUTE	DOSAGE	COMMENTS
Diazoxide	i.v./p.o.	Hypertensive crisis: 2mg/kg i.v. over 15–30s. May repeat dose until desired BP.	90% protein bound. Primary effect on arterioles. Use with caution with other antihypertensives. Sodium retention. Increases epinephrine and insulin secretion.
Diazoxide		Maximum total dose 5mg/kg. Repeat effective dose every 2–6h p.r.n.	
		Hypoglycemia: 3–8mg/kg p.o. or i.v. over 1h q8–12h p.r.n.	For hypoglycemia, give slow i.v. and monitor BP.
Digoxin	i.v./p.o.	Orally: TDD premature infant: 20–30mcg/kg over 12–24h in divided doses: 1/2 stat, 1/4 in 6–12h, and 1/4 6–12h later.	TDD = total digitalizing dose. Usually can start on maintenance dose, 10mcg/kg/day divided q12h.
		Term: 30–50mcg/kg TDD dose over 12–48h, divided doses: 1/2, 1/4, 1/4.	Observe for arrhythmias.
		Maintenance dose: 1/4 to 1/3 of TDD per day q12h; i.v.: 2/3 of oral dose	
Dobutamine	i.v.	Same as dopamine	May be more effective than dopamine.

Dopamine	i.v.	2–5mcg/kg/min Increase up to 20mcg/kg/min as indicated	Titrate BP. Dilute 3mL of 12.5mg/mL dopamine in 250mL of 5% dextrose or normal saline solution giving a concentration of 150mcg/mL. Infusion rate of 1mL/kg/h will deliver 2.5mcg/kg/min. Avoid extravasation – severe tissue damage.
Edrophonium (Tensilon)	i.v.	Give 0.05mg/kg initially. Repeat at 1 min intervals to total dose of 0.2mg/kg.	If adverse reaction, give atropine, 0.01–0.04mg/kg.
Epinephrine	i.v./i.t.	0.1mL/kg/dose using aqueous 1:10,000 solution (0.1mg/mL)	Resuscitation.
Epinephrine	i.v.	0.5–1.5mcg/kg/min infusion D5W. Run 2–6mL/kg/h.	Refractory CHF or hypotension: 4 ampules of 1:1,000 in 250mL
Erythromycin	p.o./i.v.	Infants <1 week old, 10mg/kg/dose q12h; infants >1 week old, 10mg/kg/dose q8h	May increase serum levels of theophylline and digoxin.
Erythropoietin (EPO)	i.v.	200 units/kg/day, 4–7 days per week	Provide 1–2mg/kg/day of elemental iron. Contains human albumin.
Famotidine	i.v./p.o.	0.4–1.0mg/kg/dose q8–12h to maintain gastric pH >4.0	Monitor gastric pH. Tachyphylaxis occurs.
Fentanyl	i.v.	Analgesia: 1–4mcg/kg/dose q2–4h. Minor surgery: 2–10mcg/kg. Major surgery: 20–50mcg/kg.	100 mcg is equivalent to 10mg morphine or meperidine. Nausea and vomiting occur in 50% with doses >3mcg/kg. Muscle rigidity with high doses reversible with neuromuscular blocking agents.

FORMULARY

48

48 NEONATAL DRUG FORMULARY

DRUG	ROUTE	DOSAGE	COMMENTS
Ferrous sulfate	p.o.	2mg/kg/day of elemental iron as a supplement. Up to 6mg/kg/day for infants on erythropoietin	May produce GI irritation. May reduce by dividing in 2–4 doses. Combined with amphotericin. Assess renal function. Monitor blood level (peak 50–80mcg/mL desired).
Flucytosine (5-FC)	p.o.	12.5–37.5mg/kg/dose q6h	
Furosemide	i.m./i.v.	1–2mg/kg q12h (term) to q24h (premature)	Monitor serum electrolytes.
Furosemide	p.o.	2–5mg/kg q12h	Absorption variable.
G-CSF (Granulocyte-colony stimulating factor)	s.c./i.v.	10mcg/kg q24h for 5 days	Monitor ANC.
Gamma globulin, intravenous (IVIG)	i.v.	500mg/kg/day for 2–3 days for hemolytic disease or thrombocytopenia	Administer according to manufacturer's directions.
Gentamicin	i.v.	3.0mg/kg q24h if <2000g and <1 week of age; 2.5mg/kg q12h for all other neonates; 2.5mg/kg q8h for infants >28 days of age	Monitor levels and adjust accordingly. Peak: 6–8mcg/mL; trough: <2mcg/mL.
Glucagon	i.m./i.v.	0.3mg/kg up to a total dose of 1mg	

Glycopyrrolate	i.v., p.o.	i.v.: 0.004–0.01mg/kg/dose q4–8h. p.o.: 0.04–0.1mg/kg/dose q4–8 h. Note: yes it is 10 x as much p.o.	Respiratory antisecretory. Atropine-like side effects.
HBIG (Hepatitis B immune globulin)	i.m.	0.5mL within 12 hours after delivery	For infants of HBsAg positive mothers or those untested.
Heparin	i.v.	Initial dose: 50 units/kg. Maintenance dose: 10 units/kg/h	Adjust dose to give patient 1.5–2.5 x control value. Antidote: protamine sulfate 1mg per 100 units heparin in previous 4 hours.
Hepatitis B vaccine	i.m.	First dose before hospital discharge	Refer to AAP guidelines and product brochure for dosing and schedule.
Hydralazine Hydralazine	p.o. i.v.	0.3–3mg/kg/day divided q6h. 0.15mg/kg every 10 min until drop in BP or maximum dose 1–4mg/kg/day	
Hydrocortisone	i.v./i.m./p.o.	Pharmacologic: 10mg/kg/day divided q6h. Maintenance: 1mg/kg/day.	
Indomethacin	i.v.	Doses at 12–24h intervals: see Table 48.1	Give over 10–15 seconds. Avoid extravasation. Hold subsequent doses if urine output <0.6mL/kg/h when dose is due.

48

FORMULARY

48 NEONATAL DRUG FORMULARY

DRUG	ROUTE	DOSAGE	COMMENTS
Insulin (regular)	i.v., s.c.	*For hyperglycemia:* initial 0.1 unit/kg; maintenance 0.02–0.1 unit/kg/h. *For hyperkalemia:* 0.2 units per gram of glucose, usually 0.5g/kg infused over 2h	Monitor blood glucose.
Iron dextran	i.v.	250–1000mcg/kg/day of iron	A sucrose preparation is available.
Isoniazid	p.o.	10mg/kg/day in 1–2 doses	TB prophylaxis. Pyridoxine recommended for breast-feeding infants.
Isoproterenol	i.v.	0.2–0.5mcg/kg/min (1:5,000). 2.0mg in 200mL D5W at rate of 1.0mL/kg/h delivers 0.17mL/kg/min. Titrate according to BP. Monitor for systemic vasodilatation and cardiac arrhythmias. Extravasation causes severe tissue damage.	Ampules contain 1mg/5mL.
Kayexalate	p.o./p.r.	1g/kg (25% solution = 4mL/kg) q6h	Exchange ratio: 1mEq potassium/1g of resin.
Ketaconazole	p.o.	1mL of 20mg/mL susp. q8h	Oral candidiasis.

FORMULARY

Levothyroxine	i.v./i.m./p.o.	8–10mcg/kg/day	Monitor T$_4$. Requires 4 weeks for steady state.
Lidocaine	i.v.	Loading dose 1–2mg/kg given as 1mg/kg boluses for control, then infuse at 10–50mcg/kg/min. Anti-arrhythmic.	Monitor levels if using maintenance dosage. Therapeutic levels 1–6mcg/mL. Observe for signs of toxicity, agitation, seizures.
Lorazepam	i.v.	Seizures: 0.05–0.1mg/kg/dose over 2–5min. May repeat in 10–15 min. Sedation: 0.05–0.1mg/kg/dose q4–6h	Reduce dose in hepatic disease.
Magnesium sulfate	i.v./i.m.	25–50mg/kg/dose q4–6h x 3–4 doses p.r.n.	Provided as 1g/2mL (50%) or 500mg/mL.
Mannitol	i.v.	1.0–1.5g/kg. Repeat q8–12h p.r.n.	Given as 20% solution (1g/5mL) over 20–30 min.
Methadone	i.v./p.o.	0.1–0.2mg/kg/dose q12–24h.	Wean dose 10–20% per week for treatment of opiate withdrawal.
Methyldopa	i.v.	20–40mg/kg/day divided q6–12h	For hypertensive crisis only. Dilute 1–20mg/mL and infuse over 30–60 min.
Methyldopa	p.o.	Initial: 10mg/kg/day divided q6–12h. Maximum 40mg/kg/day	
Methylene blue	i.v.	1–2mg/kg/dose over 5–15 minutes for methemoglobinemia	Has been tried in refractory hypotension.

48 NEONATAL DRUG FORMULARY

DRUG	ROUTE	DOSAGE	COMMENTS
Metoclopramide	p.o.	0.1mg/kg, 1–4 times/day to maximum 0.5mg/kg/day	
Metronidazole	i.v., p.o.	*Infants <1 week of age:* BW ≤2kg: 7.5mg/kg q24h; BW >2kg: 7.5mg/kg q12h. *Infants ≥1 week of age:* BW ≤2kg: 7.5mg/kg q12h; BW >2kg: 15mg/kg q12h	Good penetration into CSF.
Midazolam	i.v., i.m.	0.05–0.2mg/kg/dose q2–4h; or, 0.2–1mcg/kg/min continuous infusion	For sedation. Can cause respiratory depression. May be antagonized by theophylline.
Morphine sulfate	s.c./i.v.	0.05–0.2mg/kg/dose q4h p.r.n.	Has some sedative as well as analgesic effect.
Nafcillin	i.m./i.v.	<1 week, 100mg/kg/day divided q12h. >1 week, 200mg/kg/day divided q6h	Avoid extravasation – severe tissue damage.
Nalbuphine (Nubain)	i.m./i.v.	0.1–0.2mg/kg q4h for analgesia	No advantage over morphine.
Naloxone	i.m./i.v.	0.1mg/kg, repeat as necessary	May also be given intratracheally.
Neomycin	p.o.	90mg/kg/day divided q6h	

Drug	Route	Dose	Notes
Neostigmine (Prostigmine)	s.c./i.m.	0.04mg/kg/dose	Antidote: atropine, 0.01–0.04 mg/kg/dose.
Nystatin	p.o.	100,000 units q6h	Swab and swallow.
Pancuronium (Pavulon)	i.v.	0.03–0.1mg/kg q2–6h p.r.n.	Antidote: neostigmine, 0.01–0.04mg/kg/dose and atropine 0.02mg/kg (no sooner than 30min after pancuronium).
Paraldehyde	i.v.	Load: 200mg/kg, then 20 mg/kg/h	Conc: 1g/mL, half life 3–10h. Eliminated 70–80% by liver and 20% by expired air. Reserve for seizures resistant to phenobarbital, diazepam, and phenytoin. Do not expose to plastic or rubber. Avoid extravasation.
Paraldehyde	p.r.	0.3mL/kg q4–5h	Put rectal dose in vegetable oil. Do not use if solution is discolored.
Penicillin G	i.v./i.m.	<1 week, 50,000 units/kg/day divided q12h. >1 week, 75,000 units/kg/day divided q8h	
Pentobarbital (Nembutal)	i.m.	3mg/kg/dose	Sedation for procedures. Lowers pain threshold.
Phenobarbital	i.v./i.m./p.o.	Loading dose: 20mg/kg i.v. or i.m. Maintenance: 3–5mg/kg/day divided q12h	Monitor serum level to maintain 30mg/mL.

48 NEONATAL DRUG FORMULARY

DRUG	ROUTE	DOSAGE	COMMENTS
Phenytoin (Dilantin)	i.v.	Loading dose: 15–20mg/kg.	Give increments of 5mg/kg q15–20min, maximum rate i.v. = 0.5mg/kg/min. Compatible with normal saline only. Do not give i.m.
		Maintenance: 5–8mg/kg/day divided q12h	Oral doses poorly absorbed.
Pitressin, aqueous	s.c.	0.125–0.5mL/dose q6–8h	Aqueous = 20 units/mL.
Pitressin, oil	i.m.	0.2mL/dose q1–3 days	Oil = 5 units/mL (shake well). Titrate effect.
Prednisolone	p.o., i.v.	0.5–2mg/kg/day divided q6–8h	5mg = 20mg hydrocortisone.
Prednisone	p.o.	Pharmacologic, 1–5mg/kg per day divided q6h	1/5 of cortisone dose. Higher dose for short-term trial in chronic lung disease.
Procainamide	i.v.	Load: 1mg/kg i.v. q5mins to maximum of 10–15mg/kg not to exceed 100mg.	For ventricular arrhythmia, titrate dose. Monitor levels.
Procainamide		Maintenance: 20–50mcg/kg/min	Procainamide: 3–10mcg/mL. N-acetyl procainamide (the active metabolite): 5–30 mcg/mL.
Propranolol	p.o.	0.5–1.0mg/kg/day divided q6h	For ventricular tachycardia, supraventricular arrhythmias.
Propranolol	i.v.	0.1–1.2mg/kg over 10min	Toxic reaction: hypotension, bronchospasm.

Prostaglandin E$_1$	i.v.	0.01–0.05mcg/kg/min continuous infusion	Usually start at higher dose and titrate down. May cause apneic spells, rash, or elevated temperature.
Protamine sulfate	i.v.	0.5–1.0mg per 100 units of heparin given during previous 3h.	Do not exceed 50mg. Excessive doses can cause severe bleeding.
Pyridostigmine	p.o., i.m.	p.o.: 5mg/kg/24h. i.m.: 0.05–0.15mg/dose	Antidote: atropine 0.01–0.04mg/kg/dose.
Pyridoxine	i.v./i.m.	50–100mg/dose	For intractable seizures. May repeat q15min x 4.
Quinidine	i.v.	2–10mg/kg. Repeat q3–6h p.r.n.	For refractory supraventricular tachycardia, adjunctive to digoxin.
Ranitidine	i.v., p.o.	i.v.: 1–2mg/kg/day divided q8h. p.o.: 3–4mg/kg/day divided q12h	Check gastric pH for effect. Fewer side effects than cimetidine.
Rifampin	i.v., p.o.	i.v.: 5mg/kg/dose q12h. p.o.: 10mg/kg/dose q24h	Turns most secretions orange.
Sodium bicarbonate	i.v.	1–2mEq/kg/dose over 5–10min.	Commonly provided as 44mEq/50mL. Dilute 1:1 with water or D5W. '1/2 correction' (mEq) = Base deficit x 0.3 x wt (kg).
Spironolactone (Aldactone)		p.o.	1–3mg/kg/day divided q12h. Monitor for hyperkalemia.

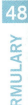

48

FORMULARY

48 NEONATAL DRUG FORMULARY

DRUG	ROUTE	DOSAGE	COMMENTS
Succinylcholine	i.v., i.m.	i.v.: 1–2mg/kg/dose. i.m.: 33mg/kg/dose	Paralysis for intubation. Pretreat with atropine. Duration of action 4–6 minutes i.v.
Theophylline	p.o.	Loading dose: 4mg/kg. Maintenance dose: 4mg/kg/day divided q6–12h	Monitor serum levels to maintain 6–13mcg/mL. Toxic effects:
Thyroxine	i.v./i.m./p.o.	8–10mcg/kg/day	Monitor T_4. Requires 4 weeks for steady state. Provided as levothyroxine.
Tolazoline (Priscoline)	i.v.	1mg/kg bolus. If no response, repeat in 10 min. If response, continue with infusion 1–2mg/kg/h	Scalp vein preferable. Generally see tolazoline flush. Monitor BP.
Trimethoprim/sulfamethoxazole (Bactrim, Septra)	i.v./p.o.	Loading dose: 3mg/kg of trimethoprim. Maintenance dose: 1mg/kg of trimethoprim every 12h. Prophylaxis: 5–10mg/kg p.o. 3 times/week.	Inj. trimethoprim & 80mg sulfamethoxazole 400mg per 5mL. Susp. trimethoprim 40mg, sulfamethoxazole 200mg per 5mL. For *Pneumocystis carinii*.
Tromethamine (THAM)	i.v.	Packaged as 0.3 mEq/mL solution. Same dose as sodium bicarbonate.	May cause hyperkalemia or hypoglycemia. Contraindicated in renal failure. Dose (mL of 0.3M THAM) = wt (kg) x (1.1) x (Base

48

Urokinase	i.v.	Large-vessel thrombosis: loading dose, 4–6,000U/kg; maintenance dose, 4–6000U/kg/h. UAC occlusion: fill lumen with solution 5000U/mL. Aspirate after 20–30 min. May repeat.	Neonates may require large doses for thrombolysis.
Vancomycin	i.v.	*Infants <1 week of age:* BW ≤2kg: 10mg/kg q12–18h; BW >2kg: 10mg/kg q8–12h. *Infants ≥1 week of age:* BW ≤2kg: 10mg/kg q2h; BW >2kg: 10mg/kg q8h	Therapeutic range: peak 20–40mcg/mL and trough 5–10mcg/mL. Infuse slowly.
Varicella zoster immune globulin (VZIG)	i.m.	125 units	Soon after delivery of woman with varicella onset 5 days before to 2 days after delivery.
Vecuronium	i.v.	Loading dose: 0.1mg/kg; i.v. infusion: 0.1–0.3mg/kg/h	Prolonged use may result in subsequent long-term muscle weakness.
Vitamin A	i.m.	2000U q48h x 14 doses	For improved healing in BPD.

48 NEONATAL DRUG FORMULARY

DRUG	ROUTE	DOSAGE	COMMENTS
Zidovudine (AZT)	p.o., i.v.	p.o.: 2mg/kg/dose q6h. i.v.: 1.5mg/kg/dose q6h. For preterm < 2 weeks of age use q12h dosing	For infants born to HIV-positive mothers.

FURTHER READING

Benitz W, Tatro D. *The pediatric drug handbook*. Chicago: Year Book; 1995.

Bhatt D, Reber D, Wirtschafter D, Parikh A, Thomas J. *Neonatal drug formulary*. Los Angeles, CA: NDF; 1997.

Gilman AG, Goodman LS, Rall TW, Murad F. *The pharmacological basis of therapeutics*, 7th edn. New York, Macmillan; 1985.

Roberts RJ. *Drug therapy in infants*. Philadelphia: Saunders; 1984.

Young T, Mongum OB. *Neofax*. Raleigh, NC: Acorn; 1997.

GLOSSARY OF ABBREVIATIONS

A

ABG	Arterial blood gas
ADH	Antidiuretic hormone
AFP	Alpha-fetoprotein
AGA	Appropriate for gestational age
Alk-Phos	Alkaline phosphatase
ALT	Alanine aminotransferase
ANC	Absolute neutrophil count
Ao	Aortic
ASD	Atrial septal defects
AST	Aspartate aminotransferase
ATN	Acute tubular necrosis
AUBC	Apparent unbound bilirubin concentration
AV	Atrioventricular

B

BAEP	Brain-stem auditory evoked potential
BCAA	Branched-chain amino acid
BP	Blood pressure
BP	Biophysical profile
BPD	Biparietal diameter
BPD	Bronchopulmonary dysplasia
bpm	Beats per minute
BUN	Blood urea nitrogen
BW	Body weight

C

CBC	Complete blood cell count
CBG	Capillary blood gas
CHF	Congestive heart failure
CIE	Counterimmunoelectrophoresis
CLD	Chronic lung disease
CMV	Cytomegalovirus
CNP	Continuous negative pressure
CNS	Central nervous system
CPAP	Continuous positive airway pressure
CSF	Cerebrospinal fluid

CST	Contraction stress test
CT	Computed axial tomography
CVH	Combined ventricular hypertrophy
CVP	Central venous pressure
CVS	Chorionic villus sampling

D

D/C	Discontinue
DES	Diethylstilbestrol
DIC	Disseminated intravascular coagulopathy
DOCA	Deoxycorticosterone acetate
DTR	Deep tendon reflexes

E

E_3	Estriol
ECMO	Extracorporeal membrane oxygenation
ECG	Electrocardiogram
ECW	Extracellular water
EEG	Electroencephalogram
ELISA	Enzyme-linked immunoabsorbent assay
EM	Electron microscopy
ESR	Erythrocyte sedimentation rate
ET	Endotracheal tube
ET	Ejection time
Et	Expiratory time

F

FiO_2	Fractional inspired oxygen concentration
FHR	Fetal heart rate
FSI	Foam stability index

G

GASA	Growth-adjusted sonographic age
GBS	Group B β-hemolytic streptococcus
GFR	Glomerular filtration rate
GGT	Gamma glutamyl transferase
GI	Gastrointestinal
GIR	Glucose infusion rate

H

HBIG	Hepatitis B immune globulin
hCG	Human chorionic gonadotropin
hCS	Human chorionic somatomammotropin

Hct	Hematocrit
HDN	Hemolytic disease of the newborn
HFV	High-frequency ventilation
Hb	Hemoglobin
HIE	hypoxic–ischemic encephalopathy
HIV	Human immunodeficiency virus
HMD	Hyaline membrane disease
HPF	High-power field
HPL	Human placental lactogen
HSV	Herpes simplex virus
H/T	Head to trunk ratio

I

ICW	Intracellular water
i.d.	Inner diameter
IDM	Infant of diabetic mother
I/E	Inspiratory-to-expiratory ratio
i.m.	Intramuscular
It	Inspiratory time
ITP	Idiopathic thrombocytopenic purpura
IUGR	Intrauterine growth retardation
i.v.	Intravenous
IVH	Intraventricular hemorrhage
IVS	Intraventricular septal thickness

K

KUB	Kidneys, ureter, and bladder

L

LA	Left atrium
LAD	Left atrial diameter
LGA	Large for gestational age
L/S	Lecithin to sphingomyelin ratio
LV	Left ventricle
LVED	Left ventricular end diastolic
LVES	Left ventricular end systolic
LVH	Left ventricular hypertrophy
LVPW	Left ventricular posterior wall

M

MPA	Main pulmonary artery
MR	Magnetic resonance

49

GLOSSARY OF ABBREVIATIONS

N

NC	Nasal cannula
NEC	Necrotizing enterocolitis
NG	Nasogastric
NICU	Neonatal intensive care unit
NJ	Nasojejunal
NPO	Nil per oram
NS	Normal saline
NST	Nonstress test

O

OCT	Oxytocin challenge test
o.d.	Outer diameter
OD	Optical density
OFC	Occipitofrontal circumference

P

PAC	Premature atrial contraction
PAT	Paroxysmal atrial tachycardia
PCR	Polymerase chain reaction
PDA	Patent ductus arteriosus
PEEP	Positive end-expiratory pressure
PEP	Pre-ejection period
PEP	Phosphoenol pyruvate
PFC	Persistence of fetal circulation
PG	Phosphatidyl glycerol
PHN	Pulmonary hypertension (of the newborn)
PIE	Pulmonary interstitial emphysema
PIP	Positive inspiratory pressure
PKU	Phenylketonuria
PMN	Polymorphonuclear
PN	Parenteral nutrition
PROM	Premature rupture of membranes
PT	Prothrombin time
PTC	Persistent transitional circulation
PTT	Partial thromboplastin time
PUBS	Percutaneous umbilical blood sampling
PVC	Premature ventricular contraction
PVS	Percussion, vibration, and suctioning

R

RA	Right atrium,
RAH	Right atrial hypertrophy
RBC	Red blood cell
RDS	Respiratory distress syndrome
ROP	Retinopathy of prematurity
RV	Right ventricle
RVH	Right ventricular hypertrophy

S

SD	Standard deviation
SGA	Small for gestational age
STI	Systolic time intervals
SVT	Supraventricular tachycardia

T

TB	Tuberculosis
TBG	Thyroid-binding globulin
TEF	Tracheoesophageal fistula
THAM	Tris-hydroxymethyl aminomethane
TORCH	Toxoplasmosis, other, rubella, cytomegalovirus, and herpes
TPN	Total parenteral nutrition
TSH	Thyroid-stimulating hormone
TT	Thrombin time

U

UAC	Umbilical artery catheter
UGI	Upper gastrointestinal
UTI	Urinary tract infection
UVC	Umbilical venous catheter

V

VLBW	Very low birthweight
VP	Venous pressure
VSD	Ventricular septal defect

W

WBC	White blood cell

49

GLOSSARY OF ABBREVIATIONS

50

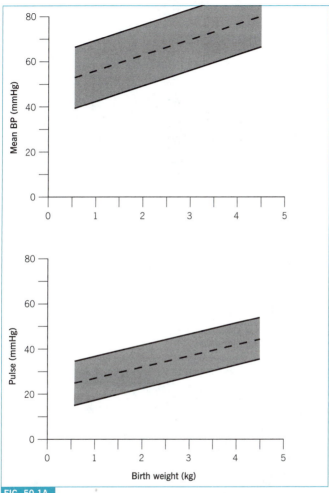

FIG. 50.1A

Blood pressure in the first 12 hours of life. Linear regressions (broken lines) and 95% confidence limits (solid lines) of systolic (top) and diastolic (bottom) aortic BP on birth weight in 61 healthy newborn infants during the first 12 hours after birth. For systolic pressure, $y = 7.13x + 40.45$; $r = 0.79$. For diastolic pressure, $y = 4.81x + 22.18$; $r = 0.71$. For both, $n = 413$ and $p < 0.001$. (From Versmold et al.[1], with permission.)

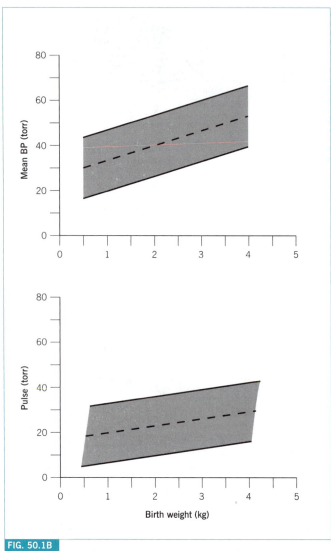

FIG. 50.1B

BP in the first 12 hours of life. Linear regressions (broken lines) and 95% confidence limits (solid lines) of mean pressure (top) and pulse pressure (systolic–diastolic pressure amplitude) (bottom) on birth weight in 61 healthy newborn infants during the first 12 hours after birth. (From Versmold et al.[1], with permission.)

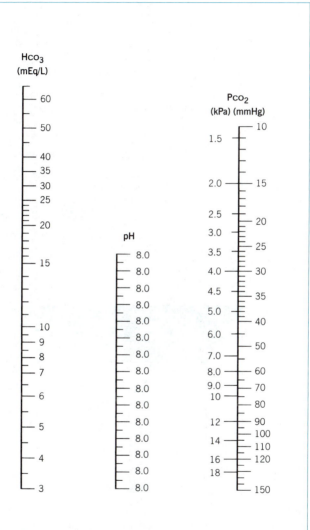

FIG. 50.2

Modified Siggaard–Anderson nomogram relating blood pH, bicarbonate (HCO$_3^-$) concentration, and PCO$_2$. (From Chatburn RL, Lough MD.[2] with permission.)

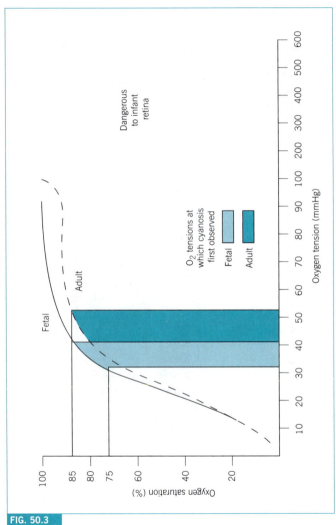

FIG. 50.3
Oxyhemoglobin dissociation curves. (From Chatburn RL, Lough MD.[2] with permission.)

TABLE 50.1

HEMATOLOGY: MEAN RED CELL VALUES DURING GESTATION

Age (weeks)	Hgb (g/L)	Hematocrit (%)	RBC (10^6/mm^3)	Mean corpuscle vol. (μm^3)	Mean corpuscle Hgb (vv)	Mean corpuscle Hgb conc. (%)	RETIC (%) (% of WBCs)	NUC RBC (% of RBCs)
12	8.0–10.0	33	1.5	180	60	34	5.0–8.0	40
16	10.0	35	2.0	140	45	33	2.0–4.0	10–25
20	11.1	37	2.5	135	44	33	1.0	10–20
24	14.0	40	3.5	123	38	31	1.0	5–10
28	14.5	45	4.0	120	40	31	0.5	5–10
34	15.0	47	4.4	118	38	32	0.2	3–10

From Oski A, Naiman JL.[1] with permission.

NUC RBC, nucleated red blood cells; RETIC, reticulocytes

50

APPENDICES

TABLE 50.2

APPROXIMATE NEUTRAL THERMAL ENVIRONMENT TEMPERATURES (°C)

Age	WEIGHT (g)			
	<1200	1201–1500	1501–2500	2500
0–12h	35.0	34.0	33.3	32.8
12–24h	34.5	33.8	32.8	32.4
24–96h	34.5	33.5	32.3	32.0
4–14 days		33.5	32.1	31.0
2–3 weeks		33.1	31.7	30.0
3–4 weeks		32.6	31.4	
4–5 weeks		32.0	30.9	
5–6 weeks		31.4	30.4	

From Scopes JW, Ahmed I[5].

TABLE 50.3

SERUM ENZYMES IN NEWBORNS

Enzymes	Age	IU/L
Acid phosphatase[a]	Birth – 1 month	7.4–19.4
Alanine amino transferase	Birth – 10 days	1.31–10.4
ALT	Birth – 1 month	0–54
Aldolase[b]	Birth – 1 month	4–24
Alkaline phosphatase	Birth – 1 month	20–225
	1 month – 3 months	73–226
Aspartate amino transaminase	Birth – 10 days	6–25
AST	Birth – 1 month	0–67
Creatinine phosphokinase (CPK)	Premature	0–210
	Birth – 3 weeks	22–267
	3 weeks – 3 months	15–134
Gamma glutamyl transferase	Premature	56–233
GGTP[c]	Birth – 3 weeks	0–103
	3 weeks – 3 months	4–111
Lactate dehydrogenase (LDH)[b]	Birth – 10 days	150–590
	1 day – 1 month	185–404
	1 month – 2 years	110–244
Leucine aminopeptidase (LAP)[a]	Birth – 1 month	29–59
	>1 month	15–50

[a]From O'Brien D, Rodgerson DO.[6]
[b]From Meites S, ed.[7]
[c]From King J, Morris MB.[8]

TABLE 50.4

WBC COUNT AND DIFFERENTIAL COUNT DURING THE FIRST 2 WEEKS OF LIFE

Age	Leukocytes		Neutrophils		Eosinophils	Basophils	Lymphocytes	Monocytes	
		Total	Segmented	Band					
Birth									
	Mean	18,100	11,000	9400	1600	400	100	5500	1050
	Range	9.3–30.0	6.0–26.0			20–850	0.640	2.0–11.0	0.4–3.1
	Mean %		61	5.2	9	2.2	0.6	31	5.8
7 Days									
	Mean	12,000	5500	4700	830	500	50	5000	1100
	Range	5.0–21.0	1.5–10.0			70–1100	0–250	2.0–17.0	0.3–2.7
	Mean %		45	6	118	4.1	0.4	41	9.1
14 Days									
	Mean	11,400	4500	3900	630	350	50	5500	1000
	Range	5.0–20.0	1.0–9.5		70–1000	70–1000	0.230	2.0–17.0	0.2–2.4
	Mean %		40	5.5	3.1	3.1	0.4	48	8.8

From Oski FA., Naiman JL.[4] with permission.

TABLE 50.5

WHITE CELLS AND DIFFERENTIAL COUNTS IN PREMATURE INFANTS DURING FIRST 4 WEEKS OF POSTPARTUM LIFE

Birth weight		<1500g			1500–2500g	
Age in weeks	1	2	4	1	2	4
Total count (x 1000/mm^3)						
Mean	16.8	15.4	12.1	13.0	10.0	8.4
Range	6.1–32.8	10.4–21.3	8.7–17.2	7.0–14.7	7.0–14.1	5.8–12.4
Percent of total						
Polymorphs						
PMN/Bands	0.11	0.11	0.11	0.13	0.16	0.13
Segmented	54	45	40	55	43	41
Unsegmented	7	6	5	8	8	6
Eosinophils	2	3	3	2	3	3
Basophils	1	1	1	1	1	1
Monocytes	6	10	10	5	9	11
Lymphocytes	30	35	41	9	36	38

From Klaus MH, Fanaroff AA.[9]

TABLE 50.6

COAGULATION FACTOR LEVELS, SCREENING STUDIES, AND FIBRINOLYSIS TIMES IN RELATION TO GESTATIONAL MATURITY

Factors	I	II	V	VII and X	VIII	IX	VI	XIII	Platelets	PT	TT	FT
	mg/100ml			Percent of normal				Titer	x 1000/mm³ (+SD)	Seconds		
<1500g (28–32 weeks)	215	21	64	42	50	–	–	–	300 (70)	21	–	326
1500–2000g (32–36 weeks)	220	25	67	37	44	–	–	1/8	260 (60)	18	14	214
2000–2500g (36–40 weeks)	240	35	66	48	67	–	–	1/8	325 (75)	17	10	214
>2500g (term)	210	60	92	56	67	26	42	1/8	325 (70)	16	9	95
Mothers of premature infants	520	92	110	178	–	–	–	–	225 (45)	14	7	–
Mothers of term infants	500	92	110	206	196	130	69	1/16	215 (41)	14	8	278

FT, fibrinolysis time.
From Klaus MH, Fanaroff AA[9].

TABLE 50.7

CEREBROSPINAL FLUID IN HEALTHY TERM NEWBORNS

	Age		
	0–24h	1 day	7 days
RBCs/mm^3	9 (0–1,070)	23 (6–630)	3 (0–48)
PMN leukocytes/mm^3	3 (0–70)	7 (0–26)	2 (0–5)
Lymphocytes/mm^3	2 (0–20)	5 (0–16)	
Proteins (mg/dL)	63 (32–240)	73 (40–148)	47 (27–65)
Glucose (mg/dL)	51 (32–78)	48 (38–64)	55 (48–66)

Color is clear or xanthochromic in each case.
Data from Naidoo BT[10], and Neches W, Platt M[11].

REFERENCES

1. Versmold H, et al. Aortic blood pressure during the first 12 hours of life in infants with birth weight 610 to 4220 grams. *Pediatrics* 1981; 67:607.
2. Chatburn RL, Lough MD. *Handbook of respiratory care*, 2nd edition. Chicago: Year Book Medical; 1990:82.
3. Chatburn RL, Lough MD. *Handbook of respiratory care*, 2nd edition. Chicago: Year Book Medical; 1990:86.
4. Oski A, Naiman JL. *Hematologic problems in the newborn*, 2nd edition. Philadelphia: Saunders; 1972.
5. Scopes JW, Ahmed I. Indirect assessment of oxygen requirements in newborn babies by monitoring deep body temperature. *Arch Dis Child* 1966; 41:25–33.
6. O'Brien D, Rodgerson DO. Interpretation of biochemical values. In: Kempe CH, Silver HK, O'Brien D (eds) *Current pediatric diagnosis and treatment*, 3rd edition. Los Altos, CA: Lange;
7. Meites S (ed). *Pediatric clinical chemistry: a survey of normals, methods, and instruments.* Washington, DC: American Association for Clinical Chemistry; 1977.
8. King J, Morris MB. *Arch Dis Child* 1961; 36:604.
9. Klaus MH, Fanaroff AA. *Care of the high risk neonate*. Philadelphia: Saunders; 1979.
10. Naidoo BT. The cerebrospinal fluid in the healthy newborn infant. *S Afr Med J* 1968; 42:933–935.
11. Neches W, Platt M. Cerebrospinal fluid LDH in 287 children, including 53 cases of meningitis of bacterial and non-bacterial etiology. *Pediatrics* 1968; 41:1097–1103.

50

APPENDICES

INDEX

INDEX

INDEX